Motor Speech Disorders

A Treatment Guide

Motor Speech Disorders

A Treatment Guide

James Paul Dworkin, Ph.D.
Private Practice
Galveston, Texas

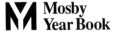 Mosby
Year Book

St. Louis Baltimore Boston Chicago London Philadelphia Sydney Toronto

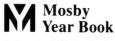

**Mosby
Year Book**

Dedicated to Publishing Excellence

Editor: David K. Marshall
Assistant Editor: Julie Tryboski
Project Manager: Linda J. Daly
Designer: Barbara Torode

Printed in the United States of America.

Mosby–Year Book, Inc.
11830 Westline Industrial Drive
St. Louis, MO 63146

Library of Congress Cataloging-in-Publication Data

Dworkin, James Paul.
　　Motor speech disorders : a treatment guide / James Paul Dworkin.
　　　　p.　　cm.
　　Includes bibliographical references and index.
　　ISBN 1-55664-223-7
　　1. Speech disorders—Treatment.　2. Speech therapy.　I. Title.
RC423.D87　1991
616.85′52—dc20
　　　　　　　　　　　　　　　　　　　　　　　　　　　　　90-85093
　　　　　　　　　　　　　　　　　　　　　　　　　　　　　CIP

CL/MY/MY　9　8　7

To my newborn daughter, McKenzie Allison,
with pride, joy, and love
and
In loving memory of
Eugene and Gloria Wolfinbarger

Foreword

It is a pleasurable chore to undertake the writing of a foreword. The pleasurable aspect is in being given a license to philoso-
phize and make lofty and profound statements. The chore, or challenge, is to attempt to express adequately to the reader the flavor,
style and utility of what is to follow. Let me say at the outset that
you hold in your hands a gem, a "keeper," whether you are an up-
per-level undergraduate major in speech-language pathology, an
advanced graduate student, an academician, or a seasoned clinician.

Specific identification and delineation of speech disorders associated with lesions of the motor system are rightly attributed to
Darley and his associates at the Mayo Clinic a quarter of a century
ago. The formalized pre- and post-doctoral fellowship programs at
the Mayo Graduate School of Medicine and the preceptorships provided by Darley, Aronson, and associates spawned a cadre of clini-
cians/investigators in the neurogenic arena, which led to a resur-
gence of interest in the understanding and detailed description of
communicative disorders associated with an array of neuropathologic conditions. More recently, during the past decade, we have
seen a proliferation of new and illuminating data relating the descriptions to treatment approaches for neurogenic communicative
disorders. Until now what has been lacking is a specific thematic
focus on therapeutic techniques.

Dr. Dworkin is eminently qualified to respond to the needs
and demands of the academic community and practicing clinicians
in presenting a current, state-of-the-art volume focusing on practi-
cality. In a cogent and readable manner he presents management
strategies that logically lead to the establishment of treatment approaches and implementation of specific therapy techniques in a
systematic and rational manner. A number of the therapeutic regimens are new and novel; however, they are not based on anecdotal
experiences, but rather are derived from quantitative empirical ev-

idence that he gathered with rigorous objectivity. These new behavioral treatment techniques are presented in an easy to follow, step-by-step procedural format. Specific guidelines for administration of these techniques are enhanced by numerous flow diagrams and tables, treatment charts for logging and tracking patient responses, and helpful algorithms. These are further complemented by clear, sequential photographs for immediate application by the novice or seasoned clinician.

Each chapter includes representative case presentations illustrative of the therapeutic approach under discussion. Dr. Dworkin has accumulated these case studies based on his rich clinical and scientific background, which ranges from having been a Fellow at the Mayo Clinic and a university professor and clinician, having directed a clinical speech physiology laboratory, and having been immersed in a private practice devoted to treating patients with communicative disorders caused by neurologic impairment.

Dr. Dworkin provides proposed solutions to the perplexing problems presented by those patients who possess communication disorders as a result of neurologic impairment in an explicit, concise and practical manner. One can rely on this much needed clinical text for practical guidance on treatment techniques and it serves as well as an essential repository of information on clinical rehabilitative procedures.

This is a signal contribution that synthesizes for the first time specific management procedures for the dysarthrias and apraxia of speech and is presented in a scholarly, stimulating and sensible fashion. I believe that university instructors will find wide use for this volume as an instructional text for students in speech-language pathology, and I anticipate that it will provoke experienced clinicians to reappraise their approaches in managing patients who possess neurogenic motor speech disorders.

Donnell F. Johns, Ph.D.
Professor of Surgery
Director, Clinical Research
Division of Plastic Surgery
University of Texas Southwestern Medical School
Dallas, Texas

Preface

The literature is replete with information on the overall characteristics of and tests for motor speech disorders. As a consequence, students of speech-language pathology and their practicing counterparts are generally well trained and experienced in conducting differential diagnostic testing of dysarthric and apractic patients. There is, however, a paucity of information on effective behavioral methods by which to treat these patients. Scanning the textbook and clinical research literature for such suggestions can be frustrating and unfulfilling.

This book was written with hopes of minimizing such frustration and maximizing the likelihood of success by providing step-by-step, sequentially ordered behavioral exercises for treating the various speech subsystem disturbances exhibited by patients with motor speech disorders. Treatment techniques that generally require the use of sophisticated laboratory procedures and instrumentation are deliberately omitted, not because they are considered unhelpful or unworthy of attention, but because the complexity of their application and high cost are usually deterrents to speech-language pathologists in average clinical settings. Whereas most of the materials that are recommended for use in this book can be found in every well-stocked clinic, some will have to be inexpensively constructed or purchased. The techniques of intervention that are covered here should therefore prove easy to administer and follow. They should not, however, be construed as an exhaustive account of feasible treatment strategies. Rather, they stem primarily from this clinician's successes and failures with apractic and dysarthric patients, and secondarily from the work of many other clinical researchers whose experiences may have been borrowed or modified to meet the objectives of each chapter.

The format chosen for this text conforms to the "How I do it" style used in many medical texts and journals. This mode of presentation enables authors to share information regarding treatment procedures that they have personally found rewarding. Such publications are generally devoid of numerous references that justify the recommended methodology of management. Instead, suggested readings are usually provided that point readers toward supportive as well as alternative treatment considerations. Inasmuch as this text ought, realistically, to be viewed as a behavioral therapeutic guide or manual, it lends itself well to this practical approach. At the end of each chapter, suggested readings are provided for further information. The inherent journalistic risks associated with this format were judged less important than the benefits that would accrue if readers were not charged with having first to sift through endless vignettes about other publications before the sum and substance of this one are unveiled.

As a therapeutic manual this text delves into intervention strategies for patients with motor speech disorders. Because readership preparation in the basic sciences of neuroanatomy, neurophysiology, and neurogenic communication disorders is presumed, only brief reviews of these topics are provided.

Chapter 1 offers a brief review of motor speech disorders, and Chapter 2 discusses the fundamental tenets underlying optional designs for their treatment. Chapter 3 provides basic ideas about improving breath support for speech purposes. Chapter 4 looks at ways of reducing hypernasality and its negative effects on speech intelligibility. Chapter 5 addresses differential clinical methods by which neurogenic voice disorders may be treated. Chapter 6 is devoted to managing articulatory proficiency through neuromuscular facilitation and phonetic practice exercises. Finally, Chapter 7 introduces techniques that may stimulate prosodic sufficiency. It may be worth noting that these chapters were arranged not by motor speech disorder headings but according to the types of communication difficulties that dysarthric and apractic patients typically exhibit. If, for example, the reader desires information on how to improve articulatory proficiency in a given patient, irrespective of the underlying differential diagnosis, Chapter 6 should be consulted. There cross-references can be made between chapter content and the patient in question so as to ferret out those treatment exercises that seem most applicable, given the patient's symptoms and diagnosis, from those that are apparently designed for another type of patient. Similar approaches should be followed using the other treatment chapters of the text.

James Paul Dworkin

Acknowledgments

The conception, development and delivery of this project required the help of many individuals to whom I am forever indebted. I would like to take a few moments to express my appreciation to each of them.

To my esteemed mentors Dr. Arnold E. Aronson and Dr. Frederic L. Darley, both of whom have struggled over the years in their attempts to wrestle me gently to the ground so that they could teach me the importance of listening to and learning from others: You have been my inspiration, and I bow with gratitude in your honor.

To my colleague and friend Dr. Donnell F. Johns, who graciously agreed to provide the foreword to this text: Whenever I have turned for assistance, advice and support you have always been there for me, through thick and thin. Learning from and working closely with you has been my pleasure.

To my colleague Ms. Terri Petrucci-Coley, with whom I had been professionally affiliated throughout this entire project: Thank you for the countless hours you devoted to providing me with invaluable editorial and substantive comments from start to finish. Your help has been indispensable.

To the many authors whose clinical research I have referenced throughout this project: Your collective wisdom and continued contributions to the literature support the foundation of our knowledge of the clinical process and patients with motor speech disorders.

To the thousands of clinicians with whom I have spoken over the years: My humble thanks to you all for representing us in the trenches, the toughest location in which to work daily. I hope that this project addresses at least some of your questions and clinical needs.

To Linda Beauchamp, who patiently typed and retyped the drafts of this project from its inception: Your penchant for detail and perfection helped ensure that only clean copies would be sent for review. I owe you, for the journey would have been much more difficult in your absence.

To Gina Scala and Linda Daly, whose editorial expertise helped erase and reconstruct several manuscript errors: Your keen professional observations and suggestions for revisions are much appreciated.

To Michael Coley, who unselfishly lent his talent and time to make possible the inclusion of the various photographs that appear in the text: The pictures you took add an important dimension to the material, and I am grateful to you for making this possible.

To my closest friends and loving family members whom I have neglected too often during the writing of this project: Your patience and loyalty are dear to my heart.

To my wife, Rebecca, who has had to sacrifice more than anyone so that I could devote the time necessary to complete this project: All these acknowledgments would have been significantly delayed without your enthusiastic support, expert advice and help with the figures, tables and charts, ongoing technical assistance with the preparation of the manuscript, and indefatigable tolerance of my work schedule. Having you by my side has made it all possible.

Last, but certainly not least, to all my patients and their families, from whom I have learned the most: Your trust in my abilities to be of help has directed my clinical focus and in large measure is responsible for this entire undertaking. I applaud your courage and strength in overcoming adversity. And I thank you for taking and holding onto my arm, even though we have stumbled in our search for answers to your pressing needs.

Contents

Chapter 1

Motor Speech Disorders

When certain components of the nervous system are damaged by injury, illness, or disease, speech motor control may be compromised. The characteristics and degree of speech difficulties that result may depend upon several factors, including the type and severity of the underlying etiology, neuroanatomic sites of involvement, coexistence of other disabilities, and the patient's idiosyncratic responses to this complex web of conditions. The diagnostic term "motor speech disorders" has traditionally been used generically to classify problems with phonation, articulation, resonation, and/or prosody that are of neuropathologic origin. Under this generic umbrella are two major subcategories: (1) apraxia of speech (from this point on, the term "apraxia" will be used instead of, but synonymously with, "dyspraxia") and (2) the dysarthrias. The possible etiologic agents of these disorders are numerous and variable, as are the differential speech and nonspeech signs and symptoms they precipitate. Here only brief overviews are presented about these agents and the motor speech disorders with which they have been causally associated. For more detailed descriptions, consult the suggested reading list at the end of this chapter.

ETIOLOGIC AGENTS OF MOTOR SPEECH DISORDERS

When considering the possible etiologies of motor speech disorders the mnemonic device "VITAMIN D" may prove helpful. These letters represent the most common causes of neurologic impairments that result in motor speech disorders. Familiarity with these agents may facilitate differential diagnoses, recommended treatments, and realistic prognoses. The "V" stands for *vascular accidents*. The "I" means *infectious processes*. The "T" symbolizes *traumatic insults* or the effects of *toxic* agents. *Allergic* or *anoxic* conditions are covered by the "A." The "M" represents *metabolic disorders*, and the other "I" paradoxically refers to *idiopathic*, which means no immediately discernible cause, or *iatrogenic* (treatment-induced). Subsumed under the "N" are *neoplasms*, and under the "D" *degenerative and demyelinating* diseases.

Victims of any one or more of these conditions may present with an assort-ment of focal or multifocal neuropathologic signs and symptoms, including limb and/or orofacial muscle paralyses, sensory disturbances, motor speech and lan-guage disorders, cognitive deficits, and psychological and neurobehavioral changes. These sequelae vary in degree, form, and combination, depending upon the nature and extent of the underlying etiology. A brief overview of each agent is presented next.

Vascular Accidents. With each contraction of the heart, roughly one-fifth of the amount of blood that is pumped into the ascending aorta is destined for the cerebral-arterial network to nourish the brain with oxygen and other nu-trients. Removal of waste products such as carbon dioxide and acid metabolites that accumulate in brain tissue is conducted by the cerebral-venous system. Cerebrovascular accidents (stroke) disrupt normal blood flow within the brain and may irreparably damage those areas that are undernourished as a result of such disruption. Of the three primary causes of strokes, *cerebral thromboses* ac-count for approximately 70 percent of reported cases. *Cerebral hemorrhages* and *embolisms* cause the remaining 20 percent and 10 percent of strokes, respec-tively. Cerebral ischemia, a diagnostic term that characterizes a deficiency of blood within the brain due to constriction or obstruction of cerebral blood vessels, commonly results from both thromboembolic conditions. Prolonged ischemia causes cerebral infarction in which affected areas of the brain die and are re-placed with scar tissue. When cerebral blood vessels rupture, on the other hand, intracranial bleeding occurs, allowing blood to flow freely and unnaturally into the surrounding areas of the brain. This flood has a softening and destructive ef-fect on the brain tissue involved.

Infectious Processes. Infectious organisms may gain entrance to the brain through the bloodstream, directly through fractures of the cranial and fa-cial bones, and through the ventricular system via cerebrospinal fluid. Meningi-tis, encephalitis, and poliomyelitis, for example, are diseases that cause diffuse inflammatory-degenerative reactions of the brain and/or spinal cord, owing to pathogenic bacterial or viral microorganisms.

Traumatic Insults. More than 500,000 severe head injuries occur annu-ally in the United States, which result in diffuse neuropathologic changes includ-ing shearing, swelling, and hemorrhaging of brain tissue. The pathophysiologic and neuropsychologic effects are usually dependent upon the areas of the brain that are damaged. If toxic agents such as insecticides, lead, and glue are ingested or inhaled, they can produce both central nervous system and peripheral nervous system signs and symptoms.

Allergic or Anoxic Conditions. Negative reactions to allergens that may invade the nervous system may cause temporary, and in some instances long-term, neurologic disturbances. Anoxia, in which oxygen supply to the brain is disrupted for a period of time, similarly is a well-known neuropathologic agent.

Metabolic Disorders. Abnormal metabolism of the nervous system can cause pathologic effects such as intracranial hypertension, brain tissue degener-ation, and disturbances in the transmission and uptake of neurotransmitter substances. A major source of such adverse metabolic reactions is dysfunctioning of one or more endocrine glands.

Idiopathic Disorders. If, at the outset of testing, the neurologic signs and symptoms presented by the patient cannot be attributed to an apparent cause, their origin may be labeled idiopathic. However, the identity of the actual etiology often unfolds over the course of time and with further diagnostic study. The emergence of signs and symptoms of tardive dyskinesia secondary to pharmacologic treatment for Parkinson's disease is an example of an iatrogenic etiology.

Neoplasms. Any type of abnormal growth such as a tumor, cyst, or vascular malformation is considered a neoplasm. When neoplasms occur within the nervous system, they may interfere with normal blood flow dynamics, and they can cause increased intracranial pressure by blocking the circulation of the cerebrospinal fluid within the ventricular system. These effects may result in widespread neuropathologic changes, including those previously outlined in the section on *vascular* etiology.

Degenerative and Demyelinating Diseases. Those degenerative diseases of the nervous system that are commonly associated etiologically with motor speech disorders include cerebral palsy, Huntington's disease, Parkinson's disease, amyotrophic lateral sclerosis, essential tremor syndrome, and muscular dystrophies. Multiple sclerosis is a demyelinating disease that also has been causally linked to difficulties with speech motor control. All these diseases, except muscular dystrophy, invade the pathways of the pyramidal and/or extrapyramidal system.

APRAXIA OF SPEECH

The effects of faulty planning are most evident in the articulatory and prosodic components of the apractic patient's speech (Figure 1–1). Articulatory breakdowns are usually of the substitution and omission types; however, distortions are also observed, and errors tend to be quite inconsistent and variable both within and between patients. Initial consonants are typically more troublesome than those in other positions, and clusters are ordinarily more difficult to produce than singletons. Multisyllabic words usually present more problems than words with fewer syllables; however, repeated trials of the same word, regardless of its length, tend to result in improved performances, sometimes called an adaptation effect. Most errors in sequencing are of the anticipatory type, in which upcoming sounds or syllables in a word, sentence, or phrase are uttered too early. Occasionally, errors of the reiterative type occur, in which the abnormal repetition of previously uttered sounds disrupts speech intelligibility. These errors may be further compounded by visible and audible groping phenomena caused by struggles or exaggerated efforts to posture correctly the articulators during ongoing speech. Some clinical researchers suggest that such behaviors are not random phenomena, but rather fragments of upcoming phonetic segments. Attempts to self-correct or avoid an error often result in dysfluent-type behaviors that resemble stut-

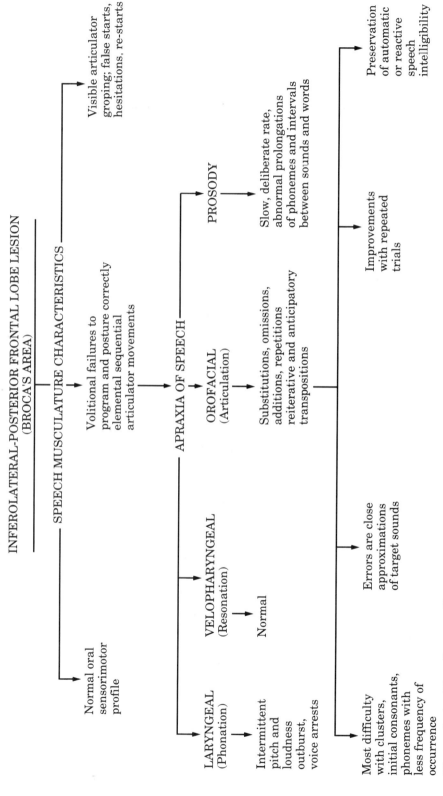

Figure 1–1. Flow diagram illustrating the overall characteristics of apraxia of speech.

tering: false starts, multiple restarts, repetitions, abnormal pausing and phrasing, and slow speech, to name but a few. Whereas unrelieved dysprosody has been considered secondary to articulatory breakdowns, more recently it has been suggested that such insufficiencies can also be primary signs of speech apraxia, particularly in those patients whose overall symptoms are moderate to severe in degree. Those with less severe involvement may, however, demonstrate extended periods of normal duration, rhythm, stress, and intonation. It is interesting that automatic and reactive speech, that is, routinely used and highly organized words and phrases, are relatively well preserved. The apractic patient, therefore, may exhibit islands of fluent and articulate speech that are embedded among dysfluent, imprecise, and effortful speech productions. Identification of this mixture of features is tantamount to differential diagnosis of speech apraxia.

Damage to the lateral aspect of the dominant inferolateral-posterior regions of the frontal lobe of the brain, otherwise known as Broca's area (Brodmann's areas 44 and 45), is thought to be the most common cause of apraxia of speech. Recently, disparate cortical and subcortical lesion sites, including the supplemental motor cortex, basal ganglia and anterior limb of the internal capsule, have also been implicated in the etiology. These zones are considered normally responsible for helping plan the postural adjustments, movements, and sequences of movements of the articulators during volitional speech production. If those areas responsible for processing language are also damaged, including the posterior and midtemporal, anterior occipital, and inferior parietal lobes of the dominant cerebral hemisphere, then the language impairments of "aphasia" may co-occur with the motor speech disturbances of apraxia. Such coexistence indeed is more the rule than the exception. However, apraxia of speech can and does occur in relatively "pure" form, that is, without a concomitant language disorder. Treatment recommendations in this text are designed for the patient with apraxia of speech whose language modalities are uninvolved. Adaptations, however, may be made to those patients who present with both apraxia and aphasia.

Many patients with speech apraxia also have co-occurring *oral apraxia*. This is a motor planning disturbance that involves one or more structures of the oral mechanism as nonspeech volitional movements are attempted. For example, if a patient were asked to pucker the lips, wiggle the tongue, puff out the cheeks, and so forth, there would be a great deal of difficulty in performing these tasks. Attempts would probably be characterized by struggling and groping to posture and program correctly the musculature responsible for such movements.

The signs and symptoms of both the verbal and the oral forms of apraxia are due to faulty neuromotor planning or programming of the structures of the speech mechanism. Upon clinical examination, the neuromuscular status of this mechanism should prove to be unaffected.

THE DYSARTHRIAS

Like apraxia of speech, dysarthria is a motor speech disorder. Unlike apraxia, however, dysarthria results from weakness, paralysis, dyscoordination, primary and secondary sensory deprivation, and alteration in the tone of the speech musculature. These neurogenic abnormalities are caused by impairments of the central nervous system, peripheral nervous system, or both, and they vary in combination from patient to patient. Considering the factors of both pathophysiology and site of involvement, five primary types of dysarthria have been classified: spastic, ataxic, hypokinetic, hyperkinetic, and flaccid. When two or more types coexist, the term "mixed dysarthria" is applied. This classification system should only be used as a guide to formulating diagnostic conclusions and treatment programs. Although there is a certain homogeneity of abnormal signs and symptoms in individuals who have been diagnosed as having the same type of dysarthria, most often such individuals exhibit heterogeneous clusters of speech and motor dyscontrol problems, thus challenging the usefulness of group classifications. In the interest of space and text objectives, however, here this commonly used system will be followed in spirit, but not law inasmuch as there are probably as many different types of dysarthria as there are patients with the diagnosis. Whereas each of the primary types will be discussed below, in the treatment chapters that follow the subtle as well as significant differences between individuals with these diagnoses will be addressed.

Spastic Dysarthria

This condition is caused by bilateral pyramidal system damage, particularly involving the corticobulbar tracts (upper motor neurons) (Figure 1–2). The characteristic speech motor dyscontrol that occurs depends upon the degree of damage to these tracts, and the resultant pathophysiologic effects, such as weakness, paresis, dyscoordination, hypertonicity, and exaggerated reflexes of involved speech musculature. Generally, articulation is imprecise and slow-labored; hypernasal resonance is prominent; phonation varies from harsh to strained and strangled; and the prosodic insufficiencies include monopitch, monoloudness, intermittent voice arrests, short phrases, and excess and equal voice inflection and syllable stress. Individuals with unilateral corticobulbar tract damage may present with an apparent unique yet mild form of dysarthria that has features of spastic dysarthria but is distinctly different. The disorder is due in part to central weakness and paresis of the facial and lingual musculature on the side opposite the lesion. This may occur because the majority of the corticobulbar tract projections to the seventh and twelfth cranial nerves, which respectively supply these muscle groups, are contralateral, thereby making the lips and tongue particularly susceptible to (hemiparetic) motor dyscontrol following unilateral corticobulbar tract damage. Phonatory signs including monoloudness, monopitch, and low pitch have been observed as well, suggesting laryngeal involvement in this disorder.

The oral neuromuscular disturbances underlying spastic dysarthria are essentially comparable to pseudobulbar palsy, because of their resemblance, albeit false, to the (flaccid) signs and symptoms of bulbar palsy, a condition caused by specific cranial nerve (lower motor neuron) damage. Many patients with spastic

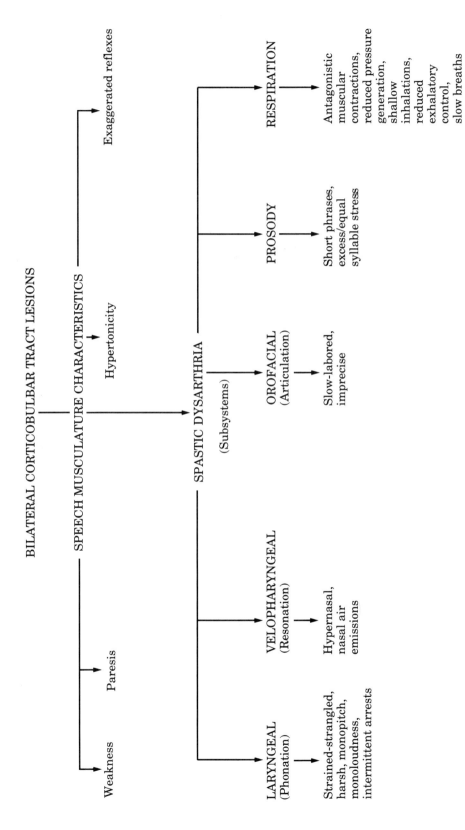

Figure 1–2.   Flow diagram illustrating the overall characteristics of spastic dysarthria.

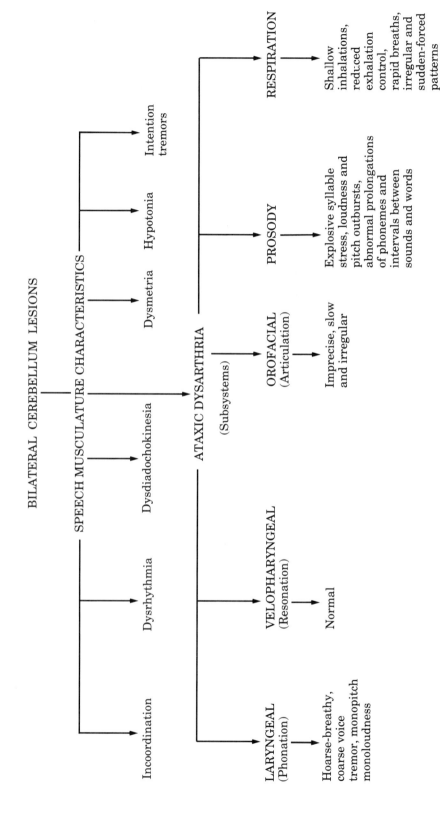

Figure 1–3. Flow diagram illustrating the overall characteristics of ataxic dysarthria.

dysarthria exhibit emotional incontinence, such as unprovoked and short outbursts of crying or laughing. They also frequently present with spastic paresis of the limb and trunk musculature as a consequence of co-existent corticospinal tract involvement.

Ataxic Dysarthria

This diagnosis is rendered when widespread disturbances in timing (dysrhythmia), synergy, speed, movement range and control (dysmetria), and coordinated and alternating forcing functions (dysdiadochokinesia) of the muscles of the speech and respiratory mechanisms cause (1) imprecise, slow, and irregular articulatory breakdowns; (2) intermittent periods of explosive inflection, syllable stress, and loudness patterns; (3) prolongation of phonemes, with accompanying respiratory dysrhythmias; (4) overall monopitch and monoloudness; and (5) hoarse-breathy phonation and mildly coarse voice tremors. Gait and limb ataxias frequently accompany these motor speech disorders. Bilateral, generalized lesions involving the deep midline nuclei and pathways of the cerebellum (Figure 1–3) usually account for the underlying cause of ataxic dysarthria. As a final caveat, it should be noted that some of the aforementioned dysprosodic features of ataxic dysarthria are observed in patients with apraxia of speech.

Hypokinetic Dysarthria

Individuals with Parkinson's disease or parkinsonian-like symptoms, due to lesions of the dopamine-rich substantia nigra (Figure 1–4), exhibit a variety of movement disorders involving the various motor subsystems.

In addition to reduced range and velocity of muscle movements (hypokinesia), the underlying pathophysiology of this disease includes marked degrees of muscle rigidity (hypertonicity) and increased stiffness, acceleration of electromyographic patterns, and tremors.

Such involvement of the subsystems of speech motor control results in hypokinetic dysarthria characterized by reduced vocal loudness with concomitant harsh-hoarse quality, slow speaking rate with intermittent bursts of rapid-fire articulation, excessive and overly long pauses, prolonged syllables, monoloudness, and reduced phonation time. Articulatory precision fluctuates greatly from periods of intelligibility to unintelligibility. The mask-like facies, shuffling gait, flexed posture of the trunk, and pill-rolling tremors of the fingers that typify Parkinson's disease may aid in the overall diagnosis.

Hyperkinetic Dysarthria

This condition results from quick and slow forms of movement disorders (Figure 1–5). Huntington's disease, ballismus, essential (organic) voice tremor and various forms of myoclonus are the most common of the quick forms, and athetosis, dyskinesias, and the dystonias generally constitute the slower forms.

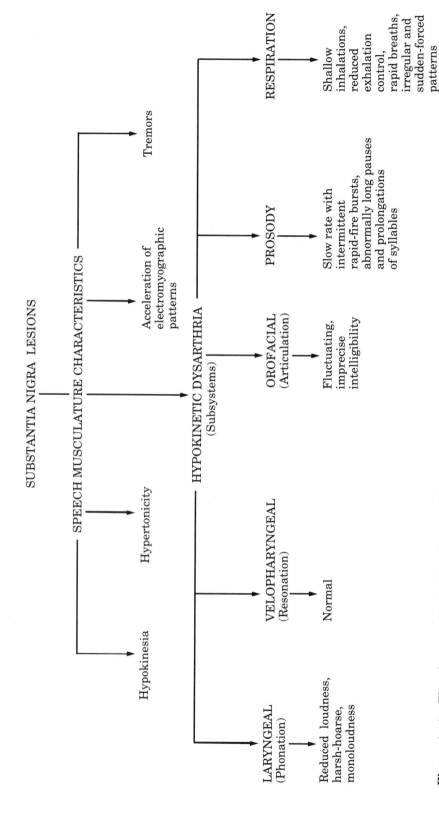

Figure 1–4. Flow diagram illustrating the overall characteristics of hypokinetic dysarthria.

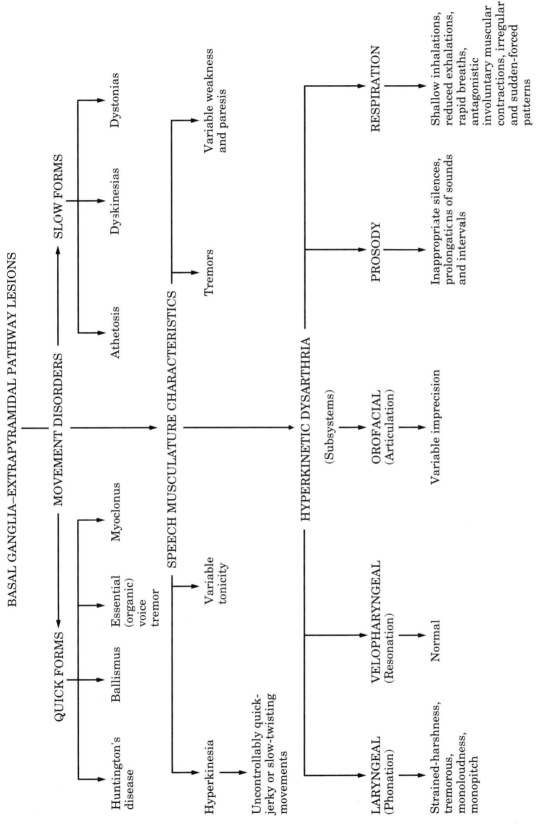

Figure 1–5. Flow diagram illustrating the overall characteristics of different patient populations with hyperkinetic dysarthria.

11

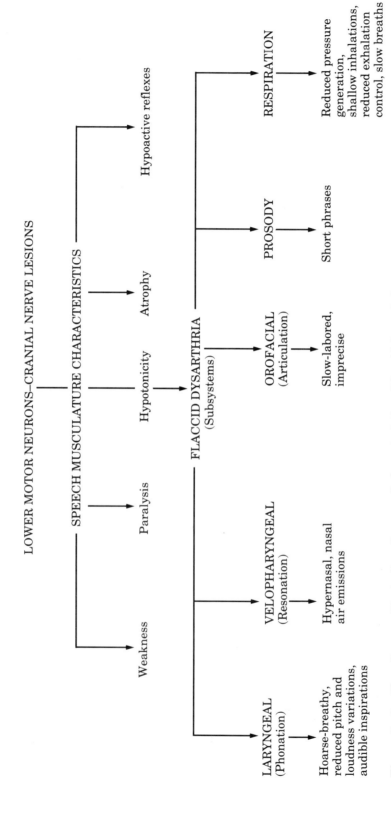

Figure 1–6. Flow diagram illustrating the overall characteristics of flaccid dysarthria.

Patients with Huntington's disease exhibit jerky, rapid, abrupt, and tic-like movements of the limb, trunk, and speech musculature that are uncontrollable, irregular, unsustained, and progressive in nature. Those with athetosis or dystonia exhibit slow, twisting, writhing, contorting, and worm-like movements of some of these same groups of muscles; such movements are similarly uncontrollable and variable. Patients with essential (organic) voice tremor or myoclonus may experience rhythmic tremors involving lingual-palatal-pharyngeal and/or laryngeal musculature; the former disorder may be accompanied by tremor of the limbs.

The hyperkinetic dysarthrias caused by these movement disorders generally are characterized by variable articulatory imprecision, vocal harshness, and prosodic abnormalities such as inappropriate silences, prolonged sounds and intervals between words, monopitch, and monoloudness. Patients with essential (organic) voice tremor, in particular, exhibit mostly voice difficulties, which along with voice tremor may include rhythmic and regular arrests of phonation that may be accompanied by periodic episodes of choking and strained voice quality. Lesions of the basal ganglia and/or their extrapyramidal projections are considered in the etiology of all these hyperkinetic disorders.

Flaccid Dysarthria

Patients with this type of dysarthria almost always present with slow-labored articulation, marked degrees of hypernasal resonance, and hoarse-breathy phonation (Figure 1–6). These characteristics are caused by paralysis, weakness, hypotonicity, atrophy, and hypoactive reflexes of involved speech subsystem musculature owing to damage to their cranial nerve supply or to inherent muscular diseases. The speech difficulties that result depend upon how many subsystems are adversely affected and the extent of their involvement, that is, which and how many cranial nerves are damaged, and whether the lesions are partial, complete, unilateral or bilateral. Injuries, diseases, or illnesses of the brain stem are among the most common causes of this peripheral nervous system condition. If involvement of the peripheral nerves is vast enough, the disturbances may be medically diagnosed as bulbar palsy.

Mixed Dysarthria

Diseases, illnesses, or injuries that cause diffuse neurologic damage may produce mixed forms of dysarthria in which a patient may present with speech and neuromuscular signs and symptoms characteristic of two or more types of the aforementioned dysarthrias.

SUGGESTED READINGS

Aronson, A. E. (1990). *Clinical voice disorders: An interdisciplinary approach.* New York: Thieme-Stratton, Inc.

Berry, N. R. (1983). *Clinical dysarthria.* San Diego, CA: College-Hill Press, Inc.

Darley, F., Aronson, A., & Brown J. (1975). *Motor speech disorders.* Philadelphia: W.B. Saunders Co.

Dworkin, J., & Hartman, D. (1988). *Cases in neurogenic communicative disorders.* Boston: Little, Brown & Co.

Gilman, S., & Winans, S. (1982). *Essentials of clinical neuroanatomy & neurophysiology.* Philadelphia: F.A. Davis Co.

Goldberg, S. (1979). *Clinical neuroanatomy made ridiculously simple.* Miami, FL: Mcd-Master, Inc.

Hartman, D., & Abbs, J. (1989). Dysarthria associated with focal unilateral upper motor neuron lesion. Paper presented at American Speech and Hearing Association Convention.

Hartman, D., & Abbs, J. (1988). Dysarthrias of movement disorders. In J. Jankovic & E. Tolosa (Eds.), *Advances in neurology* (pp. 289–306), vol. 49. New York: Raven Press.

Love, R., & Webb, W. (1986). *Neurology for the speech-language pathologist.* Stoneham, MA: Butterworths Pub.

Putnam, A. H. (1988). Review of research in dysarthria. In H. Winitz (Ed.), *Human communication and its disorders* (pp. 107–223). Norwood, NJ: Ablex Pub.

Rosenbek, J., McNeil, M., & Aronson A. (1984). *Apraxia of speech: physiology, acoustics, linguistics, management.* San Diego, CA: College-Hill Press, Inc.

Square, P. (1987). Acquired apraxia of speech. In H. Winitz (Ed.), *Human communication and its disorders* (pp. 88–166). Norwood, NJ: Ablex Pub.

Square-Storer, P., & Apeldorn, S. (1991). An acoustic study of apraxia of speech in patients with different lesion loci. In C. Moore, K. Yorkston, & D. Beukleman (Eds.), *Dysarthria and apraxia of speech: Perspectives on management.* Baltimore, MD: Paul H. Brooks, Pub.

Wertz, R., LaPointe, L., & Rosenbek, J. (1984). *Apraxia of speech in adults: The disorder and its management.* New York: Grune & Stratton.

Chapter 2

The Treatment Game: The Basics

Treatment of a patient with a motor speech disorder should be preceded by a number of obvious clinical steps. First, determine through differential diagnostic testing the overall nature and extent of speech subsystem disturbances. Second, identify the presence of specific neuromuscular abnormalities and/or motor planning deficits to which the speech difficulties presented can be logically attributed. Third, discover the underlying etiologic agent(s). Fourth, explore and understand the associated medical course and treatment needs. Fifth, hypothesize about the prognosis for speech improvement. Sixth, when it is possible, secure the cooperation of the attending physician. Seventh, develop a motor speech therapy plan with a sequential list of objectives. Eighth, prepare an intervention design to test the efficacy of the treatment plan. Ninth, assemble the tools necessary to administer the treatments, including charts to record baselines and ongoing performance. Tenth, discuss the intended game plan with the patient, and guardian if necessary, to ensure that they comprehend the treatment objectives and are as cooperative as possible at the outset. Next, each of these steps will be briefly addressed.

CLINICAL STEPS

Differential Diagnosis

Before treatments can be accurately administered, the speech subsystem disturbances must be identified and classified. For the purposes of this chapter, five subsystems will be acknowledged: (1) respiration, (2) phonation, (3) articulation, (4) resonation and (5) prosody. The diagnostic test battery used should reveal which of these subsystems are disturbed, and the characteristics and severity of their involvement.

Specific Neuromuscular Impairments

Patients who have been diagnosed as dysarthric must present with type-specific neuromuscular abnormalities of involved speech musculature, as discussed in Chapter 1. It is important that such conditions be accurately identified, classified to the extent possible, and graded so that this information can be incorporated into the treatment plan. Results of the oral mechanism examination coupled with those obtained from laryngoscopic, videofluorographic, and respirometric measurements should provide these data. Apractic patients, without coexistent dysarthria, on the other hand, usually do not present with speech neuromuscular features that require significant clinical attention.

Etiologic Agents

The underlying etiology and medical diagnoses may dictate the nature and timing of treatments as well as the overall prognosis for improvement. For example, the patient whose motor speech disorder is caused by a medically responsive neuropathology with a static clinical course usually can begin intensive speech therapy sooner and with a better prognosis than another patient with a degenerative condition that cannot be completely arrested with medical treatment. Treating patient symptoms differentially as a function of their etiology may be referred to as the type-specific approach. Treating symptoms routinely, irrespective of cause, may be labeled the symptomatological approach. Whereas employing this latter approach is tempting because these disorders, despite their diverse etiologies, are often characterized by remarkably similar speech subsystem disturbances, to do so may yield less than optimal clinical results. A patient whose velopharyngeal incompetence and associated hypernasality are caused by spastic paresis (e.g., owing to bilateral supranuclear lesions involving the corticobulbar tracts as a consequence of multiple sclerosis) usually requires a different approach clinically from that for the patient who presents with similar speech subsystem symptoms with a completely different etiology (e.g., intramedullary brainstem trauma with consequent flaccid paralysis of the velopharynx due to bilateral tenth nerve lesions). These patients are no more identical than the pathophysiologies underlying their speech subsystem disturbances: They have different medical needs, their clinical courses will differ ultimately, and their velopharyngeal incompetences will not respond in the same ways to the same treatment methodologies, as will be shown later in this text. The articulatory and prosodic disturbances of the apractic patient, as another example, respond best to treatment approaches that attack the underlying speech motor planning deficits. Moreover, even though a dysarthric patient may present with a host of similar articulatory and prosodic symptoms, the precipitating neuromuscular abnormalities demand treatments that are directed at improving the tone, strength, mobility, and/or coordination of involved speech musculature. Perhaps the most prudent clinical approach when one is working with the patient who exhibits a motor speech disorder is an eclectic one, in which the etiology, relative to causative agent, site(s) of lesion, neuromuscular features, *and* the resultant speech subsystem symptoms or disturbances all are taken into consideration when the treatment plan is being designed. The fruits of this suggestion will be illustrated later in the text when specific case studies are discussed.

Medical Course

Because motor speech disorders are induced by neurologic diseases, illnesses, and injuries, patients often require medico-surgical, pharmacologic, and/or prosthetic treatments as integral components of the rehabilitation regimen. When these treatments are prescribed, they often take precedence over speech therapy relative to timing and importance. In some cases, however, the various required treatments including speech intervention have their greatest effect when they are applied concurrently. Of course, the decision regarding the specific nature and application of appropriate treatments rests usually with the patient's attending physician, who must work closely with many different practitioners, including other physicians, speech-language pathologists (who from this point on will be called "clinicians"), dentists, and occupational and physical therapists. The patient who is judged medically stable following treatment for a head injury, for example, who may be a good candidate for a palatal lift appliance to facilitate velopharyngeal competence, will move most swiftly through the rehabilitation program if the prosthodontist and the clinician collaborate on the design and ongoing adjustments of the lift. When these practitioners work independently rather than collectively, they may not serve the patient as effectively. The patient with Parkinson's disease, as another example, will probably require a drug therapy program to improve the chances of success of other treatments prescribed. In this case, the physician in charge and the therapy team members have the patient's welfare at heart when their communication lines are free of static and open to each other. Furthermore, the patient with a degenerative disease, at some time in the treatment program, may not benefit from continued speech intervention: Further speech motor control improvements may be unlikely, and those dysfunctions that may have been successfully treated may re-emerge. In this case, the patient may be remanded to the care of the attending physician. Familiarity with the patient's medical profile and course will help the clinician orchestrate the very best strategy for interaction with other treatment team members and specific therapeutic recommendations. There may even be occasions when the clinician is first to identify certain medical needs of a patient, which must be brought to the attention of the attending physician.

Prognosis

The severity of the patient's speech subsystem disturbances as well as the underlying etiology invariably has an impact on the prognosis for improvement. When the prognosis is poor or guarded, speech intervention may best be scheduled on a trial basis to measure efficacy and obtain data to support or reject continuation of such service. Conversely, if greater success is anticipated, because the prognosis is good, a more comprehensive and long-term treatment plan may be indicated. In virtually all instances, the initial effects of such a plan should be observable within the first month. In the real clinical world, the prognosis can and does shift in either direction in concert with the medical status of the patient, which may change as time goes on, as well as with the patient's reactions to treatments applied. If and when this occurs, the focus of intervention may need to be adjusted. Other factors such as the age of the patient, general health, co-occurring language, cognitive, and psychosocial problems, family cooperation, and financial situation will influence the progress of treatment and prognosis for further improvement. Whether or not to terminate or alter the treatment program is a difficult but common question that, unfortunately, has no standard answer. Possible answers are occasionally discovered by careful review of a patient's file, which generally contains the clinician's ongoing perceptions of the effects of all treatments rendered and other relevant historical data. The opinions of other team members usually are helpful in this regard and should be sought whenever necessary and possible.

Physician Referral

Initiating speech intervention with dysarthric and apractic patients should be preceded by physician consultation, referrals and recommendations whenever possible and whenever they are required by third party payors. Not only is this good policy from a medico-legal standpoint, but also it ensures continued correspondence between primary care professionals who may become involved in the care of the patient.

Speech Therapy Intervention Plan

Patients usually move clinically at their own pace, and respond differently to (even) the same therapy. The astute clinician quickly identifies such differences between patients and accordingly tailors the focus, demands, and expectations of the intervention plan to the individual patient. Some patients may be willing and able to attend for intensive training (3 to 5 hours per week), and others may be unable to participate for more than 1 hour per week. Still others will fit in between or even beyond these frequency levels, and they may require modifications in the length of each session. Experienced clinicians all have discovered that the strategy that works beautifully with one patient may fail miserably with another. Some clinical researchers advocate that the objectives of the speech therapy intervention plan be realistic, with short-term and long-term focuses on training compensatory skills rather than on pushing patients to achieve normal speech motor control. It is not always counterproductive, however, to encourage and push certain patients to rise to levels that may be beyond their apparent physiologic potential. Some patients do much better when they are challenged to excel, even in the face of poor prognoses. The clinician must develop an appreciation of the personality differences of patients so as to set compatible treatment goals. Selection and sequencing of treatments will be addressed later in this chapter and will be illustrated with case examples in subsequent chapters.

Therapy Intervention Design

It is not sufficient merely to administer applicable treatments. Without incorporating a design to measure and test treatment efficacy, the clinician has no legitimate means of determining whether the therapy itself was responsible for significant changes made by the patient. Such determination requires that the methods employed be as objective, measurable, replicable, and empirical as possible, directed at illustrating cause-effect relationships. Familiarity with group and single-subject design strategies is a must for clinicians who wish to be able to account for and replicate significant improvements that *seem* to result from specific treatments. It is very important that clinicians, as health care providers, make improvements along these lines of accountability. Although on the surface a treatment plan may appear logical, rational, and plausible, it may not be empirically valid nor verifiable. Both group and single-subject design methodologies require use of charts to record patient performances for the purpose of pre-, para-, and post-treatment comparative analyses.

Treatment Tools

In this text, many different tools will be recommended for use with patients. Most of these tools are easy to construct or can be readily purchased at affordable prices. Information on how to construct and where possibly to purchase these materials will be provided in later chapters, as will various types of charts that should be used to record and trace treatment effects.

Treatment Preview

Before commencing with the treatment plan, it should be discussed in its entirety with the patient, significant others, and probably the primary care physician. This policy usually serves the clinician well inasmuch as it reduces the likelihood of treatment surprises that can evoke patient animosity or concern. When indicated, discussions should be held regarding the anticipated steps of the plan, the time frame for accomplishing stated objectives, and patient and family requirements to increase the chances of success. When possible, the anticipated overall costs to the patient for such services to be rendered, and office policies for fee collection should also be reviewed. If audio and videotapes of patient performances are to be collected, the clinician should be certain to obtain written permission to do so from the patient or guardian. Other types of release forms are also warranted that will enable the clinician to requisition patient data from other practitioners and to send out speech-language data upon request. These procedures should be well documented, with copies of the evaluation summary and therapy plan and policies given to the patient and family members for their information and records. If the patient was referred by another practitioner, a synopsis of diagnostic impressions and recommendations should be forwarded to that individual. Such correspondence reinforces communication with valuable referral sources, and highlights the professional protocol that is characteristic of a high-quality health care facility. In addition, progress reports that result from intervention with the patient should similarly be prepared every 4 to 6 weeks and should be reviewed with the patient, family members, and the referring practitioner. Figure 2–1 illustrates the overall flow of these recommended treatment steps.

TYPES OF TREATMENT DESIGNS

It is beyond the scope of this text to explore in detail the numerous single subject and group research designs that can be employed to test the effects of treatment. Many excellent books on these subjects are available for such information, some of which are listed among the suggested readings at the end of this chapter. Single subject treatment methodology is built on the concept of baseline logic, wherein measurements of target behaviors are repeated under at least two conditions: baseline (A) and intervention (B). Within the framework of applied behavioral analysis, there are many different variations or extensions of the basic A-B design that are popularly used by clinical researchers to demonstrate treatment efficacy. Because of time and space limitations, however, details of these single subject designs will not be addressed.

TREATMENT OBJECTIVES AND OUTCOMES

Clinicians experienced in working with dysarthric and apractic patients all know that the primary and secondary treatment objectives and outcomes can vary dramatically from one patient to the next, even when the diagnostic and etiologic distinctions are minimal. Although for each patient a hierarchy of speech subsystem exercises should be prescribed in accordance with the baseline disturbances identified, the prognosis for improvement is usually influenced by and dependent on some factors that may be beyond the clinician's control. Naturally, the severity of the motor speech disorder, the underlying etiology, and the amount of time that has elapsed since the onset, whether the disorder has been treated or not, constitutes such conditions. Any coexistent language, cognitive, intellectual, perceptual, and psychoemotional difficulties are additional factors that may temper anticipated treatment objectives and outcomes. Sometimes less obvious, but nonetheless a commonly occurring problem, is the patient's level of desire to improve. Patients may present, for example, with many different kinds of attitudes regarding their motor speech problems. Some wear a veil of denial, showing up for appointments only because they were brought into the clinic by an attendant or loved one. On the other end of the spectrum are those who are euphoric, arriving for each session with expectations of complete recovery. In be-

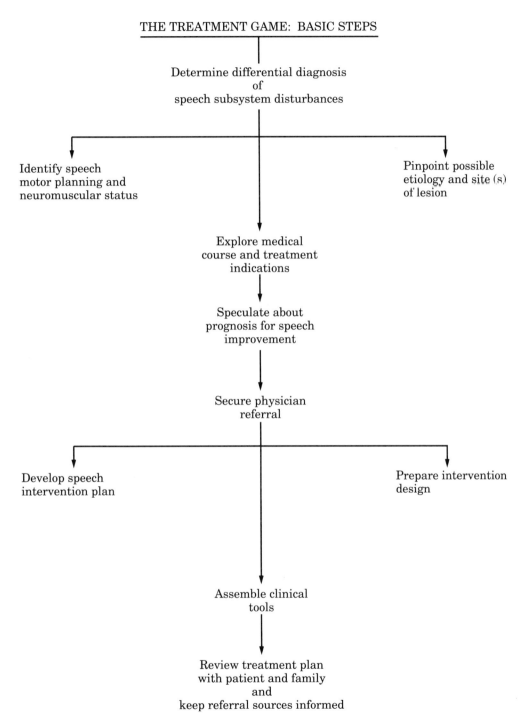

Figure 2–1. Flow diagram illustrating the overall sequential steps that may be followed when one is presented with a patient requiring evaluation and treatment of a motor speech disorder.

tween are those whose aspirations vary. The healthiest attitude, however, is a realistic one: A willingness to achieve gains gradually, which with time may add up to substantial overall improvement, and a steadfast determination to overcome treatment failures along the way can be rewarding in the end. Conversely, frustration may be facilitating in the long run, provided that through discussion and the process of self-actualization it can ultimately be channeled into positive energy and motivation.

Still other factors must be considered when the patient's treatment plan is designed. His or her age and primary medical status cannot be ignored. Cooperation and involvement of family members, guardians, or both may be essential to ensure success, and an optimal treatment schedule enables the clinician to induce potential gains in the shortest time.

In private facilities the source of funding may be an issue, at least in the minds of some administrators. Can the patient pay for the service? Will insurance coverage pick up the full tab, or the balance due? How many treatment sessions will the available funds support? Can we cover the difference between what we normally charge and what the patient or the insurance carrier will pay? If treatment needs to continue and the funds evaporate, can we carry the patient under pro bono ("free") provisions? Should we terminate the patient unable to pay, for one who can? These are examples of questions that arise in the everyday clinical world where fee for service is the rule.

In public school facilities or government agencies, such as Veterans Administration hospitals, where the source of funding is not usually a pressing daily or monthly issue, a factor such as the caseload size may have a significant impact on treatment objectives and outcome. Administrators of these institutions are known to clamor for accountability, and clinicians working under their supervision can ill afford to ignore these pleas. Frequently we must look at the patients who compose the long waiting list. It is not uncommon for the clinician to be asked whether it is justifiable to continue in treatment with patient X, who has been progressing at a snail's pace for some time, when patients Y and Z next in line on the waiting list appear poised to benefit more from the services if only they are readily admitted to the program. Decisions like these are never easy to make. They cannot emerge sporadically, injudiciously, at the expense of the long-standing patient. Nor can they be delayed indefinitely at the expense of another patient who is entitled to the same opportunities and has yet to be helped. Interestingly, in the private facility, caseload size rarely presents a problem. Additional help can often be hired to cover the overload, or referral to a sister facility can be made.

Last, but certainly not least, the factors that may ensure fulfillment of treatment objectives are the quality and accuracy of the services provided to attain these goals. Even if all the aforementioned factors were most ideally in place, inherently working in favor of the patient, substantial improvements likely would not be realized if inappropriate treatments were rendered. Patients operating in such a vacuum can and do surprise us with observable gains in spite of, never because of, misdirected therapy. Most often, however, this outcome does not come to pass.

CHARTING PROGRESS

Taxing as it may be, charting patient baseline performances and responses to specific treatments can prove invaluable. Not only will charts enable the clinician to compare and contrast pre-, para-, and post-therapeutic levels, but also they provide useful reference data in patient files. Further, trend lines may be observed on such charts that indicate the need to continue, alter slightly, or eliminate certain techniques based on the criteria and clinical objectives that were originally set for patients.

In the chapters that follow, various charts are provided and suggested for use in logging and tracking patient behaviors that are measured during baseline testing and targeted in the treatment exercises. The chart recommended for a given exercise should be used routinely. Generally, the best procedure for entering information on any one of these charts is to do so as inconspicuously as possible after each respective clinical observation so that the patient is not distracted or preoccupied with the scores rendered. Whereas ways of using these charts are suggested in later chapters, the clinician is not bound to the recommended approaches. Alterations in the design and methodology for scoring patient responses are perfectly within the purview of the individual administering the treatment. The clinician is encouraged to duplicate these blank charts for future use with all patients. These charts can be pulled for case presentation at team meetings and when accountability for services provided and fees charged must be demonstrated. If for no other reason, use of these charts helps guide the exercises administered in sequential order, thereby providing organization of the treatment program, which might otherwise be limited.

Charting behavior can be bothersome, however. It takes time to do, it can become complicated, and it presses the clinician to remain as objective as possible about the patient's progress in therapy. Clinicians have often discovered that their perceptions of how patients were progressing with treatment were challenged by chart trend lines that suggested minimal gains and the need to modify the program to achieve the stated objectives.

BASELINE BEHAVIORS

Before administering any treatment, it is best and logical to collect baseline (pre-treatment) data on the behavior to be treated. As will be discussed in subsequent chapters, for each of the exercises in this text, establishing a baseline score is recommended as the first procedural step. The thresholds or cutoff scores suggested throughout the text to help determine whether the behaviors tested require intervention are arbitrary and are not scientifically based. If they don't work well for a given patient, they should be changed to meet his or her individual needs so long as reasonable substitutes are employed. If we wish to be accountable for the services we render, we have to appreciate that baseline data are indispensable to the measurement of treatment efficacy. In addition, these data can be used strategically to shape the relative criteria for improvement that will govern movements within and between exercises.

GREAT EXPECTATIONS

The Hawthorne and Rosenthal effects may shed additional therapeutic light on perceived and actual patient progress. The former effect has essentially taught us that people tend naturally to try to do their very best when they perceive that their feelings and needs are of great concern to their supervisors. The latter effect introduced two hypotheses: (1) that the performances of people are strongly correlated with the level of expectation that is placed upon them and (2) that our expectations of how others should behave influences significantly how we may interact with them to induce that behavior.

It is obvious that such effects are likely to contribute to the results we obtain in our work with dysarthric and apractic patients. There is a growing conviction among clinicians that patients need to know that we care about them and their welfare. Also, we have to approach them clinically with an upbeat attitude. If they can be made to sense that we believe in them and their chances to improve significantly, they just may aspire to such optimistic levels. What's more, we must learn about what patients are feeling and what they wish for themselves in order for us to understand and truly believe in them.

The right chemistry between the patient and clinician can be most helpful, especially when the treatment program prescribed calls for intensive and extensive time in each other's company. Whereas good vibrations such as these do not necessarily guarantee good results in therapy, it is a safe bet that bad vibrations will most assuredly guarantee bad results. Together with a technically and methodologically sound treatment plan, warm, positive therapeutic interactions can make what might have been a good outcome an excellent one.

CRITERIA FOR TREATMENT ADVANCEMENT AND DISCONTINUATION

When planning the treatment program for the patient with a motor speech disorder, the following questions can be raised:

1. Given the patient's medical and speech-language diagnosis and status, what is the prognosis for speech improvement?
2. If treatment is to be initiated, what is the best sequence of speech subsystem exercises?
3. What research design strategy should be employed to test treatment efficacy?
4. In view of the prognosis for improvement, at what level should the cri-

teria be set for advancement and discontinuation within and between exercises?

5. To what extent will assistance from the patient's significant others be required to achieve the treatment objectives?
6. How many treatment sessions per week should be scheduled for the patient to ensure optimal results?
7. Can the clinician's schedule and the patient's financial situation accommodate the proposed therapy plan?

If after 30 consecutive trials (the definition of a trial varies with different subsystem exercises) of a given exercise the patient fails to demonstrate any *observable* trend of improvement, that treatment should be discontinued in favor of the next prescribed exercise. This guideline generally works very well in that it requires the cessation of exercises that have had no *discernible* positive effects after many attempts, and it demands the introduction of new treatment in lieu of those exercises that have failed to stimulate improved performances. In the final analysis, this cut-off technique promotes a time- and cost-efficient operation.

Clinicians should be permitted, however, to exercise their prerogative to allow clinical intuitions to overrule this discontinuation criterion when they sense that if they pushed the exercise just a little longer, maybe attempted a slightly different twist to the activity, the patient would respond favorably enough to justify continuation. The data to support this approach are weak at best, and few patients benefit from a modified plan. However, on occasion, the exceptional patient emerges who merits such consideration.

To determine when to advance to the next indicated exercise in a treatment sequence, relative criteria scales are suggested. These types of scales use the patient's own pretreatment levels of performance to measure improvement. Conversely, absolute criteria scales are more rigid because they are based on the standards of "normal" performance, without consideration of the severity of the patient's difficulties. As such, by design they may penalize the patient who is unlikely ever to improve to within normal levels of performance. By adopting relative versus absolute criteria measures, the patient is afforded the opportunity to demonstrate and be credited for significant (albeit) relative gains.

Throughout the chapters that follow, the treatment exercises are designed according to a step-by-step procedural format. At the top, baseline data are collected to determine whether the behavior tested requires intervention. For each exercise, a cut-off score, or threshold, is recommended to make this determination. It is helpful to list this score on the respective treatment chart in the cell entitled "target criterion" at the bottom of the column in which the baseline data are recorded. This listing provides a ready view of the level of performance, and whether or not treatment is indicated for the behavior tested. Because this recommendation is arbitrary, clinicians may opt to select a different level to measure whether or not treatment is indicated. As long as a reasonable scale is used for this purpose, the level chosen is relatively insignificant.

At the completion of the baseline data collection process, it is helpful to calculate the criterion for improvement that will be used to dictate advancement to the next exercise indicated. In the final step(s) of each exercise, a criterion is recommended that will govern such advancement. The criterion in most instances is not predetermined. Rather, it is based on the individual patient's baseline performances. When a percentage scale is the yardstick of measurement for a given exercise, the recommended criterion is 75 percent improvement over the baseline score or 100 percent correct, whichever is less, over "X" number of consecutive trials. Thus, if on baseline testing the patient scored 40 percent correct attempts of a particular behavior, which may be considered below threshold and in need of treatment, the relative criterion for advancement during treatment would be 70 percent correct/"X" trials (40% × 0.75% = 30 + 40 = 70%). Naturally, if the patient demonstrates the ability to make greater gains with continued practice, when no plateaus are evident, that exercise should not be terminated at 70 percent correct, even though the (minimal) criterion for improvement has been met. It is prudent to press on with the same exercise until the patient indeed reaches a plateau.

For exercises that generate perceptual scores on the seven-point interval scale, for example, the patient continues until the performances are at least 3 scale values better than the baseline score, or 1 (normal) if baseline was rated a 3 or 4 over "X" number of consecutive trials. Note that the value representing "normal" may vary across scales. Thus, if the baseline rating was a 6, indicating a severe disturbance, thereby requiring intervention, the relative criterion for improvement and advancement to the next exercise would be at least a mean perceptual rating of 3 (6 − 3 = 3). Again, if there is reason to believe that even greater gains can be realized if the exercise is continued, it should be until a plateau in performance is evident. The clinician may choose to adopt different thresholds for different patients, giving consideration to all those factors that may influence the potential success of the overall treatment program.

At the bottom of each treatment chart, there is the aforementioned row called "target criterion." The cells in this row should be used to list the calculated (target) criterion for improvement for the behavior about to be treated. Listing the target in this fashion accomplishes two primary objectives: (1) it forces the clinician to determine at the outset of intervention when the next set of treatments will be phased in, and (2) it enables the clinician to compare easily the treatment data entry on the grid of the column with the criterion listed at the bottom for quick determination of the level of progress achieved and the extent of further improvement required.

The target criterion listings across the row may vary from one exercise to the next in accordance with the baseline scores and the yardsticks of measurement used (percentile or perceptual scores, for example). Treatment usually begins following these important prerequisite procedures. It is important to note that there is nothing magical or inflexible about the proposed cut-off scores for determining the patient's need for specific intervention. The levels recommended are relatively arbitrary, but they do afford the patient some latitude from the "normal" reference before abnormal performances are considered clinically significant. Alternative thresholds can be adopted to suit the individual patient and the clinician's personal biases about when to begin treatment.

Figure 2–2 is a copy of the Speech Characteristics Chart, which should be used periodically throughout the entire treatment program to measure the overall effects of intervention on the primary parameters of speech. Specific guidelines for such use are provided in later chapters.

Figure 2–3 is a copy of a chart that should be used for retroactive measures; that is, of behaviors already subjected to treatment. Tracking the maintenance factor is very important and should be an ongoing procedure throughout the entire treatment program. Because patients can and do fail to retain learned behaviors, a chart such as this can pinpoint when and where breakdowns have occurred that may require therapeutic re-interventions. Carry-over is checked every five sessions or so to ensure that the patient is holding on to previous gains as new treatments are continuously phased into the program. When regression is identified, the current exercise regimen should be put on temporary hold until restoration of earlier attained skills is accomplished. Looking at this chart, note that both primary and secondary letters are listed in the activity symbol cell at the bottom of the column corresponding to the data entry. For example, to tag the respiration subsystem maintenance measurement of "pressure-generating" capability, place the symbol RG in this cell. The first letter represents the subsystem symbol and the second the activity being retested.

RATIONALE FOR THE TREATMENT APPROACHES TO SPEECH NEUROMOTOR REHABILITATION

Dysarthria is a neuromotor speech disorder characterized by difficulties in *executing* speech musculature events. Apraxia is also a neuromotor speech disorder, but it should be distinguished from the dysarthrias in that here the problem lies with higher level programming or planning of such events. Because of these characteristic distinctions, treatment techniques and objectives should not be identical for dysarthric and apractic patients.

Guidelines for Selection and Sequence of Dysarthria Treatments

Those patients with dysarthria may benefit from exercises aimed at facilitating the physiologic integrity of and coordination between the disturbed speech subsystems or training compensatory skills. Whereas the types and sequences of treatments used will depend upon which subsystems are malfunctioning and the nature and extent of their breakdowns, usually the treatment package includes techniques that are designed to promote (1) oral motor development in those whose dysarthria is of congenital origin; (2) adequate body and orofacial postures; (3) integration of primitive and higher-level orofacial reflexes; (4) reductions or increases in orofacial muscle tone; (5) increases in orofacial muscle strength; and (6) improvements in the range, speed, timing, and/or coordination of orofacial muscle contractions and movements. The rationale, although not without contro-

SPEECH CHARACTERISTICS CHART

Patient's name: _____

Birthdate: _____ Sex: _____

Speech diagnosis: _____

Medical diagnosis: _____

_____

Clinician: _____

Facility: _____

Address: _____

Comments: _____

_____

_____

_____

_____

_____

ACTIVITY KEY

MEASUREMENT UNIT

Feature:

1. Articulatory precision (A)

2. Resonance balance (R)

3. Voice (V)   7-Point interval scale
                  (1 = normal; 7 = most deviant)
4. Prosody (P)

5. Contextual speech (C)

Baseline (pre-treatment): B + feature symbol

Dates:

Most Deviant   7

                6

                5

← Intelligibility Ratings →   4

                3

                2

Normal   1

No. of minutes of sample activity

List A, R, V, P, C, or B + feature

Target criterion

SESSIONS

Figure 2–2. Interval scale to chart overall speech characteristics prior to, during, and following motor speech intervention.

MAINTENANCE OF TREATMENT RESPONSE CHART

Patient's name: _____

Birthdate: _____ Sex: _____

Speech diagnosis: _____

Medical diagnosis: _____

Clinician: _____

Facility: _____

Address: _____

Comments: _____

ACTIVITY KEY

Symbols

Respiration subsystem (R) + R, T, G, I, E, Q, S, P, C

Resonation subsystem (N) + H, P, V, A, W, S, C

Phonation subsystem (V) + R, Y, V, T, S, C, H, N, P, A, M, L, E+

Articulation subsystem (A) + appropriate symbol

Prosody subsystem (P) + P, L, R, S, C

Dates:

100																						
90																						
80																						
70																						
60																						
50																						
40																						
30																						
20																						
10																						
7																						
6																						
5																						
4																						
3																						
2																						
1																						
0																						
-4																						
-3																						
-2																						
-1																						

Correct per unit of Measure or Perceptual Rating

No. of trials

Activity symbol

Unit of measure

Target criterion

SESSIONS

Figure 2–3. Blank chart to be used for maintenance evaluations throughout the treatment program to determine the levels of retention of already treated behaviors.

29

versy, for these general clinical objectives has been advanced over the years by our colleagues in neurophysiology and occupational and physical therapy, who have been influenced largely by the early works of Froeschels, Kabat, Rood, and the Bobaths. We all have heard and read about neurorehabilitation treatments such as resistance isometrics, reflex-inhibiting postures, stretch pressure, icing, brushing, stroking, massaging, pushing, pulling, vibration, mass movement patterns, and dynamic slings, splints, and positioning devices that effectively support, activate, facilitate, and inhibit muscular contractions. These techniques are used to induce different, even opposing, clinical effects, depending upon the intensity, frequency, and site of their application. For example, brief and intermittent pressure application to the belly of a target muscle usually facilitates contraction. If the same pressure technique is applied to the muscle's point of insertion, however, an inhibitory response typically results. When slow, even, and rhythmic rates of sensory stimulation are presented, inhibitory reactions are generally evoked. Fast, uneven, and intermittent applications of the same stimuli are, on the other hand, facilitatory.

Another guideline taught by neurorehabilitation therapists is that any presumed facilitatory stimulus can be counterproductive and inhibitory if it is applied with enough intensity and for a long enough duration to cause a painful response. These practitioners further caution that (1) fear, anxiety, and previous experiences can alter the way in which a patient may respond to a given treatment; (2) numerous applications of the same stimulus may cause an adaptation effect, thereby lessening its subsequent neurologic penetration; and (3) frequent use of inhibitory techniques may promote an autonomic rebound or overcompensation phenomenon in which neuromuscular processes may speed up in an attempt to restore homeostasis. Naturally, not all these types of treatment modalities are applicable in motor speech rehabilitation. Many, however, may be effective adjuncts to clinical success with dysarthric (and apractic) patients. As such, the approaches to speech neuromotor therapy advocated throughout this text have, in part, been molded over the years by this author's trial and error experiences with all these techniques.

The overall goal of therapy with dysarthric patients is to improve speech motor control and intelligibility. This is best achieved when treatments that attack any underlying neuromuscular abnormalities are strategically incorporated into the exercise plan. Phonetic practice alone is simply insufficient. Rarely does a patient improve in such a vacuum.

The selection and sequence of specific treatments, of course, are dictated by the idiosyncratic signs, symptoms, and medical history presented by the patient. Generally speaking, however, treatments should begin at the patient's baseline performance levels and progress from there up the sensorimotor developmental ladder, always taking into account the speech subsystem disturbances and their functional interrelationships. If, for example, the orofacial musculature about to be treated is characterized by at least one of the following abnormalities, it is best to begin intervention with appropriate *inhibition* techniques:

1. Increased tone and any associated weakness and paresis,
2. Hyperactive reflexes,
3. Hyperkinesia, and
4. Hypersensitivity.

The successful inhibition of these types of abnormal behaviors paves the way for the facilitatory treatments that usually are indicated next to promote improved speech motor control. *Facilitation* techniques are introduced to improve functioning of those orofacial muscles with any of the following types of abnormal features:

1. Decreased tone and any associated weakness and paresis,
2. Hypoactive reflexes, and
3. Hyposensitivity.

Those patients who exhibit mixed pathophysiologic portraits may require simultaneous inhibitory and facilitatory treatments. The rationale for specific selections and sequences of such treatments will be addressed in detail in later chapters when the cases of many different dysarthric patients are presented.

The hierarchy of subsystem treatments for dysarthric patients shown in Figure 2–4 may serve as a general guideline when designing the intervention methodology. Use of this algorithm is relatively straightforward but may require a few illustrative examples.

Procedures

1. If the dysarthric patient exhibits velopharyngeal and/or respiratory musculature dysfunctions and associated hypernasality and speech breathing dyscontrol, these subsystem abnormalities should receive first-order, top-priority clinical attention. *Do not* treat subsystems on

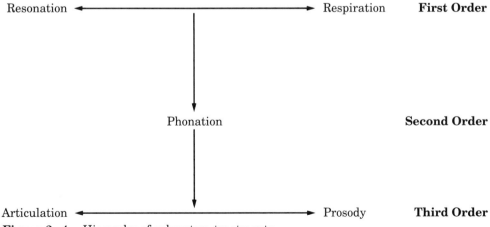

Figure 2–4. Hierarchy of subsystem treatments.

second- or third-order levels until those on the first order are treated to criteria. Treatments of first-order subsystems can be conducted simultaneously, when they are indicated and feasible.

2. If the dysarthric patient exhibits hypo- or hyperfunctioning of laryngeal musculature and associated voice abnormalities, this subsystem should be treated to criteria before intervening on third-order level disturbances. Maintenance treatments of first-order subsystems are frequently incorporated into the treatment program for these second-order disturbances.

3. If the dysarthric patient exhibits dyscontrol of articulatory musculature and associated articulation and/or prosodic imprecision, these subsystems should be treated intensively, provided that those subsystems of the first and second orders require *no* more than maintenance stimulation. Treatments of third-order subsystems can be conducted simultaneously, when they are indicated and feasible.

The hierarchy of treatments recommended here is based on a logical top-down order of physiologic interdependence between the speech subsystems. Therefore, whereas invariably there will be multiple treatments applied to each subsystem to facilitate improvement objectives, attempts to treat more than two subsystems at a time that are not on the same order can frustrate the patient and lead to failure. Exceptions to this rule do occur, however.

Guidelines for Selection and Sequence of Apraxia Treatments

Patients with apraxia of speech, without significant co-occurring dysarthria, do not require exercises designed to improve the neuromuscular integrity of the speech mechanism. Further, unless the probable co-occurring aphasia is severe, the apractic patient's speech difficulties are not generally complicated by imperceptions of the words or sounds attempted. Consequently, general language and auditory discrimination stimuli usually are not indicated. These individuals suffer from motor planning disturbances and therefore may benefit from treatments that promote voluntary control of individual and sequential articulatory adjustments for prosodically sufficient and intelligible speech production, free of struggle and groping behaviors. If dysarthria, aphasia, and/or oral apraxia coexist to degrees that demand therapeutic attention, the therapist must consider the extent to which these conditions may interfere with speech apraxia therapy. As such, the sequence of treatments may begin with focus on these coexistent disorders, and progress sequentially to the following speech motor planning activities, when they are indicated:

1. Teaching a slow-deliberate speaking rate,
2. Pairing motor gestures or external temporal pacing stimuli with speech attempts,
3. Evoking automatic-reactive speech,
4. Using melodic intonation techniques to stimulate speech output,

5. Focusing specifically on articulation imprecision,
6. Beginning phonetic training with short, reduplicating utterances, and
7. Increasing the length and complexity of phonetic stimuli, and the distance between articulatory contact points as sound sequencing improves.

The apraxia of speech case samples presented in later chapters will highlight the variable treatment methodology options, relative to task selections and sequencing and procedural strategies.

Table 2–1 provides a summary of the sequences of proposed treatment plans for the speech subsystems, segregated by type of disorder and level of severity. The hierarchy assumes the existence of the classic matrix of speech and non-

TABLE 2–1. Summary of Sequential Treatments of the Speech Subsystems Segregated by Disorder Type and Severity

Disorder/Severity	Respiration	Resonation	Phonation	Articulation	Prosody
Flaccid dysarthria					
A. Mononeuropathy:					
VIIth nerve	N/A	N/A	N/A	First	Second, if necessary
Xth nerve	N/A	First, if necessary	Second, if necessary	Third, if necessary	Fourth, if necessary
XIIth nerve	N/A	N/A	N/A	First	Second
B. Polyneuropathy:					
VIIth & Xth nerves	N/A	First	Second	Third	Fourth, if necessary
Xth & XIIth nerves	N/A	First	Second	Third	Fourth
VIIth & XIIth nerves	N/A	N/A	N/A	First	Second
VIIth, Xth, & XIIth nerves	N/A	First	Second	Third	Fourth
Spastic dysarthria					
A. Mild	First	First	Second	Second	Third
B. Moderate/severe	First	Second	Third	Fourth	Fifth
Ataxic dysarthria					
A. Mild	First	N/A	First	Second	Third
B. Moderate/severe	First	N/A	Second	Third	Fourth
Hypokinetic dysarthria					
A. Mild	First	N/A	First	Second	Third
B. Moderate/severe	First	N/A	Second	Third	Fourth
Hyperkinetic dysarthria					
A. Mild	First	N/A	First	Second	Third
B. Moderate/severe	First	N/A	Second	Third	Fourth
Apraxia					
A. Speech	N/A	N/A	N/A	First	Second
B. Phonation	N/A	N/A	First	N/A	Second

For mixed dysarthria, assume the typical combination of subsystem treatments based on the predominant and secondary components of the composite mixture.

speech signs and symptoms characteristic of that disorder type. For example, study the moderate-severe spastic dysarthria category. Note that, according to the listings across the row, "respiration" should be treated first, followed by treatments of resonation, phonation, articulation, and prosody in that order. It is implied that treatment of a given subsystem is not initiated until the entire exercise regimen for the preceding one has been administered. Thus, for this population example, at any point in time only one subsystem should be the focus of intervention. For mildly involved spastic dysarthric patients, on the other hand, two speech subsystems could be treated concurrently, either simultaneously every session or alternately every other session. This suggested approach argues that patients with moderate or severe disturbances do better when they are exposed to one subsystem treatment regimen at a time, while mildly involved patients may excel if two (or more) subsystems are treated concurrently. For those patients who do not present with the classic behavioral profile for the given motor speech disorder they exhibit, it is usually necessary to alter the sequence of treatments to be administered. This can be accomplished by simply skipping the uninvolved subsystem(s) as sequential treatments are being designed.

Table 2–2 will facilitate all exercises that involve the recommended use of a metronome as an external pacing device. The data in the table can be extrapolated for quick calculations of treatment responses, which may need to be recorded on the respective treatment chart. The examples below help illustrate the tables facilitative functions.

1. The task is an *up/down (u/d)* tongue force physiology mobility exercise, using a bite block wedge to stabilize the jaw of a spastic dysarthric patient. The metronome is set at *30 beats per minute (bpm)*. The patient is instructed to move alternately the tongue-tip to (*up,* or U) and from (*down,* or D) the alveolar ridge to the beats of the metronome. With each new beat the opposite vector is the target. If the patient can perform these movements without error for 1 full minute, the *maximum number of complete (U&D) responses* will be *15* (100 percent). If less than 1 minute is attempted, the number of correct responses can be prorated to determine the percentage that are correct.

2. The task is production of a *three-syllable word* with the metronome set at *90 bpm*. The apractic patient is instructed to produce one syllable of the word per beat, so that after three beats the entire word is produced. This speech motor planning exercise is repeated with the same word until 1 full minute has expired or until the patient signals the need to stop. The *maximum number of complete (error-free) word productions* (responses) will be *30* (100 percent), with 1 full minute of attempts or will be prorated down, depending upon the length of the trial.

3. The task is a *seven-word sentence* that contains words of varying lengths. The metronome is set at *120 bpm,* and the apractic patient is requested to produce one syllable per beat, from the beginning until the sentence is completed. This exercise is repeated again and again with

**TABLE 2–2. Index of Metronomic Levels Showing Maximum Number of
Complete Behavioral Responses Possible from Patient under Different Beats
per Minute and Treatment Task Conditions**

Task	Beats per Minute	Maximum No. of Complete Responses per Minute	% Correct
Two-vector	30	15	100
mobility	60	30	100
activity	90	45	100
(e.g., up/down)	120	60	100
	150	75	100
	200	100	100
	Variable	Variable	—
Single phoneme	30	30	100
repetitions (e.g., /aː/, /pʌ/)	60	60	100
	90	90	100
	120	120	100
	150	150	100
	200	200	100
	Variable	Variable	—
Two phoneme	30	15	100
or syllable	60	30	100
combination	90	45	100
repetitions (e.g., /pʌ-kʌ/,	120	60	100
baseball, /i-u/)	150	75	100
	200	100	100
	Variable	Variable	—
Three phoneme	30	10	100
or syllable combination	60	20	100
repetitions (e.g., tornado,	90	30	100
/pʌ-tʌ-kʌ/, /i-u-a/)	120	40	100
	150	50	100
	200	66	100
	Variable	Variable	—
Four phoneme	30	7	100
or syllable combination	60	15	100
repetitions (e.g., television)	90	22	100
	120	30	100
	150	37	100
	200	50	100
	Variable	Variable	—
Five phoneme	30	6	100
or syllable combination	60	12	100
repetitions	90	18	100
(e.g., refrigerator)	120	24	100
	150	30	100
	200	40	100
	Variable	Variable	—

the same sentence until 1 full minute has expired or until the patient signals the need to stop for a break. By the time the patient is practicing sentences like this, the scoring procedure is relatively simple: A dichotomous *correct/incorrect system* is recommended, in which the entire sentence performance is graded. If *all* syllable productions in the sentence are error free, then the patient is graded "correct." If one or more disturbances occur during syllable productions, the sentence performance is graded "incorrect." Each sentence attempt is graded independent of previous ones. New sentences can be introduced at any time. *Note:* The same principles of operation apply with the other *task* and *beats per minute* options. The important thing to remember is that *each* and *every* attempt, whether a physiologic gesture such as up, down, left, right, or so forth, or a syllable or phoneme utterance, *must* occur in tandem with a respective beat of the metronome, and *must* be performed without observable signs of difficulty, as behaviorally defined, to be considered a *"correct"* attempt: One physiologic vector per beat, one phoneme per beat, and one syllable per beat regardless of the length of the task or the set number of beats per minute. Some patients can continue for 1 full minute without the need to take a break, whereas others will need to stop sooner. The mobility treatment activities, in particular, can and do cause fatigue in much less than 1 minute, regardless of the speed of the metronome or the severity of the patient's disorder. Boredom also can influence the performance and motivation of the patient. Whenever possible, the stimulus item should be switched after each 30- to 60-second period of activity; this reduces possible order effects and boredom and is especially easy to do when speech sound productions are being treated.

Intervention cannot normally begin until the methods to be followed are carefully outlined by the clinician, as mentioned earlier. Long- and short-term objectives need to be considered as does the sequence of treatments for the deficits exhibited by the patient. When the clinician is working with patients who have disturbances of more than one speech subsystem, which is the case for virtually all individuals with motor speech disorders, the clinician must determine the sequence of treatments to be administered. In some instances, especially for severely involved patients, the aforementioned focus of intervention should be on no more than one subsystem at a time. In other cases, in particular in those patients with less severe involvements, two subsystems may be treated during each session, and the performance of each subsystem will probably improve at its own pace. Attempts to treat three subsystems at a time, however, can be unwieldy and ought to be avoided. One must remember that the underlying objective of treatment is to produce an adaptive response in the patient, in which the behavior treated becomes more productive, advanced, organized, and flexible than it was prior to such treatment. This clinical goal is less likely to be achieved or shaped if the patient is bombarded with numerous stimuli simultaneously, which

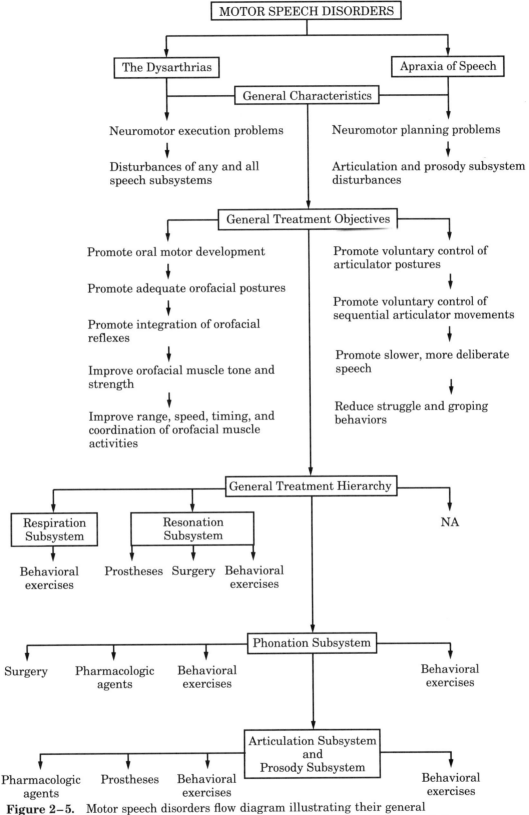

Figure 2–5. Motor speech disorders flow diagram illustrating their general characteristics, the overall objectives of speech intervention, and the top-down differential hierarchy of speech subsystem treatments. Specific descriptions of the treatment subtypes are reserved for the algorithms of Chapters 3 through 7.

might cause overstimulation and confusion. As each subsystem is improved to criteria, an untreated one can be phased in in its respective place. Naturally, treatment of each subsystem should be governed by its own set of criteria. Figure 2–5 helps summarize the proposed treatment objectives and techniques for patients with motor speech disorders.

It is important to realize that there will be some patients whose motor speech difficulties are not responsive to the treatment recommendations described in these chapters. Such individuals may be candidates for augmentation or nonoral communication systems if they do not already possess and use these types of devices. The decision to discontinue speech intervention and to initiate or focus solely on an alternative form of communication should be one that all team members agree will help the patient most. However, opting for the nonoral route of intervention before making valiant efforts to improve communication through (conventional) oral techniques may not always be in the patient's best interest, regardless of his or her clinical history.

PATIENT RESOURCES

The following associations can be contacted for information and assistance for patients, their families, and staff. Many have local or state chapters.

Alzheimer's Disease and Related Disorders
Association (ADRDA)
National Headquarters
70 East Lake Street
Chicago, IL 60601

Amyotrophic Lateral Sclerosis Association (ALS)
15300 Ventura Blvd., Suite 315
P. O. Box 5951
Sherman Oaks, CA 91403

American Heart Association (for stroke victims)
732 Greenville Avenue
Dallas, TX 75231

Ataxia Foundation (National Headquarters)
600 Twelve Oaks Center
15500 Wayzata Blvd.
Wayzata, MN 55391

Brain Tumor Research Association
6232 North Pulaski Road
Chicago, IL 60646

Dystonia Medical Research Foundation
8383 Wilshire Blvd., Suite 800
Beverly Hills, CA 90211

Epilepsy Foundation of America
4351 Garden City Drive #406
Landover, MD 20785

Head Injury Foundation (National Headquarters)
P. O. Box 567
Framingham, MA 01701

Huntington's Disease Foundation of America, Inc.
140 West 22nd Street
New York, NY 10011

March of Dimes, Birth Defects Foundation
1275 Mamoroneck Avenue
White Plains, NY 10605

Multiple Sclerosis Society (National Headquarters)
205 East 42nd Street
New York, NY 10017

Muscular Dystrophy Association
810 Seventh Avenue
New York, NY 91403

National Neurofibromatosis Foundation
70 West 40th Street, 4th Floor
New York, NY 10018

Neurometabolic Disorders Association
21707 Cheltenham
Toledo, OH 43606

Parkinson's Disease Foundation (National Headquarters)
650 West 168th Street
New York, NY

Reye's Syndrome Foundation (National Headquarters)
509 Rosemont
Bryan, OH

Spasmodic Torticollis Association (National Headquarters)
P. O. Box 873
Royal Oak, MI 48068

Spina Bifida Association of America
1700 Rockville Pike, Suite 540
Rockville, MD 20852

Tourette Syndrome Association
41-02 Bell Blvd.
Bayside, NY 11361

United Cerebral Palsy Association, Inc.
66 East 34th Street
New York, NY 10016

SUGGESTED READINGS

Costello, J. M. (1979). Clinicians and researchers: A necessary dichotomy? *Journal of National Student Speech and Hearing Association, 7,* 6–26.

Crickmay, M. C. (1966). *Speech therapy and the Bobath approach to cerebral palsy.* Springfield, IL: Charles C. Thomas, Pub.

Dworkin, J., & Hartman, D. (1988). *Cases in neurogenic communicative disorders.* Boston: Little, Brown.

Dworkin, J., Abkarian, G., & Johns, D. (1987). Therapeutic research: Can it be done? Mini-seminar at *Annual Convention of American Speech-Language Hearing Association.*

Hedge, M. N. (1985). *Treatment procedures in communicative disorders.* San Diego, CA: College-Hill Press.

Hersen, M., & Barlow, D. (1976). *Single case experimental designs.* New York: Pergamon Press.

Johns, D. F. (1985). *Clinical management of neurogenic communicative disorders.* Boston: Little, Brown & Co.

Kearns, K. (1986). Flexibility of single subject experimental designs: Part II. *Journal of speech and hearing disorders, 51,* 204–214.

McReynolds, L., & Kearns, K. (1983). *Single-subject experimental designs in communicative disorders.* Baltimore, MD: University Park Press.

Mysak, E. D. (1968). *Neuroevolutional approach to cerebral palsy and speech.* New York: Teachers College Press.

Perkins, W. H. (1983). *Current therapy of communication disorders: Dysarthria and apraxia.* New York: Thieme-Stratton, Inc.

Siegel, G., & Ingham, R. (1987). Theory and science in communication disorders. *Journal of Speech and Hearing Disorders, 52,* 99–104.

Yorkston, K., Beukelman, D., & Bell, K. (1988). *Clinical management of dysarthric speakers.* Boston: College-Hill Press, Inc.

Young, E., & Stinchfield-Hawk, S. (1955). *Motor-kinesthetic speech training.* Stanford, CA: Stanford University Press.

Chapter 3

Treatment of the Respiration Subsystem

Those patients whose motor speech difficulties are compounded by poor respiratory support present a difficult challenge for the speech clinician. Working with the speech musculature of these patients is often sufficiently frustrating. The additional task of improving respiratory support, so as to facilitate speech motor control, may prove nerve-racking, because most clinicians lack sufficient knowledge of and experience in administering breathing exercises. It is interesting that when respiratory or physical therapists are consulted for suggestions in this regard, they too are often at a loss. What is more, there is a poverty of information in the treatment literature relative to suggestions for the rehabilitation of patients with (speech) breathing difficulties. What then are clinicians to do when they are confronted with patients whose speech disorders are compounded by poor breath support and control? With no clear direction or list of proven treatment strategies, clinicians may be left to their own intuitions or ideas about management. In such a context, the information presented in this chapter is based largely on this author's trial-and-error experiences using techniques that have not yet been subjected to, nor supported by, scientific study but appear theoretically feasible and have worked well with some patients. Before commencing with any of these techniques, however, clinicians should consult with a pulmonologist for specific recommendations.

It is important to note that the pathophysiology of breathing difficulty and the prognosis for improvement may vary from patient to patient. Few patients are dependent on artificial respirators; those who are, typically, are poor candidates for the exercises that will be discussed. All others with breathing problems, however, may benefit from such exercises, provided that the specific treatments applied and the criteria set for improvement are adjusted to meet the individual patient's needs and potential. Whether to continue or terminate a treatment will usually depend upon the patient's responses and progress. After 10 sessions or fewer, the clinician should have a pretty good idea about whether that treatment has been at all helpful. If it appears to have had any degree of positive impact, it should be continued until such time that its effectiveness ceases or the clinical objectives are met. If the results have not been encouraging, however, it is probably wise to discontinue that treatment and proceed to the next step in the subsystem treatment sequence. The prognosis for further improvement from this point on, however, depends upon where in the treatment sequence the patient failed to improve. Whereas failures at the very top of the treatment ladder generate a very poor prognosis, those at or near the bottom are not usually as binding. Experienced clinicians all have learned that attempts to improve coexistent phonatory, articulatory, and/or resonatory disturbances that are plagued by significant and intractable breathing problems are often unsuccessful. Nonetheless, the therapy focus should shift to the speech exercise components of the regimen, with hopes that some clinical success may still be possible.

GENERAL RULES OF THUMB

It has been well established that the amount of air needed for speech production is no greater than that required for normal breathing activities at rest. This amount of air, however, must be managed efficiently to promote adequate speech breathing activities. Several clinical researchers have advanced the idea that if the patient can steadily generate subglottal air pressure of 5 cm H_2O for 5 seconds or longer, the respiration system may be sufficient enough to support speech efforts. This pressure-generating capability can be misleading, however. Many patients with neuromuscular respiratory difficulties may prove able to perform this static type of task but unable to coordinate the more dynamic and complex respiratory maneuvers that are required for speech breathing events. Thus, measures of both static and dynamic respiratory skills of the patient may prove diagnostically indispensable.

Table 3–1 was designed to highlight, using "X" marks, the kinds of respiration subsystem disturbances that are most commonly observed in the dysarthric populations. This table may serve as a comparative diagnostic guide during differential appraisal of the subsystem.

The types of exercises utilized with a patient may need to be varied in accordance with the underlying pathophysiology of the respiratory difficulty. Those patients with spastic-hypertonic musculature, for example, may require treatments that will facilitate air pressure–generating capability, relaxation and reciprocal and forceful contractions of inhalatory and exhalatory musculature. Those patients whose breathing problems are caused by hyperkinesia and abnormal posturing of the respiratory musculature may also benefit from relaxation exercises and possibly braces or girdles for abdominal support. More important, however, activities that train control of involuntary movements and promote the performance of purposeful respiratory adjustments may prove most helpful for such patients. Ataxic patients usually need to improve the balance, sense of position, and synchronization of inspiratory/expiratory chest and abdominal wall excursions. Exercises designed to accomplish such aims, in particular, may be most indicated for these patients. Patients with flaccidity of the respiratory musculature may need exercises that increase the strength and reciprocal forces of in-

TABLE 3-1. Differential Respiration Subsystem Disturbances in Dysarthric Patients

Dysarthria Type	Poor Posture	Neck and Trunk Rigidity	Reduced Pressure-Generating Capability	Shallow Inhalations	Reduced Exhalation Control	Rapid Breaths	Slow Breaths	Antagonistic Muscular Contractions	Involuntary Muscular Contractions	Irregular Patterns	Sudden-Forced Inhalations/ Exhalations
Spastic	X	X	X	X	X		X	X			
Ataxic				X	X	X				X	X
Hyperkinetic	X	X		X	X	X		X	X	X	X
Hypokinetic	X	X		X	X	X				X	X
Flaccid	X		X	X	X		X				

43

spiratory/expiratory musculature contractions. Severe flaccid paralysis of the breathing apparatus often requires artificial respiration for life-supporting purposes. Finally, for those patients who possess a mixture of neuromusculature difficulties that involve the respiration subsystem, exercises that take into consideration each of the underlying pathophysiologic components may be indicated.

PRECURSORS TO INTERVENTION

If the functioning of the dysarthric patient's respiration subsystem is suspect, it is important that the nature and extent of any existing incompetence be determined. It is just as important to identify and measure the degree to which disturbances in coexistent laryngeal and/or velopharyngeal musculature either compound the difficulty of the respiration subsystem or mask its overall potential and capability. Differential appraisal of these speech subsystems will enable the clinician to judge accurately the existence of both primary and secondary conditions that have an adverse impact on speech breathing efforts and treatments. This chapter focuses exclusively on treatment strategies for "primary" respiration subsystem disturbances. Despite their potential influence on the results of these techniques, treatment recommendations for the other speech subsystems will be reserved for later chapters.

Clinical judgments of respiration subsystem dysfunctions can be made as the patient performs some basic speech and nonspeech respiratory aerodynamic maneuvers. As discussed in the previous chapter, disturbances of the respiration subsystem should receive top priority in the treatment plan. Improvements in the functioning of this subsystem will enhance the chances for success with the treatment of other subsystem abnormalities, for without adequate respiratory support the performances of the remaining speech subsystems invariably will be compromised. To determine the characteristic respiration subsystem abnormalities, the Respiration Subsystem Behavioral Treatment Chart (Figure 3–1) can be used to record the patient's pre-treatment abilities on various evaluation tasks. Note on Figure 3–2 that on 4/12/89 the spastic dysarthric patient illustrated underwent testing of all nine key respiratory activities. In the comments section of the chart, note that a noseclip was used for all test components, owing to significant velopharyngeal incompetence that would, if it were overlooked, camouflage inherent respiration subsystem capabilities. Also note in this section that variable degrees of vocal fold hyperfunctioning were perceived during those measures that required vocalizations—pathophysiologic behaviors that usually disrupt translaryngeal airflow and can similarly yield inaccurate and misleading data regarding the performances of the respiration subsystem itself. Thus, this laryngeal phenomenon must be and was weighed in the final analyses of these measures and in the recommendations for treatment.

Column 1 on this chart highlights that the patient presented with a very mild degree of head, neck, and trunk stiffness (score of 6). In column 2 her "0" score signified poor postural status. Column 3 reveals that she could not sustain 5 cm H_2O for 5 seconds over five trials. This minimal pressure-generating capabil-

RESPIRATION SUBSYSTEM BEHAVIORAL TREATMENT CHART

Patient's name:

Birthdate: Sex:

Speech diagnosis:

Medical diagnosis:

Clinician:

Facility:

Address:

Comments: Note here any nasal air emissions and/or lip seal difficulties that needed adjustments for these measures. Also note value during measures.

ACTIVITY KEY

Feature:

1. Relaxation (tonal) status (R)

2. Postural (tonal) status (T)

3. 5 cm H_2O/5 seconds pressure generating capability (G)

4. Prolonged inhalation (I)

5. Prolonged exhalation (E)

MEASUREMENT UNIT
No. correct, or
Hypotonic–Normal–Hypertonic
$0 \longleftarrow 2 \longrightarrow 5 \longrightarrow 7 \longrightarrow 10$

Poor = 0;   Adequate = 1;
Good = 2;   Excellent = 3

No. correct

No. of seconds

No. of seconds or no. correct

Feature:

6. Max. No. of quick breaths possible in 20 seconds (Q)

7. Inhalation/exhalation synchrony (S)

8. Isolated sound productions (P)

9. Connected speech breathing (C)

Baseline (pre-treatment): B + activity symbol

MEASUREMENT UNIT
No. breath cycles

No. correct

No. of seconds or no. correct

No. of syllables/breath

Dates:

Average No. per Unit Measured

30
20
15
10
9
8
7
6
5
4
3
2
1
0

No. of trials

Activity symbol

Measurement unit

Target criterion

SESSIONS

Figure 3–1. Respiration Subsystem Behavioral Treatment Chart to be used to track patient responses to therapy.

RESPIRATION SUBSYSTEM BEHAVIORAL TREATMENT CHART

Patient's name: Jane Doe

Birthdate: 5/3/67 **Sex:** Fe

Speech diagnosis: Spastic Dysarthria

Medical diagnosis: Pseudobulbar palsy due to CHI

Clinician: Dworkin

Facility: XYZ

Address: Anywhere, USA

Comments: Note here any nasal air emissions and/or lip seal difficulties that needed adjustments for these measures. Also note value during measures.

Severe oral and velopharyngeal seal incompetence required compensatory adjustments for virtually all exercises: manual assistance to promote lip seal and a noseclip to eliminate nasal air escape. Vocal fold hyperfunctioning during some of the "speech" breathing tasks was evident.

ACTIVITY KEY

Feature:	MEASUREMENT UNIT
1. Relaxation (tonal) status (R)	No. correct, or Hypotonic-Normal-Hypertonic $0 \leftarrow 2 \longrightarrow 5 \longrightarrow 7 \longrightarrow 10$
2. Postural (tonal) status (T)	Poor = 0; Adequate = 1; Good = 2; Excellent = 3
3. 5 cm H_2O/5 seconds pressure generating capability (G)	No. correct
4. Prolonged inhalation (I)	No. of seconds
5. Prolonged exhalation (E)	No. of seconds or no. correct

Feature:	MEASUREMENT UNIT
6. Max. No. of quick breaths possible n 20 seconds (Q)	Vo. breath cycles
7. Inhalation/exhalation synchrory (S)	No. correct
8. Isolated sound productions (P)	No. of seconds or no. correct
9. Connected speech breathing (C)	No. of syllables/breath

Baseline (pre-treatment): B + activity symbol

	BR	BT	BG	BI	BE	BQ	BS₁	BS₂	BP₁	BP₂	BC₁	BC₂
Activity symbol	BR	BT	BG	BI	BE	BQ	BS₁	BS₂	BP₁	BP₂	BC₁	BC₂
No. of trials	2 min.	N/A	5			3 min.	6	30	3	10	30	3
Measurement unit	0-10	0-3	Correct	# Sec.	# Sec.	# Breath	Correct	Correct	# Sec.	# Sec.	# Syll./breath	# Syll./breath
Target criterion	5	1	3 of 5	10	10	5	4 of 6	21 of 30	15	7	20	10

Baseline scores (Dates: 4/12/89), Average No. per Unit Measured — values plotted: BR = 6, BT = 0, BG = 1, BI = 5, BE = 6, BQ = 2, BS₁ = 1, BS₂ = 10, BP₁ = 9, BP₂ = 5, BC₁ = 8, BC₂ = 5.

SESSIONS

Figure 3–2. Respiration subsystem baseline scores obtained from spastic dysarthric patient. Note that she did not achieve any target criterion, indicating the need for intervention across the board.

ity was measured using a simple glass jar that was filled with water and marked off in 1-cm units, as described in 1982 by Hixon and his associates. Columns 4 and 5 illustrate, respectively, that the patient's inhalatory and exhalatory prolongation controls averaged less than 10 seconds each. On several quick breath cycles, each lasting 5 seconds, she was able to achieve a mean of two inhalatory/ exhalatory maneuvers, as shown in column 6. Columns 7 and 8 illustrate poor synchronization of inhalatory/exhalatory muscle contractions. Columns 9 and 10 show the baseline results of breath support for isolated vowels and vowel sequences, which fell short of threshold. Finally, her contextual speech was analyzed for average number of syllables per breath. The results of these baseline measures appear in columns 11 and 12, which also fell below threshold requirements. Note that across the bottom row of the chart, for each baseline measure a target criterion for improvement is listed. This listing is based on the recommended degree of improvement for that particular behavioral exercise, as will be detailed a little later when we review the various exercises. As suggested in the preceding chapter, it is a good idea to calculate these criteria following the baseline data collection process and to enter these figures on the treatment chart prior to initiating the respective exercises. In this way, quick glances at the chart enable determination of the patient's ongoing degrees of improvement and the extent to which additional treatment is needed to reach target objectives. Figure 3–5, *A* to *C*, helps illustrate this point.

Note: For this patient all baseline measures were made prior to the initiation of the entire treatment plan. Retrospectively, such measures should have been collected throughout the plan to determine the actual need for each exercise administered. Baseline scores are therefore best documented immediately before an anticipated treatment to establish a platform against which to test the efficacy of therapy.

In the succeeding section, differential strategies for intervention with patients who present with respiration subsystem disturbances will be explored in detail.

TREATMENT APPROACHES

Manipulations of the breathing mechanism *should* be cleared by those professional allies who know best about such clinical procedures. This conservative approach reduces sharply the liability issue and, more important, ensures better chances for success than operating in a vacuum without such input. Notwithstanding this warning, the suggestions in this chapter will afford clinicians at least a good starting point in their discussions with such allied professionals and in their work with dysarthric patients who exhibit associated respiratory difficulties.

Figure 3–3 is an algorithm that offers a general guide to treatment sequencing. This diagram can be very helpful in directing the sequence of treatments in a logical order. Thus, it is this order that will be used later to focus on specific treatment techniques that can be employed to combat the various types of

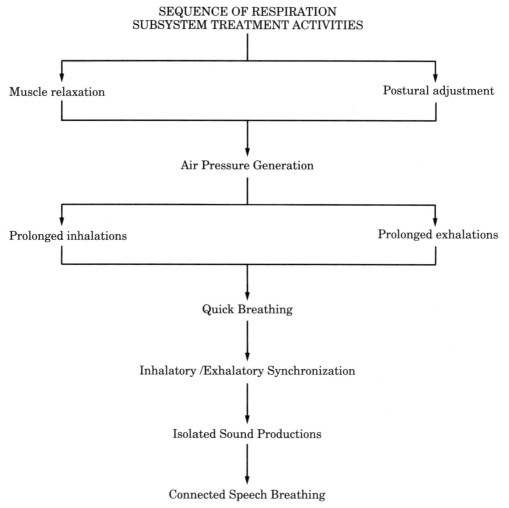

Figure 3–3. Recommended hierarchy of respiration subsystem treatment parameters.

respiration subsystem disturbances that are differentially depicted in Table 3–1. As can be seen from the top-down flow diagram, the treatment sequence begins with relaxation/postural adjustment techniques and progresses through general, nonspeech, isolated speech, and contextual speech breathing exercises. Depending upon their baseline respiration subsystem disturbances and overall neuromuscular status, patients will vary relative to where in the sequence they should begin the program and which, if any, of the steps can be omitted as their travels through this course are being designed and administered. Matching the patient's baseline data against the recommended treatment steps should help guide the clinician in making such decisions.

Notwithstanding these suggestions, the methodology chosen by the clinician to measure treatment effects will largely dictate the procedures that must be followed when one implements this recommended intervention sequence.

Before proceeding with the treatment strategies section of this chapter, suggestions about how best to proceed and use the Respiration Subsystem Behavioral Treatment Chart (Figure 3–1) are in order here. First, the section on patient history should be completed. Second, in the comments section, note any velopharyngeal and/or labial valve dysfunctions that require compensations prior to these treatments. Third, list the improvement criteria that will dictate progress within and between treatment steps. Naturally, the criterion may be changed for any step, at any time, as deemed facilitative. Often, use of both absolute and relative rating scales are required. That is to say, depending upon the patient's baseline scores, the effects of some treatment tasks may best be measured with predetermined threshold criterion levels. Other treatments, perhaps those that address grave deficits, may better be evaluated less stringently as a function of the patient's prognosis for change. Fourth, list at the top of the column the date of the treatment session, and in the respective cells at the bottom of the column record the treatment activity symbol and the measurement unit from the "Activity Key." Fifth, enter the number of trials of treatment for the session in the appropriate cell in the column. Sixth, mark the patient's average score for the session along the y-axis. Seventh, when the patient achieves the criterion for the first treatment indicated in the sequence of treatments shown in Figure 3–3, or no greater progress is anticipated if such intervention were continued, begin entering data accordingly for the second set of indicated treatments, and so on.

Depending upon the number of treatments necessary and the speed with which the patient travels through to criteria, several charts may be required to record all treatment data sequentially collected and to observe trendlines in patient performances. Whenever it is necessary, possible, and potentially helpful, the clinician should demonstrate the task for the patient to ensure comprehension and to provide a basis for comparison.

TREATMENT MATERIALS

The clinician will need to assemble the following materials in order to carry out the various and sundry exercises recommended in this section:

1. *See-Scape Device** (Figure 3–4)
2. *Standard metronome,* which can be purchased for under $20 at most music stores
3. *Noseclip,* which can be purchased at most sporting goods or hospital supplies outlets
4. *Box of paper clips* (28 mm)
5. *Regular drinking straws*
6. *Box of facial tissues*
7. *Respiration Subsystem Behavioral Treatment Chart* (see Figure 3–1)

*See-Scape Device. Pro-Ed, 8700 Shoal Creek Blvd., Austin, TX 78758 (512-451-8542).

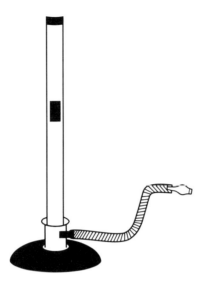

Figure 3–4. See-Scape device (Pro-Ed) showing the Styrofoam float within the test tube and the plastic nasal olive connected to the rubber hose.

Let's now focus on specific treatment strategies from this point forward. The techniques provided are ordered according to the sequential-step diagram shown earlier in Figure 3–3.

RELAXATION AND POSTURAL SUPPORT TECHNIQUES

At the top of the treatment sequence ladder we find techniques aimed at improving the tone and posture of the respiration subsystem, if such therapy is indicated in a given dysarthric patient. Table 3–1 reveals that spastic, hyperkinetic, and hypokinetic dysarthric patients frequently evidence postural and tonal disturbances of the head, neck, and trunk that adversely influence speech breathing activities.

Relaxation Exercises

To try to reduce stiff or rigid (hypertonic) characteristics of the head, neck, and/or trunk musculature, relaxation therapy may be helpful. Ordinarily, relaxation exercises are designed to reduce body tension and (increased) resistance to manipulation through inhibitory techniques involving stretch pressures and passive movements of joints, as will be seen in later chapters. However, because the basic anatomy of the breathing mechanism does not lend itself well to such applications, alternative approaches to relaxation are necessary.

Long ago, Froeschels reminded us that the greatest relaxation of muscles is accomplished by complete rest, and that methods used to induce relaxation of any muscle group should incorporate specific types of breathing exercises. Individuals familiar with the tenets of meditation and Yoga appreciate the role of breathing dynamics in the attainment of overall body relaxation. The following treatment sequence may prove most effective.

Exercise No. 1

Step 1. To establish baseline head, neck, and trunk musculature tonal status, stand behind the patient and passively manipulate the head backwards, forwards, and from side to side. Perform these movements for at least 1 minute, and render a perceptual rating from 0 to 10 regarding the tonal status. Scores of "0 to 4" represent varying degrees of *hypotonicity,* a "5" indicates *normal* tone, and scores of "6 to 10" are suggestive of increasing degrees of *hypertonicity.* If the patient can stand up, assess truncal tonicity by requesting him or her to touch the toes without bending at the knees, and to bend at the hip alternately from side to side and forwards and backwards several times. As the patient performs these tasks, observe the fluidity of the movements and render an additional perceptual rating, using the aforementioned scale. Average these two ratings and enter this baseline result on the y-axis grid of the Respiration Subsystem Behavioral Treatment Chart, making certain to list the date, number of trials (in minutes), activity symbol (BR_1), and measurement unit (0–10 scale) in the corresponding cells of the data column. Proceed with this exercise (Steps 2 to 6) and the next three exercises in the sequence if this score is at least "2" scale values above or below "5" (normal). Otherwise, advance to the Postural Exercises subsection.

Step 2. To facilitate abdominal diaphragmatic musculature support for speech, the patient should be placed in a supine position, on either a tabletop or the floor, in a quiet environment free from distractions. This technique induces relaxation of the limb and trunk musculature and restricts movements of the thoracic wall. Because these patients may also benefit from improvements in thoracic posturing, an upright or standing position (which induces chest wall activity) may be attempted later, in concert with speech breathing exercises.

Step 3. Once the patient is placed in a supine position so as to relax the trunk musculature, he or she should be instructed to breathe in and out through the nose as effortlessly, steadily, and deeply as possible. Both the inhalatory and the exhalatory cycles should be practiced each to the count of five, in an even, rhythmic pattern so as to prevent hyperventilation.

Step 4. As this breathing pattern is established, the clinician should place the patient's hands on the abdominal wall so its respective lifting and lowering movements during inhalation and exhalation can serve as a source of respiratory biofeedback. The patient is instructed to try to accomplish these types of abdominal wall excursions that are consistent with each phase of the breathing cycle.

Step 5. Use the See-Scape device, which permits observations of airflow dynamics using rubber tubing interfaced with a test tube containing a small Styrofoam float, to provide yet another means of biofeedback to the patient during this relaxation exercise. Connect the nasal olive to the rubber tubing, gently position it in either nostril of the patient, and place the test tube in comfortable view for visual feedback of inhalatory and exhalatory airflow characteristics. Request that the patient continue with the breathing patterns practiced, noting that during the deep and protracted inhalation phase, the float should remain perfectly still at the very bottom of the test tube, signaling the vacuum effect of lung-thorax expansion with air intake. Periodically check that the float is "free-floating" inasmuch as condensation in the tube may cause it to stick. The patient should be instructed to try to maintain this float position throughout the count of five by the clinician. Any oppositional exhalatory behaviors should be readily visible as the float moves upwards in the test tube in concert with such airflow. The patient can use this facilitatory feedback to develop more relaxed airflow dynamics. During the exhalation phase of this exercise, the float should rise rapidly to the very top of the test tube, with the goal being that it remain there without fluctuation until inhalation is requested by the clinician after the count of five. Again, any involuntary-oppositional movements during this exhalatory cycle will be revealed by coincident downward deflection of the float. Each cycle, 5 seconds inhalation/5 seconds exhalation, constitutes one trial. Rate the trial as either correct or incorrect. A "correct" score is rendered if the float activity is suggestive of uninterrupted airflow control during both the inhalatory and exhalatory phases of the cycle. Use a notepad to record each score, and repeat this procedure with periodic rest periods until the patient performs 30 consecutive trials correctly, at which time advance to the next exercise.

After each set of 30 trials, tally the number of correct scores from the notepad and enter the result on the treatment chart, making certain to list the number of trials (30), the activity symbol (R_1), and the absolute criterion figure (30) in the respective cells of the data column. If after 30 consecutive trials the patient does not demonstrate any observable trend of relaxed breath cycles, discontinue this exercise and advance to the next one.

Note: If the patient is unable to perform this activity without an open mouth posture, the nasal olive or tubing itself can be placed in the corner of the *mouth* (provided that the lips can be adequately approximated and sealed) for airflow feedback. It is also important to note that laryngospasms and other hyperfunctional vocal fold behaviors that may occur during this exercise can interrupt translaryngeal airflow and give the false impression of an inhalation maneuver as the float remains at the bottom of the test tube. The clinician should monitor the patient for such occurrences by listening carefully for the sounds of airflow with each breath cycle. The patient can then be instructed as to the presence of such interruptive behaviors and their effects on the position of the float as they occur. The patient too can be requested to listen for and promote unobstructed airstreams during this relaxation breathing exercise.

Step 6. If the See-Scape device is unavailable, for the time being the clinician can use an ordinary facial tissue, which should be folded in half and placed directly over the mouth of the patient for best results. Fasten a noseclip on the patient and instruct him or her to perform the aforementioned inhalatory/exhalatory activities, to the respective counts of five, breathing through the mouth so as to enable observations of the tissue as it flutters outwards during exhalation and flattens against the mouth opening during inhalation. As with the See-Scape device, the tissue will provide aerodynamic feedback to the patient, which can be used to demonstrate smooth and relaxed versus erratic, oppositional and other abnormal respiratory musculature contractions during this ongoing relaxation breathing exercise. Follow exactly the same scoring, charting, and advancement methods as those detailed in Step 5.

Exercise No. 2

Step 1.   Follow exactly the same baseline procedures as those detailed in Exercise no. 1. Be certain to use the activity symbol "BR_2" to tag these data, however, on the treatment chart.

Step 2.   Place the patient in a supine position as in the preceding initial exercise regimen, and instruct him or her to tighten muscles in the neck, thorax, and abdomen with simultaneous inhalation effort.

Step 3.   After establishing and maintaining this increased tonal state for a count of five, the patient is then instructed to release slowly such tone with steady and relaxed exhalatory airflow to another count of five by the clinician. Repeat this procedure for 10 minutes, allowing rests when necessary. At the completion of each 10 minutes of practice, retest head, neck, and trunk tonal status following the baseline methods, and enter the perceptual rating on the treatment chart accordingly. Continue with this approach until the patient achieves a perceptual rating that is at least "3" scale values improved over baseline, or a "5" if the baseline rating was "2," "3," "4," "6," "7," or "8," over 10 consecutive minutes of practice, at which time, advance to the next exercise. Calculate this target criterion according to the baseline score, and enter the figure in the respective cell at the bottom of the anticipated treatment data column.

Step 4.   After each set of 10 minutes of practice, enter the rating rendered on the treatment chart, using the activity symbol "R_2" to tag this impression. Discontinue the exercise if after 30 consecutive minutes of practice there is no discernible trend of improvement over the baseline level to justify continuation. Advance to the next exercise, nonetheless.

Exercise No. 3

Step 1.   Follow exactly the same baseline procedures as those detailed in Exercise no. 1. Be certain to tag these data with the activity symbol "BR_3" on the treatment chart.

Step 2.   If possible, have the patient sit upright in a comfortable chair without arms, and request that he or she lean over from the waist, allowing the arms to hang loosely at the sides of the chair.

Step 3.   With the patient in this position, stand behind him or her and slowly, gently, and passively lift and lower the head to respective counts of 10. Then passively manipulate the head to the left and right, also to counts of 10, as the patient remains bent at the waist with arms loosely at the sides of the chair. Theoretically, this exercise may facilitate a tonic labyrinthine response, which has been reported in the neurorehabilitation literature to promote relaxation of head, neck, and trunk musculature.

Step 4. Follow the same perceptual rating, scoring, charting, and advancement methods detailed in Step 3 of the preceding exercise, except that here be certain to use the activity symbol "R_3" when tagging the data entries on the treatment chart.

Exercise No. 4

Step 1. Again, follow the same baseline procedures as those in the preceding three exercises. Tag these data with the activity symbol "BR_4" on the treatment chart.

Step 2. The patient is next instructed to sit up so as to imitate the floppy body parts of a "rag doll." Instruct him or her to allow the head alternately to fall forward, backward, and to the sides in as loose and smooth a fashion as possible. The patient who has trouble initiating and controlling such attempts can be assisted by the clinician, who may stand behind and gently manipulate the head in these directions to respective counts of 10, as the patient remains as still, relaxed, and cooperative as possible.

Step 3. The clinician can passively elevate the patient's arms above the head, requesting that when they are released they be allowed to fall down loosely to the sides like that which would happen with the "rag doll."

Step 4. Repeat these procedures for 10 minutes, permitting a rest periodically, and follow the scoring, rating, charting, and advancement methods recommended in Exercise no. 2, Step 3. When entering these perceptual ratings on the treatment chart be sure to use the activity symbol "R_4" to represent the data.

Postural Exercises

Whether confronted with the flexed trunk of the patient with Parkinson's disease, the twisted and contorted head, neck, and trunk alterations of patients with spasmodic torticollis or athetoid cerebral palsy, or the overall slumped posture of patients who may be wheelchair bound as a consequence of any number of pathophysiologic conditions, clinicians must consider improving postural status before compensatory speech breathing training is initiated.

If postural support is to be improved, it may be best achieved through the use of prosthetic devices such as head, neck, chest and/or abdomen straps, braces and girdles that may prop and maintain the patient in an upright or sitting position and add stiffness to an otherwise flabby mechanism. Whereas this type of patient may require a therapeutic increase in postural tone and balance, spastic, hyperkinetic, and hypokinetic dysarthric patients, as previously mentioned, may benefit from exercises that diminish muscle tone and train better postural support for speech breathing activities. The following postural adjustment treatment sequence, when it is coupled with the preceding relaxation exercises, if indicated, may prove most effective. Before proceeding, however, render a rating from 0 to 3 to designate the perceived head, neck, and trunk postural status, in which "0" symbolizes poor, "1" adequate, "2" good, and "3" excellent posture. Administer the exercises below only if the patient is rated "0." Otherwise, skip the next three exercises and advance to the next indicated subsection.

Exercise No. 1

Step 1. Patients who are wheelchair bound, irrespective of cause, may achieve better respiration subsystem control if certain adaptive alterations are made to the chair that actually neutralize abnormal postures and facilitate neuromuscular activity. The canvas seat and back found on most wheelchairs provide little or no head support and promote abnormal rotation of the trunk, hips, and legs. Tailored construction of a wooden seat, with an adjoining seatback that extends from the buttocks region of the patient to the C7 vertebral level, are adaptations that will immediately afford the patient better postural support for speech breathing. If head support is also needed, the seatback can be extended higher than the C7 level for such purposes. Foam rubber and upholstery can be used to make comfortable this newly designed chair.

Step 2. Static head and trunk supports and slings can also be attached to the new seat for those patients who are prone to involuntary postural shifts, as well as those with very poor volitional head and/or trunk control.

Step 3. A lap tray may also prove helpful for those patients with poor trunk posture and support. If this tray is padded in the area facing the patient's trunk, it may be used to induce abdominal musculature contractions during speech breathing efforts. The observant clinician should be able to distinguish between those patients who need these types of wheelchair adaptations and those who do not. However, for the ultimate design and construction of this equipment, a physical therapist or biomedical engineer is usually indispensable, not only for the proper fitting of the chair, but also its successful use.

Note: If these procedures were followed, test their effects by re-evaluating postural status following the baseline procedures. These data, however, are tagged with the activity symbol "T_1" on the treatment chart.

Exercise No. 2

Step 1. Those patients with weak belt muscles may benefit from wearing an elastic strap or girdle that can provide abdominal support for speech breathing activity. Before the clinician applies such a device, however, he or she should first experiment with systematic manual compression forces to augment or help drive the exhalatory airstream. This approach requires the clinician to use an open hand to pump forcefully against the patient's abdomen as various speech and nonspeech exhalation maneuvers are attempted upon command. If significant assistance is observed as a consequence of this technique, the patient may be a good candidate for the aforementioned strap or girdle, which can provide ongoing aid.

Step 2. Positioned around the abdomen below the lower thorax region, such devices can be tightened to desired yet comfortable levels so as to maximize their effects. Experimentation with tension alternatives should illustrate the best fit for the patient, as respiratory output may vary with such adjustments. If this technique was employed periodically, measure its effects by re-evaluating postural status using the baseline procedure. Be sure to tag these perceptual ratings with the activity symbol "T_2" on the treatment chart.

Exercise No. 3

Step 1. When it is not too burdensome for the patient to stand, whether assisted or not, this position should be incorporated into the respiration subsystem exercises prescribed for that individual. Working closely with pulmonologists, this author has learned that this posture often promotes better results with both speech and nonspeech treatments. Periodically test the effects of this approach by re-evaluating postural status in the usual way using the symbol "T_3" on the chart.

Finally, the rehabilitation literature is replete with methods for inducing muscle relaxation and improving overall body posture. Although the use of tranquilizing and muscle relaxing drugs will probably continue for years to come, of late the therapeutic spotlight has shifted focus somewhat onto other alternatives. We now hear of techniques such as Rolfing, which involves deep massaging of stiffened muscle groups, hemi-synch music stimulation that portends promotion of an expanded form of consciousness, creative visualization and self-actualization exercises that purportedly teach ways of monitoring and altering degrees of body tension, and meditation and Yoga, which for years have been hailed by some to be excellent ways of achieving inner peace and total body relaxation. The scope of this text does not, however, permit reviews of these procedures, though the interested clinician may wish to consult the references provided at the end of the chapter for further information.

PRESSURE-GENERATING EXERCISES

Of all the dysarthric patients we encounter clinically, those with spastic and/or flaccid diagnoses are the ones who most often present with reduced air pressure–generating capability, as shown in Table 3–1. Consequently, the following exercises generally aim at these individuals, although they may prove sequentially appropriate for others in that their purpose is to teach low pressure exhalations, controlled over a period of time, which may prove beneficial for many different dysarthric patients. When these exercises are indicated, they should be administered *following* the necessary relaxation and postural adjustment procedures that were previously discussed.

Before commencing with specific exercises to improve subglottal air pressure dynamics, however, it is imperative to segregate out the nonrespiration subsystem disturbances that may have contributed to the patient's pressure-generating difficulty. Invariably those spastic and flaccid dysarthric patients who present with such difficulty exhibit coexistent incompetence of the velopharyngeal and oral musculature valves. If the consequent nasal and oral seal leakages are significant, they must be taken into consideration in the design and administration of the exercises suggested in this section. Whereas these exercises need not necessarily be delayed until the disturbances of these subsystems are successfully treated, they should be administered with such anticipated treatments in mind. As methods for improving functioning of the resonation subsystem are being explored or developed, such as the fitting of a palatal-lift appliance, the clinician can reduce the adverse influence of velopharyngeal incompetence on the patient's performances during pressure-generating exercises by using a noseclip. Faulty valving of the lips during these exercises can similarly impair patient performances. Although treatments of the articulation subsystem may not be introduced until later in the rehabilitation program, the clinician may facilitate success by enabling the patient to compensate for oral seal incompetence using manual assistance to achieve lip closure during pressure-generating exercises.

Note: If these compensatory adjustments result in the immediate ability to sustain subglottal air pressure of 5 cm H_2O for 5 seconds or longer, the exercises that follow probably are not indicated for the patient because at least minimally sufficient (respiratory) pressure-generating capability for speech purposes already exists.

Exercise No. 1

Step 1. To establish baseline subglottal air pressure–generating capability, use the See-Scape device (see Figure 3–4). Remove the rubber cap, and drop four 28-mm paperclips into the tube on top of the Styrofoam float. Remove the nasal olive from the rubber hose and insert in its place a piece of drinking straw that extends about 2 inches from the end of the hose. To simulate the effects of a bleed valve, poke a hole about the size of a dull pencil point into the wall of the straw about halfway between the mouth of the rubber hose and the free end of the straw.

Step 2. Put a noseclip on the patient, if velopharyngeal incompetency exists, and instruct him or her to blow steadily into the straw with the objective of raising the float and paperclips to the top of the tube and *maintaining* them in this position for 5 seconds with controlled exhalatory effort.* Allow the patient five trials, with a 15-second rest between each attempt. The dichotomous correct/incorrect rating scale is used here, in which "1" is rendered if the patient correctly achieves the aforementioned criterion, and "0" (incorrect) is awarded if the

---

*Through experimentation, it has been discovered that this adapted use of the See-Scape device roughly simulates 5 cm H_2O displacement, as may be measured with a water manometer or the "around the house" device reported by Hixon et al. (1982). Clinicians may prefer the See-Scape adaptation over the latter measurement tool inasmuch as it affords the patient continuous visual feedback regarding ongoing and changing exhalation control, whereas the latter device provides only visual feedback when the patient achieves and maintains the designated level of water displacement (cm H_2O).

performance falls short of the objective. Each trial is rated individually. Tally the correct scores, and if the result is equal to or less than "3" proceed with this exercise. Otherwise, advance to the next indicated exercise. Enter the result on the treatment chart, using the activity symbol "BG$_1$" to represent these data.

Step 3.   Continue practicing the same procedure, listing on a notepad after each trial whether the patient correctly or incorrectly performed the task objective. Repeat the procedure until the patient demonstrates the ability to perform the task correctly over 10 consecutive trials, at which time advancement to the next exercise is indicated.

Step 4.   At the completion of each set of 10 trials, tally from the notepad recordings the number of correct performances, and enter the result on the treatment chart in a separate column, making certain to list the appropriate activity symbol (G$_1$) and the target criterion (10). Discontinue this exercise if after 30 consecutive trials the patient fails to demonstrate any observable trend of improvement over baseline to justify further practice. Advance nonetheless to the next indicated exercise.

Note: Over many trials, there is a tendency for a mild amount of condensation to form in the See-Scape tube, which can retard float action. A rolled-up facial tissue can be threaded through the tube periodically to wipe dry its interior and to ensure uninterrupted float excursions with subsequent use.

Regardless of the homemade device used to improve subglottal air pressure–generating capability, the ultimate objective is to train the patient to increase the amount of air pressure from reduced baseline levels to the minimum target of 5 cm H$_2$O over 5 seconds duration. There really is no good reason to push the patient beyond this threshold level for speech purposes. Naturally, some patients will not make significant improvements, leaving only the residual strength and coordination of the respiration subsystem upon which the clinician must try to capitalize as subsequent treatments become the focus. As discussed earlier in this chapter, when the patient experiences failure at or near the top of the subsystem treatment ladder, as would be the case with this exercise regimen, the prognosis for improvement during the treatments indicated next in the sequence is generally quite poor. The clinician may wish to press on, nonetheless, with hopes that the subsequent exercises may promote gains great enough to have made some sort of difference clinically. To quit without attempting other indicated treatments can prove premature. Failures at one task do not necessarily generalize to all succeeding exercises.

PROLONGED INHALATION/EXHALATION EXERCISES

As can be seen from Table 3–1, shallow inhalations and failures to control variably prolonged exhalations are features that may be observed in all the dysarthrias. The exercises in this section are not designed to alter substantially the patient's vital capacity, inasmuch as little is known about the possible influence of such change on speech breathing capability. Rather, they were developed with two primary purposes in mind for those patients whose baseline data show deficits in these speech breathing dimensions.

The first objective is to improve lung volume so that as much air as possible is available for talking; the second is to improve the strength and coordination of the muscles used voluntarily to control inhalation and exhalation so as to maximize the amount of syllables that can be successfully uttered per breath. Moreover, Table 3–1 also highlights that ataxic, hyperkinetic, and hypokinetic patients, in particular, are prone to exhibit quick (rapid-fire) breathing patterns that invariably contribute to their motor speech difficulties. The following sequence of intervention techniques is recommended not only to help obtain the aforementioned objectives but also to teach patients that improvements in inhalatory/exhalatory controls may yield positive effects on breathing rates as well. Finally, the exercises that follow may similarly prove helpful in modifying upper thoracic and/or clavicular breathing patterns, which are especially prevalent in patients with spastic dysarthria.

Inhalation

Exercise No. 1

Step 1.   To establish baseline inhalation prolongation capability request that the patient breathe in as long and as steadily as possible. Use a stopwatch or the second hand of a wristwatch to time the length of the inhalation. To ensure that the patient is inhaling, request that the airstream be made audible. This may be accomplished by breathing in through the mouth with the lips puckered to create an associated friction noise. Repeat this procedure five times, and list on the treatment chart the mean number of seconds achieved, making certain to tag these baseline data with the activity symbol "BI_1." A score less than 10 seconds indicates the need for intervention. Therefore proceed with the exercise. Otherwise advance to the next indicated exercise subsection.

Step 2.   To improve the strength of diaphragmatic contractions and, therefore, air intake potential, have the patient sit upright in a comfortable armless chair, if possible. Patients who cannot shift from their wheelchairs should not be excluded, however. Instruct the patient to take as deep a breath as possible and hold it. During this breath-holding phase, apply varying degrees of light counterforce with an open hand against the distended abdominal wall, as the patient is instructed to try to oppose these deflating compression forces by maintaining strong diaphragmatic contractions until the need to exhale.

Step 3.   Repeat this technique for 10 minutes, permitting rest periods judiciously. At the completion of this time frame, test the effects of this exercise by re-evaluating prolonged inhalation skills, following precisely the baseline method of Step 1. However, enter this result on the treatment chart with the corresponding activity symbol "I_1." Continue with the procedure until the patient achieves a score that is at least 75 percent improved over the baseline score, or

10 seconds, whichever is less after 10 minutes of practice, at which time advance to the next exercise. Calculate the target criterion according to the baseline score, and enter the figure in the respective cell at the bottom of the anticipated treatment data column. As always, invoke the discontinuation rule if after 30 consecutive minutes of practice no discernible trend of improvement is demonstrated to justify further practice. Advance to the next exercise nonetheless.

Exercise No. 2

Step 1. Repeat exactly the same baseline methods as those in the preceding exercise, except that here the activity symbol "Bl$_2$" should be used to tag the data on the treatment chart. Advance as indicated.

Step 2. Following this recording, use the See-Scape device for this exercise. It should be noted beforehand that the objective here is to improve lung volume without exacerbating any underlying weakness and incoordination of the inhalatory and exhalatory musculature. Therefore, the mid-volume level is targeted, at which the patient may most benefit from practice.

Step 3. Remove from the tube any paperclips that may have been placed for pressure-generating exercises. Substitute a piece of drinking straw about 2 inches long for the nasal olive, and poke a small hole about the size of a dull pencil point into the wall of the straw between the mouth of the rubber hose and the free end of the straw. Turn the tube upside down so that the float rests at the top rather than the bottom. Make sure that it is free-floating. The best float action occurs when the clinician holds the tube off of the tabletop during this exercise.

Step 4. Fasten a noseclip on the patient, and instruct him or her to position the straw between the lips and prolong an inhalation as long and steadily as possible. Upon inhalation, the float will rise to the (inverted) bottom of the tube and remain there for feedback as long as the patient maintains the air-intake cycle. Cessation or interruption of this cycle, which may result from exhalation, laryngospasms, and/or breath-holding maneuvers, will be evident as the float immediately reverses its upward route at a speed commensurate with the aerodynamic characteristics of the oppositional behavior. Either counting out loud or providing a stopwatch to cue the patient about the length of each effort is an acceptable form of feedback. As an additional form of feedback, the patient may occasionally place a hand on the abdomen during this exercise to feel the distention that occurs with each inhalation effort.

Step 5. On a notepad, record the number of successful seconds achieved by the patient. Allow 15 seconds of rest, and repeat the procedure until the patient achieves a score that is at least 75 percent improved over the baseline score, or 10 seconds, whichever is less, after 10 consecutive trials, at which time advance to the next indicated subsystem exercise. Calculate the target criterion according to the baseline score, and enter the figure in the respective cell at the bottom of the anticipated treatment data column.

Step 6. After each set of 10 trials, calculate the mean number of seconds from the notepad recordings, and enter the result on the treatment chart in the usual way, making certain to tag these data with the activity symbol "I_2." As always, invoke the discontinuation rule if necessary after 30 consecutive trials with no evidence of improvement to support further practice.

Note: If the See-Scape device is unavailable for use here or in other exercises recommended below, the clinician can try using a 3-inch square piece of facial tissue and a 3-inch piece of drinking straw. After clipping the nose of the patient, the clinician should position the straw in the mouth of the patient and the tissue directly in front of the free end of the straw. Upon inhalation, the tissue will be sucked into the mouth of the straw; exhalation, on the other hand, will cause the tissue to flutter outwards in concert with the degree and length of air emission through the straw. Tissue actions can serve as feedback for the patient.

Exhalation

The ultimate purpose of the following exercises is to help the patient learn how to regulate exhalations so that speech phrasing may become less irregular and may be accompanied by more controllable vocal volume.

Exercise No. 1

Step 1. To establish baseline exhalation prolongation capability, request that the patient breathe out for as long and as steadily as possible. Follow the same basic methods as those employed in Inhalation Exercise no. 1, Step 1, except that here the task is exhalation and the activity symbol to be used to tag the data collected is "BE_1." Advance as indicated.

Step 2. This exercise uses the same See-Scape modifications as those in the preceding inhalation exercise, except that the device should be positioned in its normal upright position on the tabletop at which the patient is comfortably seated. Instruct the patient to place the straw lightly between the lips, take a deep breath in, and then prolong an exhalation as long and steadily as possible. Upon exhalation, the float will rise to the top of the tube and remain there for feedback as long as the patient continues to exhale. Any disruption in such airflow will cause the float to drop toward the bottom of the tube for performance feedback. The clinician can either count aloud or use a stopwatch to signal the patient regarding the length of the effort.

Step 3. Have the patient periodically place a hand on the abdomen during this exercise to feel its retraction throughout the exhalation cycle. Point out any abnormalities in float activity as the patient attempts this task.

Step 4. On a notepad, record the number of seconds that the patient successfully prolonged exhalation. Allow 15 seconds of rest. Follow exactly the same scoring, rating, charting, and advancement methods as those detailed in Step 5 of the preceding inhalation exercise. Here, however, the data collected and recorded on the treatment chart are tagged with the activity symbol "E_1."

Exercise No. 2

Step 1. Follow the same baseline procedures as those in the preceding exercise, except that here the activity symbol "BE_2" is used to tag the data on the treatment chart.

Step 2. Following this recording, the same basic exercise can be reintroduced, except that here the length of each exhalation will vary in concert with clinician commands. First, once the straw is positioned between the patient's lips and the noseclip is fastened, request a deep inhalation and then an exhalation for 5 seconds. When 5 seconds have elapsed, signal the patient to hold his or her breath for approximately 2 seconds to permit the float to move slowly downwards to within 1 inch of the bottom of the tube. At that point, instruct the patient to exhale once again and to prolong the airflow for an additional 5 seconds. At the conclusion of this trial, allow the patient to rest for 30 seconds.

Step 3. Repeat the task, except that this time the first exhalation should last for 3 seconds and the second one for 7 seconds, with the same 2-second pause time between exhalations.

Step 4. After another rest period of 30 seconds, repeat the task again. However, this time vary the exhalation requirements from those preceding this trial: 6 seconds for the first one and 4 seconds for the second one, with the same pause time.

Step 5. Three exhalations on one breath may be attempted next in the following way. Instruct the patient to take a deep breath and then to exhale continuously through the straw for 3 seconds. After this exhalation, the breath is held until the float slowly drops to within 1 inch of the bottom of the tube. The float is then sent immediately upwards again with the next exhalation, which is to be prolonged for another 3 seconds. After this 3-second period, the patient needs to hold the breath one more time, until the float moves to the near-bottom position of the tube. At this point, a final exhalation is prolonged for 3 more seconds.

Step 6. Repeat these four exercises three times each for a total of 12 trials per session. Of course, the clinician is not bound to these recommended time frames for each exhalation attempt. Patients will vary with respect to their abilities to perform these tasks, and such variance ought to govern the individual designs used in treatment. It is important to note that this exercise is most ideally performed without interruptive inhalatory maneuvers during the exhalation cycle. Should such disruptions occur during a given trial, they will evoke an abrupt downward movement of the float to the very bottom of the tube. This drop will serve as visual feedback for the patient and may facilitate, with clinician instructions, performance modifications on subsequent trials.

Step 7. After each set of 10 minutes of practice, test the efficacy of these exercises by re-evaluating exhalation prolongation capability according to the same methodology as that employed for baseline analysis. Enter the result obtained on the treatment chart in the usual way, using the activity symbol "E_2" to represent these treatment data. Continue with this regimen until the patient achieves a score that is at least 75 percent improved over the baseline score, or

10 seconds, whichever is less, after a set of 10 minutes of practice, at which time advance to the next indicated exercise. Calculate the target criterion according to the baseline score, and enter the figure in the respective cell at the bottom of the anticipated treatment data column. Discontinue the exercise if after 30 consecutive minutes of practice no discernible trend of improvement is demonstrated to justify additional drilling.

QUICK BREATHING EXERCISE

Table 3–1 reveals that among the many respiratory subsystem difficulties exhibited by spastic and flaccid dysarthric patients, slow speech breathing rates are frequently observed. The exercise in this section is designed to treat the patient whose baseline data reveal the need for intervention to quicken this rate by learning how to inhale more often, with hopes of improving ultimately the slow-labored characteristics that typify the speech profiles of these patients.

Exercise No. 1

Step 1. To establish baseline breathing speed capability request that the patient breathe in and out continuously and as quickly as possible for 5 seconds. Record on a notepad the number of complete cycles (inhalation/exhalation = 1 cycle) demonstrated, and repeat the task four more times, allowing rests of 15 seconds between trials. Calculate the mean number of cycles achieved, and enter the result on the treatment chart, making certain to tag these data with the activity symbol "BQ_1." If the patient scores less than "5" proceed with the exercise. Otherwise advance to the next indicated exercise.

Step 2. The See-Scape apparatus modifications made for the preceding set of exercises should be prepared for this exercise. Seat the patient comfortably at a table upon which the See-Scape unit is placed, fasten the noseclip in the usual manner, and position the straw in the patient's mouth in preparation for the exercise to follow.

Step 3. Instruct the patient to inhale through the straw for 2 seconds, then exhale for 2 seconds, then inhale for 2 seconds, then exhale for 2 seconds, and so on until 20 seconds have elapsed, which constitutes one trial. A stopwatch can be used to cue the patient that the next cycle is due and when time is up for that trial. Allow a 1-minute rest period, and repeat the 20-second trial again. Follow this approach until 12 trials are accomplished. Note that with each inhalation the float should remain still at the bottom of the tube; each exhalation should force the float to remain at the top of the tube until the next inhalation pulls it swiftly to the bottom, and so on.

Step 4. At the completion of 12 trials, test the possible effects of such practice on breathing rate control by requesting that the patient perform the baseline task described in Step 1. Enter the mean result on the treatment chart, using the activity symbol "Q_1" to represent these data.

Step 5. Continue with the exercise in the same fashion until the patient achieves a mean score that is at least 75 percent improved over the baseline level (Step 1) or "5," whichever is less, after 24 consecutive trials of practice. Calculate the target criterion according to the baseline score, and enter the figure in the respective cell at the bottom of the anticipated treatment data column. Discontinue the exercise if after 30 consecutive minutes of practice there is no observable trend of improvement to justify further drilling.

INHALATORY/EXHALATORY SYNCHRONIZATION EXERCISES

The last four columns of Table 3–1 differentiate the various forms of inhalatory/exhalatory asynchrony that are frequently observed in patients with dysarthria. The exercises in this section aim to effect harmonious contractions of the normally opposing muscle groups of the respiratory subsystem. If this primary objective can be accomplished, airflow should be more readily available for speech activities.

Exercise No. 1

In the Speech Physiology Laboratory, the Respitrace apparatus has been very helpful in illustrating the nature and degree of inhalatory/exhalatory subsystem excursions during nonspeech as well as speech breathing events. Because few clinicians have this instrument at their disposal, the following technique may be a useful alternative.

Step 1. To establish baseline inhalatory/exhalatory synchronization characteristics request that the patient prolong inhalations and exhalations alternately, each lasting roughly 5 seconds, continuously for 1 full minute. Each cycle represents one trial. In this time frame, six complete trials are possible. Record on a notepad the total number of trials that were characterized by synchronous inhalatory/exhalatory behaviors; that is, free of any abnormal, interruptive, oppositional, and/or dysrhythmic respiratory features. Repeat the procedure four more times, allowing a rest between efforts, and calculate the mean number of correct trials performed by the patient. Enter this result on the treatment chart, making certain to list the activity symbol "BS_1" to tag these baseline data. If the score is less than "4" (out of a possible maximum mean score of "6") proceed with the exercise. Otherwise advance to Exercise no. 2 below.

Step 2. Place the See-Scape device on the table at which the patient is seated comfortably. Note that for this exercise, connect the plastic nasal olive that is supplied with the device to the rubber hose. Place the olive in the most patent nostril of the patient and tape it to the bridge of the nose so that it remains in place without having to be held. Request that the patient perform all breathing tasks through the nasal passage with the mouth shut, if possible.

Step 3. Instruct the patient to prolong an inhalation for 5 seconds, and then prolong an exhalation for 5 seconds, and so on for 1 minute for a total of 6 full cycles or 6 complete trials. A stopwatch can be used to time each command to the patient. Have the patient observe the float during each breath. It should move swiftly to the bottom of the tube and remain there during inhalations and, upon exhalations, travel up to and remain fixed at the very top of the tube. From cycle to cycle the float's movements should signal airflow that is consistent in timing, rate, and degree.

Step 5. Abnormalities in cycle characteristics that can be caused by the types of respiration subsystem disturbances that are highlighted in the last four columns of Table 3–1 should be recorded on a notepad. The clinician should treat each cycle independently: if the patient struggles within a given cycle, that cycle is scored incorrect, and if no breakdowns occur in the cycle, it is graded correct. The clock is stopped when such breakdowns occur, to permit discussion. It resumes when the patient is instructed to continue, and it is stopped ultimately when 1 minute has elapsed. At the completion of each full minute of practice, keep a running total of the number of correct trials. Remember that a maximum of "6" is possible in any given minute.

Step 6. Repeat the procedure 10 times, with a 30-second break between the full-minute sets of trials. At the completion of these 60 trials, calculate the mean number of correct cycles performed. Enter this result on the treatment chart, making certain to tag these data with the activity symbol "S_1." Continue with the exercise in this fashion until the patient achieves a mean correct score that is at least 75 percent improved over the baseline score or "6," whichever is less, over 60 consecutive trials. Calculate the target criterion according to the baseline score, and enter the figure in the respective cell at the bottom of the anticipated treatment data column. Discontinue the exercise if after 120 consecutive trials there is no observable trend of improvement to justify further practice. In either case, advance to Exercise no. 2.

Exercise No. 2

Step 1. To establish again baseline inhalatory/exhalatory synchronization this time request that the patient take a short breath and upon exhalation prolong the /m/ consonant for 2 full seconds, then take another breath and prolong the /m/ again for 2 more seconds, and so on until 10 complete trials are attempted. Rate each trial individually as either correct or incorrect. A "correct" score is rendered when the inhalation is quick and is immediately followed by a smoothly produced /m/ for 2 seconds. Repeat this procedure two more times for a total of 30 trials, and calculate the total number of correct scores. Enter the result on the treatment chart, tagging these baseline data with the activity symbol "BS_2." Proceed with the exercise if this score is less than "21." Otherwise, advance to the next indicated exercise regimen.

Step 2. Assemble the See-Scape device in the same way as that for the preceding exercise. Request that the patient perform the same task as that in Step 1 above. Discuss, however, that with each inhalation the float mechanism should rush to, and remain at, the bottom of the tube, and that each time the /m/ is prolonged, the float should rise to, and remain fixed at, the top of the tube.

Step 3. As in Exercise no. 1, explain the adverse airflow effects of antagonistic and asynchronous respiratory musculature contractions, as can be measured and observed by deviant float dynamics during the present exercise.

Step 4. At the completion of each set of 10 trials, tally the total number of correct scores, following the rating method discussed in Step 1 above. Repeat the procedure until 30 trials have been accomplished, at which time tally the sum total of correct scores and enter this result on the treatment chart, tagging the entry with the activity symbol "S_2" in the appropriate cell at the bottom of the data column. Continue with this procedure until the patient achieves a total correct score that is at least 75 percent improved over baseline or "30," whichever is less, over 30 consecutive trials. Calculate the target criterion according to the baseline score, and enter the figure in the respective cell at the bottom of the anticipated treatment data column. Discontinue the exercise, as always, if after 60 consecutive trials no discernible improvement is evident to justify further practice. In either case, advance to the next indicated exercise.

Exercise No. 3

Note: This is basically the same exercise as Exercise no. 2 above, only here the duration of prolongations of the /m/ consonant should be 1 second each. The baseline data entry is tagged with the activity symbol "BS_3," and the treatment data are represented by the "S_3" symbol.

Exercise No. 4

Note: Follow basically the same method here as that adopted for Exercise nos. 2 and 3, except that for this exercise, following each shallow inhalation, the patient will be instructed to prolong the /m/ for variable amounts of time. The first /m/ will last for 10 seconds, the second for 4 seconds, the third for 6 seconds, the fourth for 2 seconds, the fifth for 8 seconds, the sixth for 1 second, the seventh for 3 seconds, the eighth for 7 seconds, the ninth for 9 seconds, and the tenth for 5 seconds. Be certain to point out to the patient deviations in the aerodynamics of the float that may have been precipitated by the aforementioned types of respiration subsystem disturbances.

As in Exercise no. 1, score each trial on a notepad independently, using the "correct/incorrect" dichotomous scale, in which if the patient struggles within a given trial (which is defined as a short breath followed by a prolonged /m/ consonant) that trial is rated incorrect. No such breakdown in the trial, on the other hand, is graded correct. At the completion of 30 trials, tally the total number of "correct" scores that the patient achieved, and enter the score on the treatment chart in the usual way. Follow the same charting and advancement methods as those detailed in Exercise no. 2, Step 4. Remember that for the baseline data the activity symbol "BS_4" is used, and for the treatment data the "S_4" is used on the treatment chart.

ISOLATED SOUND PRODUCTION EXERCISES

The exercises in this section are indicated either for those patients who initially present with adequate nonspeech respiration subsystem capabilities but fail to transfer such skills to speech breathing activities, or for those patients who have progressed to this point in the treatment sequence after having shown substantial improvements on the preceding (nonspeech) breathing exercises. The primary purpose of the following exercises is to help the patient learn how to incorporate underlying respiration subsystem potential into motor speech activities. We begin with isolated sounds because for most dysarthric patients this requirement is easier than complex strings of sounds, thereby ensuring some degree of success in coupling breath control and speech output in virtually all patients from the outset. Note that if and when a patient struggles with any of the following exercises, the clinician should attempt to facilitate performances using gentle manual compression force against the patient's abdomen in concert with the exhalation requirement of the task.

Exercise No. 1

Step 1. To establish baseline sound prolongation ability, request that the patient say the vowel /i/ for as long and as steadily as possible. Time the length of this production, and have the patient repeat the task with the /u/ vowel. As a final trial, use the /o/ vowel, and repeat the task. Calculate the mean number of seconds achieved over these three trials. Enter this result on the treatment chart, tagging this finding with the activity symbol "BP_1." If the score is less than 15 seconds, proceed with the exercise. Otherwise, move on to Exercise no. 2.

Step 2. Use the See-Scape device for this exercise. Replace the nasal olive with a 2-inch piece of drinking straw (without a bleed hole) and connect the straw to the rubber hose. Once the patient is seated comfortably at the table upon which this device is situated, he or she may be fitted with a noseclip if necessary and then instructed to position the free end of the straw between the lips so that it rests lightly against the labial surfaces of the central incisor teeth.

Step 3. Instruct the patient to take a deep breath and then prolong the vowel /u/ as long and steadily as possible. Note that at the onset of voicing for this sound, the float will rise to the top of the tube and remain there for the duration of the production, provided that the integrity of vowel articulation is preserved throughout the trial. Using a stopwatch, the clinician should time the isolated vowel production, informing the patient beforehand that the clock starts when the float reaches the top of the tube and irrevocably stops when the float descends more than 1 inch from that position.

Step 4. On a notepad, record the number of seconds achieved, and repeat the task 20 times, allowing a break of 30 seconds between trials. To reduce the potential for boredom, alternately use any one of the following three vowels only: /u/, /i/, and /o/.

Step 5. At the completion of the 20 trials, tally the total number of seconds recorded on the notepad, and divide the sum by 20 to derive the mean. Enter this score on the treatment chart, making certain to tag the data with the activity symbol "P_1." Continue with this procedure until the patient achieves a mean score that is at least 75 percent improved over the baseline score or 15, whichever is less, over 20 consecutive trials, at which time advancement to Exercise no. 2 is indicated. Calculate the target criterion according to the baseline score, and enter the figure in the respective cell at the bottom of the anticipated treatment data column. Discontinue this exercise if after 30 consecutive trials no observable trend of improvement is evident to justify further practice. Move on to the next exercise nonetheless.

Exercise No. 2

Step 1. To establish baseline breath support for sound sequencing tasks, instruct the patient to take a deep breath and then prolong the vowel train /i-u-o/ as long and steadily as possible, giving roughly equal amounts of time to each component of the sequence. Thus, if the patient can prolong voiced exhalation only for 10 seconds, the /i/ would occupy the first 3 seconds, the /u/ the next 3 seconds, and the /o/ the last 4 seconds or so. Explain to the patient that the transition from one vowel to the next has to be smooth relative to respiratory support, and that an equal amount of time must be awarded to each vowel produced. If these criteria are met, the trial is rated "correct." Otherwise, it receives an "incorrect" rating. Allow 10 trials and tally the total number of correct trials. Enter this score on the treatment chart, tagging these baseline data with the activity symbol "BP_2." If this score is equal to or less than "7," proceed with the exercise. Otherwise, advance to Exercise no. 3.

Step 2. Use the See-Scape device again. It is to be used in the same way as that discussed in the preceding exercise. Once the straw is in position, request that the patient perform the same task as that in Step 1 above. Explain to the patient that normally when this vowel sequence is steadily prolonged, with shifts occurring from one sound to the next in equal time intervals, the float will remain at the top of the tube, with virtually no fluctuation from that position upon the shift from /i/ to /u/, and will descend only momentarily to a minimal degree on the shift from /u/ to /o/, provided that the ongoing integrity of the vowel productions is preserved. Upon completion of the trial, rate it either correct or incorrect, using the criteria adopted for the baseline measurement above.

Step 3. Continue with this procedure until the patient achieves a total correct score that is at least 75 percent improved over the baseline score or "10," whichever is less, over 10 consecutive trials. Calculate the target criterion according to the baseline score, and enter the figure in the respective cell at the bottom of the anticipated treatment data column. After each set of 10 trials, tally the total number of correct trials and enter this result on the treatment chart, tagging these treatment data with the activity symbol "P_2." Advance to Exercise no. 3 as indicated. As always, discontinue this regimen if after 30 consecutive trials there is no observable trend of improvement to justify further practice. Move on to Exercise no. 3 nonetheless.

Note: To reduce the potential for boredom and possible order effects, the three-vowel train can be periodically changed to any one of the six possible combinations.

Exercise No. 3

Step 1. Establish baseline breath support for vowel repetitions by requesting that the patient repeat continuously the vowel /u/ for 10 full seconds, separating each production by 1 second. On a notepad keep score of the number of correct productions achieved according to this criterion. Allow the patient three trials, 10 seconds each, and tally the total number of correct repetitions. Enter this baseline score on the treatment chart, tagging the data with the activity symbol "BP_3." If this score is less than "21," proceed with the exercise. Otherwise, advance to Exercise no. 4.

Step 2. Set up the See-Scape device as in the preceding exercises, and fasten the noseclip on the patient, irrespective of velopharyngeal status.

Step 3. Set the metronome to beat at 60 beats per minute (bpm). As the patient (or clinician) holds the end of the straw lightly against the incisor teeth as in the preceding exercises, instruct him or her to prolong the vowel /u/. As soon as the float rises to the very top of the tube, set the metronome in motion and instruct the patient to repeat this sound to the beat of the metronome, one utterance per beat, with the objective of never allowing the top of the float to drop more than 1 inch from the top of the tube throughout 10 full seconds of vowel repetitions. Illustrate for the patient that in order to prevent the float's descent during this exercise, inhalations must be voluntarily inhibited. Any inhalatory maneuver will cause the float to descend rapidly and extensively, which will be visually evident as a form of feedback.

Step 4. Once the patient understands the task, record on a notepad how many of the 10 required repetitions (1 per second [60 bpm] for 10 seconds) the patient performed without error, as previously defined. Upon completion of three trials, 10 seconds each, tally the total number of correct repetitions achieved and enter this score on the treatment chart, tagging these treatment data with the activity symbol "P_3." Continue with this procedure until the patient achieves a score that is at least 75 percent improved over the baseline score or "30," whichever is less, over 30 consecutive repetitions, at which time advance to Exercise no. 4. Calculate the target criterion according to the baseline score, and enter the figure in the respective cell at the bottom of the anticipated treatment data column. Discontinue this regimen if after 30 consecutive minutes of such practice there is no observable trend of improvement to justify further practice. Advance to Exercise no. 4 nonetheless.

Exercise No. 4

Note: To stimulate speech respiration rates that approximate (more) normal levels, experimentation with faster metronomic speeds is recommended.

Step 1.   This is exactly the same exercise as the preceding one except that this time the speed of the metronome is increased to 90 bpm.

Step 2.   Follow the same scoring procedure as that in Exercise no. 3, noting that here the required number of repetitions is 15 over the 10-second trial period.

Step 3.   Follow the same data entry procedure as in Exercise no. 3, using a separate column on the treatment chart and making certain to list the activity symbol as P_4. Baseline entry is tagged with the activity symbol "BP_4."

Note that with the patient whose prognosis is good for gains at faster metronomic speeds, experimentation with 120 and 150 bpm may prove worthwhile and motivating. Then move on to the next exercise.

Note: The following six exercises provide excellent practice material. Clinicians may choose to establish their own criteria for scoring, charting, and advancement within and between these programs.

Exercise No. 5

Step 1.   Assemble the See-Scape device again. Use the straw instead of the nasal olive, fasten a noseclip on the patient, and position the end of the straw close enough to the patient's lips so that upon production of the consonant /f/ the float readily and abruptly rises to the top of the tube.

Step 2.   Instruct the patient to take in a deep breath and then prolong the /f/ as long and steadily as possible, noting that the clock begins as soon as the float reaches the top of the tube and irrevocably stops once the float drops more than 1 inch from this position. Allow the patient 10 trials, with a 30-second break between attempts. On a notepad record the number of seconds achieved for each trial, and divide the sum by 10 to derive the mean.

For additional articulation practice, and to reduce the potential for boredom, other continuant sounds such as /s/ and /ʃ/ may be alternately introduced into this regimen, whenever feasible. However, the position of the straw may need to be adjusted slightly for the best aerodynamic feedback.

Exercise No. 6

Step 1.   This is the exact same program as that in Exercise no. 3 above except that here we use a continuant sound such as /ʃ/, /s/, or /f/, whichever is easiest for the patient, instead of a vowel. Clinicians may wish to follow the same scoring and data entry procedures as those in Exercise no. 3, remembering, however, that the activity symbol here would be "P_6" for the record.

Exercise No. 7

Step 1. This is the exact same program as that in Exercise no. 4, only here the continuant sound is used, not the vowel. Again, clinicians may wish to follow the same scoring and data entry recommendations as those in that exercise, remembering that the activity symbol here would be "P_7" for the record.

Exercise No. 8

Step 1. Use the See-Scape device, the metronome, and the noseclip. Substitute the straw, once again, for the nasal olive, fasten the noseclip on the patient, and set the metronome to 30 bpm.

Step 2. Position the straw between the patient's lips so that the open end lightly touches the central incisors, set the metronome in motion, and instruct the patient to take a deep breath and repeat the word /pi/ to the beat, allowing only one consonant-vowel (CV) syllable per beat for 10 full seconds. Illustrate for the patient that with such productions you want the float to rise to and remain relatively fixed at the top of the tube, and that to accomplish this objective the vowel must be prolonged on each production. Also inform and demonstrate for the patient that any inhalatory maneuvers that occur within the 10-second trial will be evidenced by quick descent of the float; a downward shift of the float that exceeds 1 inch from the top of the tube will be rated an error in performance.

Step 3. On a notepad record how many of the five required repetitions (one every 2 seconds [30 bpm] for 10 seconds) the patient performed without error. Allow a total of 10 trials for 10 seconds each, with a rest period of 30 seconds or so between trials.

Step 4. At the completion of these trials, tally the total number of correct CV syllable repetitions recorded on the notepad and divide by 10 to derive the mean.

Use of the /ʃ/, /f/, and other consonants that may be within the patient's articulatory repertoire may also be coupled to the /i/, /o/, and/or /u/ vowels for this exercise so as to expand motor speech practice. Slight adjustments in the position of the straw may be necessary with such CV alternatives to ensure the best float aerodynamics.

Exercise No. 9

Step 1. This is the same exercise, only this time the metronome will be set at 60 bpm for the CV syllable repetitions.

Step 2. Follow the same scoring procedures as those in Exercise no. 8, noting that here there is a required 10 repetitions (1 per second for 10 seconds) per trial.

Note that with the patient whose prognosis is good for improvement at faster metronomic speeds, experimentation with 90 bpm and higher may prove valuable.

Exercise No. 10

Step 1. Prepare a long list of real and nonsense CVC, CVCV, and CVCVCV words, making certain to use only the /i, o, and u/ vowels and only plosive, fricative, and affricative consonants that are within articulatory reach of the patient, inasmuch as these types of sounds activate the float with the greatest consistency. Randomly list these words on index cards, roughly 15 words per card.

Step 2. Assemble the See-Scape set-up as in the previous exercise, fasten the noseclip on the patient, and position the end of the straw gently between the lips so that it rests lightly against the central incisors.

Step 3. Place a prepared index card on the tabletop in front of the patient and instruct him or her to take a deep breath in and then begin reading aloud, one at a time, the words on the card until the next inhalation is required. The overall objective is to complete as many words as possible per breath, noting that the float should rise to the top of the tube upon production of the very first word and remain within 1 inch of this position with all subsequent productions. Any inhalatory maneuver that occurs will cause the float to descend below this 1-inch threshold toward the bottom of the tube, at which point the trial is considered over. It is important to ensure that the patient knows and can read the names of the words prior to scoring, such that errors cannot be attributed to task confusion or reading difficulty.

Step 4. On a notepad record how many words the patient produced per breath. Remember that speech breathing control, not articulatory precision, is the target, especially because from the start the straw may interfere with intelligibility.

Step 5. Allow a total of 10 trials, with a rest of 20 seconds between trials. At the completion of these, tally the total number of words produced and divide the sum by 10 to derive the mean.

Here are some suggested words that can be used in this exercise, depending upon the articulatory capability of the patient: (1) she, (2) show, (3) shoe, (4) fee, (5) foe, (6) see, (7) sew, (8) sue, (9) pea, (10) key, (11) chew, (12) tea, (13) toe, (14) two, (15) doe, (16) do, (17) bee, (18) bo, (19) boo, (20) sheet, (21) beat, (22) pope, (23) poop, (24) feat, (25) coat, (26) cheap, (27) eat, (28) oat, (29) bootie, (30) bee-bee, (31) bobo, (32) boobie, (33) Phoebe, (34) beefy, and (35) boo-boo. Note that many other nonsense bi- and tri-syllable words can be made using any combination of the single syllable words listed here.

CONNECTED SPEECH BREATHING EXERCISES

The exercises that compose this section are designed to help the patient who is having difficulty in either transferring gains made in preceding respiration subsystem treatments or extending inherent subsystem capabilities to connected speech efforts. It should be noted that anticipated results with these exercises are likely to be hampered by coexistent disturbances of other subsystems. For this reason, the clinician must be lenient in establishing the criteria for improvement and advancement to the next treatment indicated for the patient. That is to say, the untreated difficulties with articulation, phonation, and/or prosody, for example, that may plague the connected speech breathing exercise performances should not be factored into the scoring system during such practice. Rather, the clinician must see through the potentially camouflaging effects of other speech subsystem difficulties that have yet to be treated successfully. The clinical focus should be on whether or not the patient is learning to expand consistently the number of syllables (however imprecisely uttered) that can be produced per breath during connected speech and to improve the timing and coordination of these breath groups.

For those patients with marked to severe degrees of dysarthria involving multiple subsystems, connected speech breathing exercises may prove fruitless until gains are made with resonation, phonation, articulation, and/or prosody treatments. Thus, even if factoring out such coexistent disturbances still limits the usefulness of respiration exercises, then these exercises should be delayed until the "climate" is more accommodating, perhaps following successes with the other subsystem treatments.

Exercise No. 1

Step 1. To establish baseline breath support during connected discourse, use the See-Scape device and use a 2-inch piece of drinking straw rather than the nasal olive. Place a thin piece of tape around the tube at approximately the halfway mark, and prepare the following 10 sentences on one or two index cards for the patient to read aloud. (Note that these sentences contain certain sounds that will activate the float for biofeedback.)

1. Today is Tuesday.
2. Pete threw the baseball to Sue.
3. Two plus four is six.
4. Be sure to chew your food.
5. This exercise is to help us breathe better.
6. The boy kicked the football for three points.
7. She stopped by the shop for cookies.
8. The professor wore a tie to all his classes.
9. She applied for the position at the school.
10. Happy birthday to you, happy birthday to you, happy birthday dear Phoebe, happy birthday to you.

Step 2. After fastening a noseclip on the patient (regardless of the status of the velopharyngeal mechanism) position the free end of the straw gently between the lips so that it rests lightly against the labial surfaces of the central incisor teeth. Instruct the patient to read Sentence no. 1 aloud, noting that speech output causes the float to rise above the tape threshold and remain at a high level in the tube as long as the patient neither pauses for an abnormally long time nor inhales during the sentence production. Pausing will result in a slow descent of the float, perhaps through the tape threshold, but inhalation will cause an abrupt and decisive return of the float to the bottom of the tube, which in either case provides good visual feedback regarding connected speech breathing activity. For this task, only the inhalatory maneuvers will be scored, to allow calculation of the number of syllables per breath.

Note: Those patients who present with reading difficulties may need coaching from the clinician to perform this exercise, which would certainly have an impact on the validity of the end results.

Step 3.   Once the patient understands that the task is to produce as many syllables per breath as possible during each sentence production, instruct him or her to take a deep breath and read Sentence no. 1 again. On a notepad, record the number of breaths required to complete the sentence. Repeat the procedure for each of the 10 target sentences individually, with a 15-second break between trials and allowing the patient to take a breath before reciting each new sentence. Note that at the completion of the 10 sentences, a total of 100 syllables will have been attempted by the patient.

Step 4.   Permit the patient three trials per sentence.

Step 5.   Tally the total number of breaths taken by the patient, and divide 300 by this result to derive the baseline number of syllables per breath. The best score possible on this task, as it is set up, is 30 syllables per breath (one breath at the beginning of each of the 30 sentence attempts).

Note: To reduce the potential for boredom and possible order and familiarity effects on performances, other sentences containing the same sound classes as used in the 10 target sentences can be constructed by the clinician and introduced when desired, depending, of course, upon the articulatory proficiency of the patient.

Step 6.   After the number of syllables per breath has been calculated, enter the baseline result on the Respiration Subsystem Behavioral Treatment Chart, making certain to tag these data with the activity symbol "BC_1." If this score is less than "20," proceed with this exercise. Otherwise, advance to Exercise no. 2.

Step 7.   Follow exactly the same procedure as that in the preceding steps, and continue such practice until the patient achieves a score that is at least 75 percent improved over the baseline score or "30," whichever is less, over 30 consecutive sentence attempts. Calculate the target criterion according to the baseline score, and enter the figure in the respective cell at the bottom of the anticipated treatment data column. At the completion of each set of 30 attempts, calculate from the notepad scores listed the number of syllables per breath, and enter the result on the treatment chart in the usual way, making certain to tag these data with the activity symbol "C_1." Discontinue this exercise regimen if after 30 consecutive minutes of such practice no discernible evidence of improvement is observed. In either case, advance to Exercise no. 2.

Exercise No. 2

Step 1. To establish baseline breath support during connected discourse, again use the same set-up and methodology with the See-Scape as those in the preceding exercise. However, here prepare the following paragraph on an index card, which contains a total of 100 syllables that will facilitate airflow visual feedback, for the patient to read aloud:

> Today I will practice this paragraph. Each word was picked to help with breath control feedback as I speak. Each word produced should cause the float to stay above the tape threshold. Pauses cause the float to drop slowly toward or below this threshold. A quick drop of the float occurs if I take a breath. The objective is to produce a lot of words with each breath. But if I should choose to pause or take a breath, that is okay.

Step 2. After familiarizing the patient with the previously described dynamics of the float, relative to its rise and fall during speech output and pauses or inhalations, respectively, instruct the patient to read aloud the paragraph with the objective of producing as many syllables as possible between breaths. As in Exercise no. 1, only inhalations will be scored.

Step 3. On a notepad record the number of breaths required to complete the reading. Remember, the clinical focus here is on the patient's control of the respiration subsystem output. Disturbances of other subsystems must be overlooked to the maximum degree possible during the scoring procedure. Permit the patient three trials.

Step 4. At the completion of these trials, tally the total number of breaths taken during the readings and divide 300 by this result to derive the number of syllables per breath. To reduce boredom and familiarity effects, as noted previously, other paragraphs containing similar sound classes as those constructed in the target paragraph for See-Scape feedback should be substituted periodically.

Step 5. After the number of syllables per breath has been calculated, enter the result on the treatment chart, tagging these baseline data with the activity symbol "BC_2." If this score is less than "10," proceed with this exercise. Otherwise, advance to the next speech subsystem in the sequence that requires treatment.

Step 6. Follow exactly the same procedure as that in the preceding steps, and continue such practice until the patient achieves a score that is at least 75 percent improved over the baseline score or "21," whichever is less, over 10 consecutive trials of the entire paragraph. Calculate the target criterion according to the baseline score, and enter the figure in the respective cell at the bottom of the anticipated treatment data column. At the completion of each set of three trials, calculate from the notepad scores the number of syllables produced per breath, and enter the result on the treatment chart, in the usual way, making certain to tag these data with the activity symbol "C_2." Discontinue this exercise regimen if after 30 consecutive minutes of such practice no discernible evidence of improve-

TABLE 3–2. Differential Respiration Subsystem Treatments, Objectives, and Methods for Dysarthric Patients

Sequence of Respiration Subsystem Treatment Exercises	Speech Breathing Objectives	Techniques
Relaxation	Reduce stiffness, tension, and rigidity of head, neck, and trunk musculature	Supine breathing exercises using See-Scape device for airflow feedback Alternate tightening and relaxing of respiration subsystem muscular contractions in supine position Passive manipulation of head and neck in sitting position Rag doll exercise Alternatives: Drugs, rolfing, meditation, Yoga, creative visualization, self-actualization
Postural support	Augment and reinforce respiration subsystem musculoskeletal framework	Adaptive alterations of wheelchair Elastic straps, girdles, slings Alternating sitting and standing positions
Pressure generation	Train low-pressure exhalations, controlled and maintained over time	Adaptive alteration of See-Scape device for subglottal air pressure generation practice at 5 cm H_2O/5 seconds
Prolonged inhalation	Improve lung volume Improve strength/coordination of inhalatory/exhalatory musculature Maximize no. of syllables/breath Facilitate rate control	Manual compressions of abdominal wall as breath is held firmly to combat deflating forces Inverted See-Scape device for feedback practice of prolonged inhalations
Prolonged exhalation	Modify upper thoracic and clavicular breathing patterns	Prolonged steady exhalations using See-Scape device for feedback practice Variably prolonged exhalations using See-Scape device for feedback
Quick breaths	Improve rate alternatives	Multiple quick breaths using See-Scape device for feedback
Inhalatory/exhalatory synchronization	Train cooperative, synchronous contractions of opposing muscle groups	Regularly timed inhalatory/exhalatory maneuvers, using See-Scape device for feedback Repetitions of the consonant /m/ for variably prolonged time intervals, using See-Scape device for feedback
Isolated sounds	Improve coupling of respiration subsystem controls with speech motor output	Isolated vowel prolongations Vowel train prolongations Fricative prolongations } Using See-Scape device for feedback Real and nonsense word productions Vowel and fricative repetitions CV syllable productions at various rates } Using See-Scape device and metronome for feedback
Connected speech	Increase no. of syllables/breath in connected discourse	Sentence productions, using See-Scape device for feedback Paragraph productions, using See-Scape device for feedback

ment is observed. In either case, the respiration subsystem treatment regimen is officially completed at this point.

Table 3–2 provides a synopsis of the sequence of respiration subsystem treatments, their objectives and methods.

FINAL COMMENTS AND ILLUSTRATIVE CASE SAMPLE

That there will be some patients for whom the treatments in this chapter are indicated but unsuccessful in improving functional control of the respiration subsystem is important for the clinician to realize up front. These patients may need to be taught to establish the best controls possible and to accept the fact that very few syllables per breath may be all that can be achieved. Compensatory phrasing techniques, however, may help minimize the effects of such limited subsystem control.

Upon graduation from this exercise program, the patient is advanced in the sequence to treatments directly aimed at improving motor speech production. However, inasmuch as the success that may be accomplished with subsequent treatments depends on the ongoing cooperation of the respiration subsystem, maintenance speech breathing exercises should be periodically introduced throughout the duration of the overall intervention program.

The following case sample helps illustrate some of the procedures that have been recommended throughout this chapter.

Illustrative Case

The patient is a 22-year-old female with a history of closed head injury (CHI) that was sustained at the age of 16 years. In addition to resultant severe cognitive deficits, she exhibits severe spastic dysarthria with the classic pathophysiologic characteristics that typify widespread involvement of the speech subsystems. Figure 3–2 illustrates the results of baseline testing of the respiration subsystem, which revealed severe degrees of (1) hypertonicity, (2) air pressure–generating difficulty, (3) inhalatory/exhalatory prolongation and synchrony breakdowns, and (4) dyscontrol during isolated and connected speech efforts. Although evaluations of the other subsystems showed severe weakness, hypertonicity, and forcing dysfunctions of the laryngeal, velopharyngeal, and articulatory musculature with consequent strained-strangled phonation, hypernasality, and slow-labored articulatory imprecision, because the respiration subsystem is significantly involved it receives top priority along with the velopharynx in the treatment sequence. At the onset of the following treatment program the patient was simultaneously evaluated and fitted for a palatal-lift appliance that was constructed, modified for the best fit possible, and worn continuously throughout the total intervention program. For the record, the lift was only moderately effective in reducing abnormal nasal air emissions and hypernasality.

Figure 3–5, *A, B,* and *C* represents the patient's responses to air pressure and inhalatory/exhalatory prolongation subsystem treatments administered over

RESPIRATION SUBSYSTEM BEHAVIORAL TREATMENT CHART

Patient's name: Jane Doe

Birthdate: 5/3/67 Sex: Fe
Speech diagnosis: Spastic Dysarthria
Medical diagnosis: Pseudobulbar palsy due to CHI

Clinician: Dworkin
Facility: XYZ
Address: Anywhere, USA

Comments: Note here any nasal air emissions and/or lip seal difficulties that needed adjustments for these measures. Also note value during measures.

Severe oral and velopharyngeal seal incompetence required compensatory adjustments for virtually all exercises: manual assistance to promote lip seal and a noseclip to eliminate nasal air escape. Vocal fold hyperfunctioning during some of the "speech" breathing tasks was evident.

A

ACTIVITY KEY

Feature:
1. Relaxation (tonal) status (R)

2. Postural (tonal) status (T)

3. 5 cm H_2O/5 seconds pressure generating capability (G)

4. Prolonged inhalation (I)
5. Prolonged exhalation (E)

MEASUREMENT UNIT
No. correct, or
Hypotonic-Normal-Hypertonic
$0 \leftarrow 2 - 5 - 7 \rightarrow 10$

Poor = 0; Adequate = 1;
Good = 2; Excellent = 3

No. correct

No. of seconds
No. of seconds or no. correct

Feature:
6. Max. no. of quick breaths possible in 20 seconds (Q)
7. Inhalation/exhalation synchrony (S)
8. Isolated sound productions (P)
9. Connected speech breathing (C)

Baseline (pre-treatment): B + activity symbol

MEASUREMENT UNIT
No. breath cycles

No. correct
No. of seconds or no. correct
No. of syllables/breath

Dates:	6/6/89		6/7		6/13		6/15		6/21	
30										
20										
15							X*			
10							X			
9					X					
8				X						
7					X					
6		X								X
5	X	X		X					X	X
4		X						X	X	X
3										
2								X		
1	X	X					X	X		
0										

Average No. Per Unit Measured

SESSIONS

No. of trials	10					10			12	10
Activity symbol	G_1					I_1	I_1	E_1	E_1	E_1
Measurement unit	# Correct					# Seconds				
Target criterion	10					9	9	10	9	10

Figure 3–5. A to C, Spastic dysarthric patient's responses to pressure-generating (G) and prolonged inhalation/exhalation (I/E) treatments. Note that the

78

RESPIRATION SUBSYSTEM BEHAVIORAL TREATMENT CHART

Patient's name: Jane Doe (continued)

Birthdate: ___ Sex: ___
Speech diagnosis: ___
Medical diagnosis: ___

Clinician: ___
Facility: ___
Address: ___

ACTIVITY KEY

Feature:
1. Relaxation (tonal) status (R)

2. Postural (tonal) status (T)

3. 5 cm H_2O/5 seconds pressure generating capability (G)

4. Prolonged inhalation (I)

5. Prolonged exhalation (E)

MEASUREMENT UNIT
No. correct, or
Hypotonic-Normal-Hypertonic
$0 \leftarrow 2 — 5 — 7 \rightarrow 10$
Poor = 0; Adequate = 1;
Good = 2; Excellent = 3

No. correct

No. of seconds
No. of seconds or no. correct

Feature:
6. Max. no. of quick breaths possible in 20 seconds (Q)

7. Inhalation/exhalation synchrony (S)

8. Isolated sound productions (P)
9. Connected speech breathing (C)

MEASUREMENT UNIT
No. breath cycles

No. correct

No. of seconds or no. correct
No. of syllables/breath

Baseline (pre-treatment): B + activity symbol

Comments: Note here any nasal air emissions and/or lip seal difficulties that needed adjustments for these measures. Also note value during measures.

Dates:	6/21	7/5				7/6				7/10				7/11				7/13		
30																				
20																				
15																				
10																				
9																				
8																X				
7														X						X
6												X							X	
5			X			X				X					X					X
4				X													X			
3									X											
2							X					X								
1	X												X							
0				X																
No. of trials	12	10	10	12		10		12		10		12		10		12		10		12
Activity symbol	E_1	I_1	E_1	E_1		I_1		E_1		I_1		E_1		I_1		E_1		I_2		E_2
Measurement unit	# Sec																			
Target criterion	10	9	9	10		9		10		9		10		9		10		9		10

Average No. Per Unit Measured

SESSIONS

B

Figure continues on following page.

Figure 3–5. *Continued.*

79

RESPIRATION SUBSYSTEM BEHAVIORAL TREATMENT CHART

Patient's name: Jane Doe (continued)

Birthdate: Sex:
Speech diagnosis:
Medical diagnosis:

Clinician:
Facility:
Address:

Comments: Note here any nasal air emissions and/or lip seal difficulties that needed adjustments for these measures. Also note value during measures.

ACTIVITY KEY

Feature:	MEASUREMENT UNIT
1. Relaxation (tonal) status (R)	No. correct, or Hypotonic-Normal-Hypertonic $0 \leftarrow 2 - 5 - 7 \rightarrow 10$
2. Postural (tonal) status (T)	Poor = 0; Adequate = 1; Good = 2; Excellent = 3
3. 5 cm H_2O/5 seconds pressure generating capability (G)	No. correct
4. Prolonged inhalation (I)	No. of seconds
5. Prolonged exhalation (E)	No. of seconds or no. correct

Feature:	MEASUREMENT UNIT
6. Max. no. of quick breaths possible in 20 seconds (Q)	No. breath cycles
7. Inhalation/exhalation synchrony (S)	No. correct
8. Isolated sound productions (P)	No. of seconds or no. correct
9. Connected speech breathing (C)	No. of syllables/breath

Baseline (pre-treatment): B + activity symbol

Average No. Per Unit Measured: 30, 20, 15, 10, 9, 8, 7, 6, 5, 4, 3, 2, 1, 0

Dates: 7/13/89 → 7/18 → 7/20 → 7/25 → 7/27 → 7/28 →

No. of trials	12	10	12	10	12	10	12	10	12	10	12	10	12	10
Activity symbol	E_2	I_2	E_2	I_2	E_2	I_2	E_2	I_2	E_2	I_2	E_2	I_2	E_2	E_2
Measurement unit	# Sec.													→
Target criterion	10	9	10	9	10	9	10	9	10	9	10	9	10	10

SESSIONS

Figure 3–5. *Continued.*

several sessions. Her baseline data pointed first to the need for relaxation exercises, which were conducted with moderate success prior to the initiation of these highlighted treatments.

Air Pressure–Generating Therapy

The top of column 1 in Figure 3–5, A reveals that the first treatment session was on 6/6/89. Of the 10 trials attempted, she correctly achieved just one. The remaining adjacent columns illustrate the patient's ongoing responses to this intervention technique. Note that on 6/13/89 she achieved the criterion for improvement and advancement, which was arbitrarily set at 10 correct performances over 10 consecutive attempts. As can be seen from the comments section of the treatment chart, the patient was permitted to use her fingers to assist lip seal during this blowing task, and a noseclip was fastened for each trial owing to persistent nasal air escape despite use of the palatal-lift appliance.

Inspiratory/Expiratory Prolongation Exercises

Figure 3–5, A through C illustrates the patient's responses to the second indicated treatments—inspiratory/expiratory prolongations—which began on 6/15/89 and continued until 7/28/89.

Note that an asterisk denotes a performance that met or exceeded the criterion level set for the task. These exercises were administered simultaneously for this patient. Note that on 7/11, we advanced to the second exercises (I_2/E_2), owing to the failure to achieve the criteria set for the first exercises. On 7/28 we discontinued the exercise regimen because there was no observable trend of improvement to justify further practice of inhalatory/exhalatory synchronization. When stable trendlines like this are observed, it is often best to move on to the next indicated exercise.

Notwithstanding the fact that at this point in time she still was short of the target criteria set for these exercises, gains over baseline levels were achieved. We moved on from here to the next treatments in the sequence as dictated by the patient's baseline data.

Quick breathing, inhalatory/exhalatory synchronization, isolated sound production, and connected speech breathing exercises all were administered. The patient moved steadily through this sequence of treatments over the course of 1 month at three to five 50-minute sessions per week. In the interest of time and space the individual chart formations drawn during this time frame have been omitted. For the record, however, the patient struggled the most with virtually all the speech breathing exercises. We calculated her baseline data relative to syllables per breath at a mean of 2.25. At the completion of these exercises, she achieved an average just shy of 4 syllables per breath. Content with these results, we continued from here with treatments aimed at her resonation and phonation disturbances.

The next chapter focuses on treatments to facilitate functioning of the resonation subsystem, which is positioned alongside the respiration subsystem in the treatment priority hierarchy. The suggested references that follow are relevant for those clinicians interested in more information on the respiration subsystem.

SUGGESTED READINGS

Bernthal, J. E., & Beukelman, D. R. (1978). Intraoral air pressure during the production of /p/ and /b/ by children, youths, and adults. *Journal of Speech and Hearing Research, 21,* 361–371.

Crickmay, M. C. (1966). *Speech therapy and the Bobath approach to cerebral palsy.* Springfield, IL: Charles C. Thomas.

Darley, F. L., Aronson, A. E., & Brown, J. R. (1975). *Motor speech disorders.* Philadelphia: W. B. Saunders Co.

Farber, S. D. (1982). *Neurorehabilitation: A multisensory approach.* Philadelphia: W. B. Saunders Co.

Froeschels, E. (1952). *Dysarthric speech: Speech in cerebral palsy.* Magnolia, MA: Expression Co.

Fugl-Meyer, A. (1974). Relative respiratory contributions of the rib cage and abdomen in males and females with special regard to posture. *Respiration, 31,* 240–251.

Hixon, T. J. (1987). Respiration function in speech and song. San Diego, CA: College-Hill Press.

Hixon, T. J., Hawley, J. L., & Wilson, J. L. (1982). An around-the-house device for the clinical determination of respiratory driving pressure: A note on making simple even simpler. *Journal of Speech and Hearing Disorders, 47,* 413–415.

Hixon, T. J., Mead, J., & Goldman, M. (1976). Dynamics of the chest wall during speech production: Function of the thorax, rib cage, diaphragm and abdomen. *Journal of Speech and Hearing Research, 19,* 297–356.

Hixon, T. J., Putnam, A. H. B., & Sharp, J. T. (1983). Speech production with flaccid paralysis of the rib cage, diaphragm, and abdomen. *Journal of Speech and Hearing Disorders, 48,* 315–327.

Hoit, J., & Hixon, T. J. (1987). Age and speech breathing. *Journal of Speech and Hearing Research, 30,* 351–366.

Kabat, H., & Knott, M. (1953). Proprioceptive facilitation techniques for treatment of paralysis. *Physical Therapy Review, 33,* 53–60.

Kreitzer, S., Saunders, N., Tyler, H., & Ingram, R. (1978). Respiratory muscle function in amyotrophic lateral sclerosis. *American Review of Respiratory Disease, 117,* 437–447.

McCool, F. D., Loring, S. H., & Mead, J. (1985). Rib cage distortion during voluntary and involuntary breathing acts. *Journal of Applied Physiology, 58,* 1703–1712.

Murdoch, B. E., Cheney, H. J., Bowler, S., & Ingram, J. C. (1989). Respiratory function in parkinson's subjects exhibiting a perceptible speech deficit: A kinematic and spirometric analysis. *Journal of Speech and Hearing Disorders, 54,* 610–626.

Netsell, R., & Hixon, T. J. Noninvasive method for clinically estimating subglottal air pressure. *Journal of Speech and Hearing Disorders, 43,* 326–330.

Putnam, A. H. B., & Hixon, T. J. (1984). Respiratory kinematics in speakers in motor neuron disease. In M. McNeil, J. Rosenbek, & A. Aronson (Eds.), *The dysarthrias* (pp. 37–67), San Diego, CA: College-Hill Press.

Rood, M. (1954). Neurophysiological reactions as a basis for physical therapy. *Physical Therapy Review, 34,* 444–451.

Chapter 4

Treatment of the Resonation Subsystem

CANDIDATES FOR TREATMENT

Of all the different types of patients with motor speech disorders, those with spastic or flaccid dysarthria or with mixed conditions including at least one of these types are most prone to experiencing difficulty with functions of the resonation subsystem, as was discussed in Chapter 1. Table 4–1 illustrates that whereas the pathophysiologic conditions underlying such difficulty are different in these dysarthric patients, the end results are quite similar. That is, in each case in which the patient presents with clinically significant involvement of the resonation subsystem, hypernasal resonance and concomitant abnormal nasal air emissions plague motor speech efforts. The primary neuromuscular signs and symptoms that account for these motor speech disturbances in most patients with spastic dysarthria (pseudobulbar palsy) include weakness, paresis, incoordination, and increased tone and reflex activity of the velopharyngeal musculature. Abnormal tongue posturing and overall hypertonicity and weakness of the muscles that compose the articulation subsystem are secondary factors that may also contribute to the resonance imbalance in this population. These primary and secondary conditions result from bilateral corticobulbar tract lesions. Patients with flaccid dysarthria, on the other hand, who have sustained damage to the pharyngeal plexus (ninth and tenth cranial nerves), whether unilateral or bilateral, are ridden with coincident weakness, paralysis, atrophy, and decreased tone and reflex activity of the velopharyngeal musculature. These patients may present with coexistent weakness and hypotonicity of the muscles of the articulation subsystem if other cranial nerves are also involved, which may secondarily compound resonance imbalance. Medically, the pathologic effects of select cranial nerve lesions are diagnosed as bulbar palsy. It should be noted that patients with mixed pathophysiologic portraits, in which at least one component of the mixture is characteristically "spastic" or "flaccid" in nature, also may suffer from resonation subsystem difficulty. We observe this fact in patients with amyotrophic lateral sclerosis (ALS), who most often present with mixed spastic-flaccid dysar-

TABLE 4–1.   Differential Resonation Subsystem Signs, Symptoms, and Treatments in the Two Types of Dysarthric Patients Who Most Commonly Exhibit Velopharyngeal Incompetency

	Flaccid Dysarthric Patient	Spastic Dysarthric Patient
Lesion sites:	Unilateral or bilateral ninth and tenth cranial nerves	Bilateral corticobulbar tracts
Medical diagnosis:	Bulbar palsy	Pseudobulbar palsy
Pathophysiologic velopharyngeal musculature signs and symptoms*:	Unilateral or bilateral weakness; unilateral or bilateral paralysis; hypotonicity; hypoactive gag reflex	Bilateral weakness; bilateral paralysis; hypertonicity; variably hyperactive gag reflex
Motor speech effects:	Hypernasality; excess nasal air emission; reduced intraoral air pressure and associated articulatory impreciseness	Hypernasality; excess nasal air emission; reduced intraoral air pressure and articulatory imprecision
Treatment considerations†:	*Behavioral management:* improve velopharyngeal valving competency and institute speech resonation exercises *Prosthetic appliance:* palatal lift *Surgical intervention:* pharyngeal flap, or muscle implantation	*Behavioral management:* normalize reflex through touch pressure and massage techniques; normalize tone through touch pressure and massage techniques; improve velopharyngeal valving competency through nonspeech and speech exercises *Prosthetic appliance:* palatal lift *Surgical intervention:* pharyngeal flap, or muscle implantation

*Degree will vary commensurate with extent of neurologic involvement.
†Sequence and number of applications will vary, depending on the severity of the incompetence and the patient's responses.

thria, and in patients with multiple sclerosis, who frequently exhibit a blend of signs and symptoms that yield the speech diagnosis of spastic-ataxic dysarthria. Moreover, on occasion, patients with other types of dysarthria emerge with clinically significant involvement of the resonation subsystem. However, this occurrence is the exception, not the rule.

INDICATIONS FOR TREATMENT

Rarely does hypernasality occur in isolation. Rather, it usually coexists with many other motor speech disturbances that the dysarthric patient exhibits. Examining the degree to which such coexisting conditions may possibly influence one another, clinicians have discovered that neurogenic incompetency of the velopharyngeal valving mechanism both directly results in resonance imbalance and secondarily places increased burden on the respiration, phonation, and articulation subsystems. Consequently, the experience of many clinicians has proved that successful management of such incompetency, whether it is a constant and severe condition or an intermittently mild one, not only improves resonance balance but also provides an enhanced physiologic backdrop that generally fosters success with other speech subsystem treatments. Therefore, along with the insidious effects of breathing difficulties on speech motor control (as discussed in Chapter 3), the hypernasal resonance and nasal air emission abnormalities caused by velopharyngeal incompetency should receive top priority in the intervention plan hierarchy.

PRECURSORS TO TREATMENT

It is not trite to caution that differential diagnosis is essential prior to initiating treatment for perceived disturbance of the resonation subsystem. Routinely, clinicians will proceed first to engaging the would-be patient in extemporaneous conversation, then to requesting the reading aloud or repetition of selected sounds, consonant-vowel (CV) syllables, words, sentences, and paragraphs so as to gather sufficient motor speech data relative to the balance of the resonation subsystem. If hypernasality is perceived, usually accompanied by signs of excessive nasal air emissions particularly during pressure consonant productions and possibly compensatory facial postures, an in-depth oral mechanism examination is performed. With this examination, the clinician appraises the anatomic and physiologic status of the velopharyngeal valving mechanism, enabling clinical descriptions of the type and extent of dysfunctioning, and speculations about the nature of the underlying pathophysiologic condition (e.g., bilateral, severe spastic or flaccid weakness and paresis) as well as the possible lesion site(s) based on the observed signs and symptoms (e.g., bilateral corticobulbar tracts or bilateral ninth and tenth cranial nerves). Knowledge of the medical history and other pertinent data may aid in the completion of the diagnostic portrait with a suspected etiologic agent (e.g., spastic dysarthria due to early signs of ALS, or flaccid dysarthria as a consequence of bulbar palsy following brainstem trauma).

In the speech physiology laboratory, clinical speech aerodynamics testing is usually conducted to measure the functional status of the velopharyngeal musculature in those patients whose clinical examination results suggest incompetency of this valving mechanism. This pre-treatment procedure normally incorporates the aid of airflow and pressure transduction systems that produce quantifiable data regarding subglottal and intraoral air pressure and glottal, oral, and nasal airflow dynamics. Generally speaking, if the patient generates nasal airflow velocities that consistently exceed 100 cc/second during non-nasal speech sound productions, and concomitant intraoral air pressures that fall below 4 cm H_2O, these subthreshold values are signs of velopharyngeal dysfunctioning to which perceived hypernasality and speech unintelligibility may be at least partially attributed. When results of such testing confirm such dysfunctioning, multiview videofluorographic study and/or nasopharyngeal videoendoscopy of the valving mechanism should be conducted next. This will afford observations of the full extent of neurogenic incompetency.

Notwithstanding the intrinsic value of quantitative analyses of velopharyngeal dysfunctioning, in the real world most clinicians do not have access to a speech scientist and a speech physiology laboratory for assistance. Therefore, they are left with the results of the clinical speech and oral mechanism examinations they have administered to determine the actual degree of resonation subsystem difficulty. When the clinician is fortunate enough to be able to arrange for the patient to undergo videofluorographic study, the information generated usually couples well with the clinical measurements obtained, making the differential diagnosis that much more convincing.

Clinicians outside of the laboratory setting may wish to consider adding a few simple measures of nasal airflow and subglottal and intraoral air pressure to their clinical examination battery, which may offer relatively objective differential diagnostic data against which treatment effects ultimately can be compared. To gather these data the See-Scape apparatus, described in the preceding chapter (see Figure 3–4), will be required and can be used for such purposes in the following ways:

First, to measure the degree of nasal airflow during non-nasal speech sound productions, which normally is negligible, position the nasal olive in one nostril of the patient as he or she repeats or reads aloud the following:

1. Isolated pressure consonants (p, t, k, s, f, ʃ, tʃ, dʒ, sp, st, sk)
2. Isolated CV syllable repetitions (pʌ, tʌ, kʌ, and so on),
3. Isolated words (puppy, paper, tape, cookie, cheese, fish, ship, potato chips), and
4. Sentences ("Put the paper plate beside the couch;" "Pet the puppy;" "Check the store for strawberry shortcake;" "The shirt with flowers is pretty;" "She wore a dress to church").

Note the degree to which the Styrofoam float travels upwards in the test tube; ideally, it should remain perfectly still at the bottom of the tube throughout production of all these sounds, syllables, words, and sentences. Next, drop one 28-mm paper clip into the tube and note whether the degree of float movement is significantly reduced as the patient performs all the aforementioned speech elements again. Repeat this procedure, but this time place two paper clips in the tube. Continue systematically to place additional clips into the tube until such time that the accumulated weight of the paper clips completely retards movement of the float as the patient attempts to produce the speech elements. Along the way keep accurate notes regarding the relative degree of float movement under each measurement condition.

Second, to measure *subglottal air pressure*–generating capability, which normally for speech purposes should be at least 5 cm H_2O over 5 seconds, as discussed in the preceding chapter, place four 28-mm paper clips in the See-Scape tube, substitute a 2-inch-long piece of drinking straw with a bleed hole for the plastic nasal olive, and request that the patient blow into the straw as hard and steadily as possible in order to try to elevate the float to the top of the tube and keep it fixed there for at least 5 seconds. The ability to perform this task adequately is roughly equated with the threshold of 5 cm H_2O/5 seconds that can be measured more traditionally and accurately with a water manometer, for example. Note the degree to which the patient achieves this objective with this modified See-Scape technique. Several trials should be attempted in order to obtain an accurate appraisal. Finally, put a noseclip on the patient, permit two or more trials, and note whether the criterion was met under this condition. If the patient still is unable to achieve the objective, it may be safe to assume that there exists a combination of resonation and respiration subsystem disturbances that contribute to faulty subglottal air pressure–generating capability.

Third, to obtain measurements of *intraoral air pressure,* which normally for pressure consonant productions range from 5 to 10 cm H_2O or greater, put a noseclip on the patient, substitute a 2-inch-long piece of drinking straw for the plastic nasal olive (note that for patients with significant lip seal difficulty a plastic tube of smaller diameter may need to be threaded through the straw to ensure better lip seal for this measurement technique), place four 28-mm paper clips in the See-Scape tube, and position the straw between the lips so that the open end rests lightly between the central incisor teeth in the vicinity of the alveolar ridge. If the patient has significant lip seal difficulty, allow him or her to facilitate closure with manual assistance. Next, request the patient to recite the following, noting whether and when the paper clips rise to the top of the tube during productions: (1) /a:pa:/, (2) /i:pi/, (3) pop, (4) pope, (5) peep, (6) pup, (7) puppy, (8) paper, (9) hope, (10) cope, (11) happy, and (12) pet the puppy.

Allow at least three trials per stimulus. If the paper clips consistently rise to or near the top of the tube upon the /p/ productions, the four-clip condition becomes the ultimate treatment challenge. If the patient cannot generate enough intraoral pressure to cause the four paper clips to reach the top of the tube despite the nose being clipped, remove one clip and have the patient repeat the aforementioned sounds and words again. If the patient meets the criterion under this condition, the three–paper clip condition becomes the treatment target. If the patient still cannot achieve the criterion, despite the presence of the noseclip, have him or her again repeat the sounds and words with only two paper clips in the tube.

Again, if the patient achieves the criterion of driving the paper clips to or very near the top of the tube upon the /p/ productions, the two–paper clip condition is set as the treatment objective, and so on. As a last resort, if the patient still fails, remove the last paper clip, make certain the noseclip is on, have him or her repeat the speech elements once again. Whether the float rises to the top of the tube or not during this trial period, treatment will begin with this condition as the intraoral air pressure goal. Next, for the baseline record, request that the patient perform the same intraoral air pressure tasks again, except that this time the sounds and words are attempted without the noseclip or paper clips within the tube. If the patient consistently drives the Styrofoam float to the top of the tube upon the /p/ productions, have him or her repeat the sounds and words again, but this time with one paper clip in the tube. If the float still rises consistently to the top of the tube, repeat the procedure with two paper clips and so on until the patient cannot impound enough speech-generated intraoral air pressure to cause the weighted float to rise to the top of the tube. These data will play an important role in determining the extent to which any treatments administered influence intraoral air pressure—generating capability.

During baseline testing in the speech physiology laboratory, this clinical researcher has discovered that dysarthric patients with signs and symptoms of severe velopharyngeal valving incompetency were consistently unable, without assistance, to generate more than 1 or 2 cm H_2O of intraoral air pressure, and produced abnormal nasal airflow velocities that at times well exceeded 1000 cc/second. Even those patients with mild incompetency failed consistently to achieve pressures greater than the minimally acceptable 4 cm H_2O or nasal flows less than 100 to 200 cc/second. Experimenting with the See-Scape device, as suggested earlier, demonstrated that patients with severe velopharyngeal incompetency without significant respiratory subsystem involvement (1) generated at least 5 cm H_2O/5 second subglottal air pressure when the nose was clipped; (2) exhibited nasal airflows on the aforementioned speech elements that consistently propelled one paper clip up to the top of the tube, two clips up to the three-quarter mark, three clips up to the halfway mark, and four clips up ever so slightly; and (3) generated intraoral air pressures, with a noseclip on, during production of the previously listed speech elements that consistently propelled three paper clips up to the top of the tube, but could not generate substantial speech oral pressures without the noseclip to propel even one paper clip up to the top of the tube. Those patients with less severe velopharyngeal involvement demonstrated on baseline measures various ability levels, usually highly correlated with the degree of their incompetency. However, none of these individuals was able to produce the non-nasal sounds and words (1) without nasal flows that consistently propelled the *unanchored* float to the top of the tube and (2) with sufficient intraoral air pressures to propel the float anchored with three paper clips to the top of the tube (without a noseclip).

The final pre-treatment step involves employing a system that can be used to rate and record perceptions of the resonation and other possible speech subsystem disturbances exhibited by the patient. Figure 4—1 is a copy of the speech characteristics chart introduced in Chapter 2, which may be used for such ratings. Formatted according to a seven-point equal-appearing interval scale often used in the literature on motor speech disorders, this chart enables the clinician to assign a numeric rating to perceived speech motor control difficulties exhibited by the patient. Although the use of interval scales has been criticized by some clinical researchers, most clinicians find them helpful, especially when collateral ratings of the patient, made by clinical associates, demonstrate good to excellent inter-rater reliability scores. Once these baseline data are gathered, they will serve the clinician well, since accurate measures of forthcoming treatment effects are virtually impossible without such comparative information.

The date on which a given rating is awarded should be entered on the top

SPEECH CHARACTERISTICS CHART

Patient's name: J. M.

Birthdate: 11/15/55 Sex: M

Speech diagnosis: Flaccid Dysarthria

Medical diagnosis: Bulbar palsy owing to brainstem injury involving cranial nerves IX and X (bilaterally) and VII and XII (unilaterally).

Clinician: Dworkin

Facility: Private Practice

Address: Anywhere, USA

ACTIVITY KEY

MEASUREMENT UNIT

Feature:
1. Articulatory precision (A)
2. Resonance balance (R)
3. Voice (V)
4. Prosody (P)
5. Contextual speech (C)

} 7-Point interval scale (1 = normal; 7 = most deviant)

Baseline (pre-treatment): B + feature symbol

Comments:
1. Articulation is severely imprecise;
2. Resonation is severely hypernasal with nasal air emissons on all speech tasks requiring substantial intraoral air pressure;
3. Phonation is breathy-hoarse and wet-gurgly in quality;
4. Prosody has monopitch and monoloudness features with short phrases and severely slow-labored syllable combinations;
5. Connected speech is severely unintelligible.

SPEECH RATINGS

	Dates: 10/14/76													
Most Deviant	7		X											
	6	X		X	X	X								
	5													
← Intelligibility Ratings →	4													
	3													
	2													
Normal	1													
No. of minutes of sample activity		5	5	5	5	5								
List A, R, V, P, C, or B + feature		BA	BR	BV	BP	BC								
Target criterion		1	1	1	1	1								

SESSIONS

Figure 4–1. Interval chart used to log overall speech characteristics prior to, during, and following motor speech intervention.

row of the chart corresponding to the column in which the speech subsystem or activity is being rated. It is best to use one column per activity rating. Note that in Figure 4–1, column 1, the flaccid dysarthric patient depicted was judged on 10/14/76 to exhibit severe baseline disturbance of articulation (BA) after a 5-minute sample. Columns 2, 3, 4, and 5, respectively, show that the baseline ratings of resonance (BR), voice (BV), prosody (BP), and connected speech (BC) yielded similar perceptual ratings of severe to marked abnormalities, also collected on 10/14/76. For the record, this young man did not suffer from respiration subsystem difficulties. In fact, he was quite athletic. Thus, the initial treatment focus was on his marked degree of resonation subsystem incompetency, which resulted from complete, bilateral paralysis of the velopharyngeal musculature.

The remaining columns on the chart may most effectively be used, in this case, to rate the patient's ongoing responses to treatment. Such ratings can be made following each treatment session or after intervals of predetermined length. It may prove most economical, in the long run, to use one chart per speech feature undergoing treatment so that improvement over treatment sessions can be observed without the camouflaging or interruptive effects of data points that represent patient responses to other treatments that may be under simultaneous administration. In the bottom row of the chart, the criterion being used to dictate movement within the treatment plan should be specified, as discussed in Chapter 2. In a given patient's treatment file, there may exist numerous speech characteristics charts that enable the clinician to record and track responses to specific articulation, phonation, resonation, prosody, and/or contextual speech treatments.

Figure 4–2 summarizes the factors and procedures that should be considered and implemented prior to initiating treatment of resonation subsystem disturbances in dysarthric patients.

TREATMENT PROCEDURES

Regardless of the type, extent, and etiology of neurogenic resonation incompetency, the overall objective of any form of treatment is to improve the adequacy of velopharyngeal valving so as to reduce hypernasality and nasal emission and improve intraoral air pressure–generating capabilities during speech. There are three primary approaches to such treatment: (1) behavioral management techniques, which include various nonspeech and speech velopharyngeal musculature exercises, with accompanying aerodynamic biofeedback; (2) fitting of a palatal-lift prosthesis; and/or (3) surgical intervention, including (a) nasopharyngeal muscle augmentation using Teflon, silicone rubber, and silastic pillows, and (b) pharyngeal flap procedures. Review of the latter two approaches will be provided first, followed by extensive coverage of differential behavioral management techniques that may be administered either in lieu of or as an adjunct to prosthetic or surgical treatments.

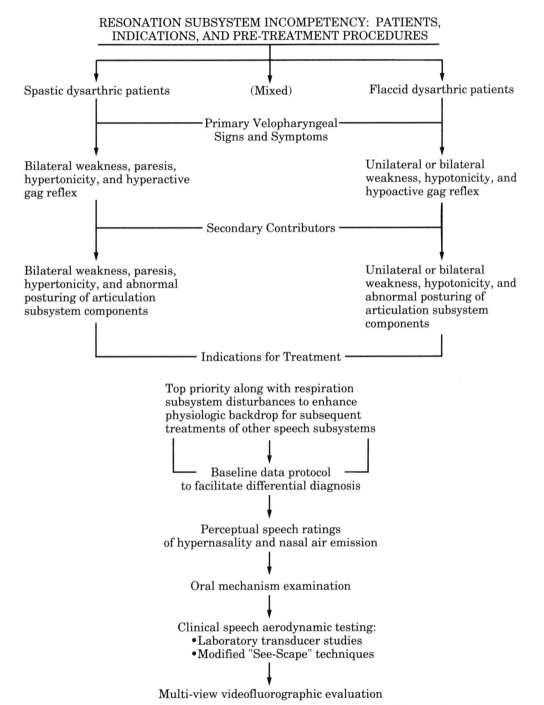

Figure 4–2. Flow diagram illustrating the pre-treatment sequential procedures for patients with suspected velopharyngeal incompetency.

Prosthetic Appliances

Objectives

Generally speaking, any dysarthric patient who is diagnosed as having moderate to severe velopharyngeal paralysis and consequent valving incompetency may be an excellent candidate for immediate fitting of a *palatal-lift* prosthesis. The lift is designed to do what neurologically the patient is voluntarily incapable of achieving; that is, to facilitate velopharyngeal closure by mechanically displacing the velum upwards and backwards toward the posterior pharyngeal wall, where contact would normally occur. Typically made of light acrylic-resin material with metal hooks for dental retention, this type of prosthetic appliance is usually designed and constructed by a prosthodontist. It is tailor-made and modified to the individual patient's oropharyngeal anatomy and can be altered based on ongoing speech perceptual and aerodynamic evaluations. The ultimate objective for prescribing a palatal-lift appliance is to effect velopharyngeal closure significant enough that the hypernasality and excess nasal emission features are substantially reduced, and intraoral air pressure–generating capability is increased so as to improve the aerodynamic backdrop for articulatory precision, particularly on pressure consonants. Whereas successful achievement of these treatment objectives is not necessarily predictable for this type of patient, experienced clinicians have discovered that without such intervention, the likelihood of promoting improvement through intensive behavioral exercises alone is rather remote. Only a successful surgical procedure may serve usefully in lieu of prosthetic management. However, the risks and expenses associated with such an option are frequently high enough to delay this decision until later in the treatment plan, if all other more conservative methods fail to bring about the desired results. In some instances, a palatal lift is fitted to start the treatment sequence. Next, behavioral management is introduced to augment the possible effects of the lift. Finally, surgical intervention may be recommended for patients who either prefer not to wear a prosthesis, cannot tolerate it, or have fallen somewhat short of expectations with alternative nonsurgical treatments.

Contrary Indications

Any dysarthric patient who presents initially with mild velopharyngeal paralysis and coincident resonation subsystem imbalance, highlighted primarily by a similar degree of hypernasality, nasal emission, and articulatory imprecision, may not be the best candidate for quick fitting with a palatal-lift appliance. Instead, the more conservative treatment route of behavioral management techniques ought first to be attempted with this would-be patient. If such exercises fail to promote the degree of speech improvement expected or desired, alternative prosthetic and/or surgical methods of intervention may be explored secondarily to provide the needed physiologic and aerodynamic boosts.

Factors Influencing Success

To increase the chances of successful fitting with a palatal-lift prosthesis, the patient selection process is critical. Those patients who suffer from severe intellectual, cognitive, and language disturbances, and who are generally uncooperative and noncompliant, are poor candidates for such treatment. If the family support system is deficient, this too can serve as a deterrent to success, inasmuch as the prosthesis requires a modicum of care by the patient, which oftentimes is facilitated by the encouragement and assistance of the patient's loved ones.

The chance for success with palatal-lift treatment can sometimes be impeded if the clinician inadvertently and erroneously prompts the patient to expect unrealistic outcomes following the fitting. Almost always, unreasonably high expectations are rooted in the notion that this type of treatment is a panacea that will correct all the problems for which it is prescribed. Even under the best of circumstances, following a good fitting, neither the clinician nor the patient should expect restoration of *"normal"* resonance balance, voice quality, and articulation proficiency. Rather, it is more realistic to forecast and eventually hail the successful fitting as an indispensable precursor to any degree of improvement that may be achieved with subsequent speech treatments.

Another factor that usually has an impact on the likelihood of success with palatal-lift prescriptions is the degree to which resonation incompetency is plagued by coexistent motor speech disturbances. Those patients with concomitant neuromuscular involvement of the respiratory apparatus, larynx, tongue, mandible, and/or lips generally benefit less from a good fitting than their counterparts whose speech motor control difficulties result largely from focal velopharyngeal incompetency.

Patients who are edentulous are often difficult subjects for the prosthodontist because of the obvious problem with good retention of the palatal lift. Yet, another possible contraindication to successful fitting is the tonal status of the velum itself. Excess tone associated with spasticity or a brisk pharyngeal reflex may counter or retard the elevating force of the lift as well as potentially place undue stress on the dentition. Spastic dysarthric patients, in whom such negative factors are most commonly observed, may also present with associated hyperactivity of the pharyngeal reflex, which exacerbates the problem with a successful fit. Treatments to normalize the tone and reflex reactions of the velar musculature, coupled with a gradual time adaptation approach to the wearing of the lift, are therapeutic procedures that may increase the opportunity ultimately for a successful outcome, and should be administered first and foremost prior to lift considerations. The flaccid dysarthric patient usually does not present with passive mechanism resistance to the lift, owing to inherent velopharyngeal musculature hypotonicity and a hypoactive pharyngeal reflex. Techniques aimed at accomplishing such behavioral modifications will be presented later in the chapter.

One final note of caution relative to clinical success or failure with prosthetic management has to do with the potential negative effects of the palatal lift on oral hygiene and resting salivary flow rate. Like a denture, the lift must be cared for by the patient or a care provider. Halitosis, initial and possibly prolonged irritation of the delicate mucous membranes against which the lift exerts constant pressure, gingivitis, and increased salivation are possible side effects that may individually or collectively contraindicate protracted use of the lift.

Illustrative Case No. 1

Figure 4–3 is an example of a light-weight acrylic palatal-lift appliance that was tailor-made for the 22-year-old patient with flaccid dysarthria whose record was shown in Figure 4–1, whose clinical and videofluorographic examinations disclosed total velopharyngeal paralysis with resultant marked degrees of hypernasality and nasal air emission. This, along with coincident involvement of the articulation and phonation subsystems, collectively rendered him virtually unintelligible. Clinical speech aerodynamics testing revealed (estimates of) maximum subglottal air pressure–generating capability at 10 cm H_2O/15 seconds when his nose was clipped to prevent nasal air escape, intraoral air pressures that failed to exceed 2 cm H_2O without the noseclip, and nasal airflows that consistently exceeded 1250 cc/second during attempts to perform various non-nasal motor speech tasks. It is fortunate that respiration was not significantly compromised. Thus, initially the treatment program focused solely on the pathophysiologic resonation disturbances. If there were clinically significant signs of respiration difficulties, the sequence of speech breathing exercises recommended in Chapter 3 would have been scheduled simultaneously with the resonation treatment program.

Because of the extent of the patient's velopharyngeal incompetence, the prognosis for speech aerodynamic improvements was very poor. Nonetheless, following differential diagnostic testing, he was fitted with the palatal lift. Some prosthodondists purposely like to design the lift a bit short of the target length and width for the first fitting. As the patient develops a tolerance to its presence,

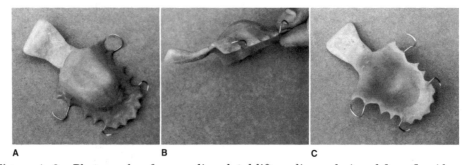

A   B   C

Figure 4–3. Photographs of an acrylic palatal-lift appliance designed for a flaccid dysarthric patient with bilateral paralysis of the velopharyngeal mechanism. Note the upward tilt and unusually wide width at the distal end to compensate for the severe degree of incompetency of both the velar and the lateral pharyngeal wall musculature.

graduated adjustments are made, usually allowing a week between necessary modifications until the best (aerodynamic) fit possible is achieved and tolerated by the patient. For this patient, three adjustments were ultimately required to achieve the threshold fit. Between adjustments, speech aerodynamic testing and perceptual ratings were performed to decipher the possible therapeutic effects of the lift. Whereas significant improvements were not identified during any of these evaluation sessions, the patient was still instructed to continue to wear the appliance at all times, except during meals, at bedtime, or when a short break was desired. The rationale behind this requirement, supported in part by years of clinical experience as well as research data found in the medical literature, is that the static elevating pressure of the lift against the velar tissue may serve mechanically to induce or stimulate velopharyngeal musculature activity, which may improve the chances of success with the behavioral management treatments, which for this patient were delayed until this point in the clinical treatment course.

Not all palatal lifts need to be as long or wide as the one depicted in Figure 4–3. In some cases, the length is as much as a full centimeter shorter and the width 33 percent narrower, yet maximum results are obtained without further adjustments. In these cases, experimentation with additional modifications often leads to the complications of mouth breathing and denasal resonance, which prompt their own set of unexpected and undesirable drawbacks.

Note from Figure 4–3 the upward tilt of the velar portion of the appliance, designed specifically to displace the palate and assist velopharyngeal closure. Also note that the total length of the lift is 8.6 cm, and at the velar end the width is 2.4 cm. Initially, the lift was merely 7 cm long and 1.9 cm wide at the velar tip. Referring the patient back to dentistry to make the necessary length and width adjustments can be time consuming and inefficient. With the help, in-service training, and supervision of a prosthodontist, the clinician may learn how to perform such modifications. By being able to alter readily the anatomy of the palatal lift, the clinician can quickly determine the patient's tolerance level and make on-the-spot measurements of resonation subsystem reactions to such alterations. The procedures are relatively simple and worth reviewing below.

Steps to Follow to Make Palatal-Lift Adjustments

Step 1. Materials needed include (1) approximately one cup of boiling water, (2) light-fibered repair material powder,* (3) Fastray Liquid Hardener,† (4) K-Y Lubricating Jelly, (5) a single-edge razor or cutting knife, and (6) a sheet of waterproof silicon carbide fine wet sandpaper.

Step 2. In a clean, small dish or tray, place about one-quarter of a level teaspoon of repair material. Next, add to this powder substance two or three eye-

*Repair Material (Powder)-Light Fibered (680027), Dentsply/York Division, Dentsply International, Inc., York, PA.
†Fastray liquid hardener for individual trays, Harry J. Bosworth Co., Skokie, IL.

drops of the liquid hardener, and mix thoroughly with a wooden tongue depressor until the material becomes putty-like, which takes roughly 15 to 30 seconds.

Step 3.   Place a few drops of K-Y Jelly on the tips of the thumb and index and middle fingers of one hand. With the tongue depressor transfer the putty from the dish to the distal end of the lift, and then use the lubricated fingers to mold the putty into a desirably long extension on the end of the lift. The lubricant prevents sticking and facilitates shaping.

Step 4.   Be careful not to add more than a total of 5 mm to the length or 2½ mm to the width of each side during any one session. Gradual adjustments are better tolerated by the patient, and oftentimes a slight increment in length or width is all that is required to achieve maximum velopharyngeal assistance.

Step 5.   Once the lift is smoothly molded into the desired extension shape, and excess material is cut off, immerse the remodeled end in the boiling water to hasten the hardening process. This usually takes about 1 minute.

Step 6.   Once the extension has hardened, it is ready to be sanded. Working at a sink, wet the sandpaper and begin sanding the rough prominences and edges to a smooth finish. The razor blade or knife may be helpful if large pieces need to be carved away.

Step 7.   Next, rinse off the lift, apply a little K-Y Jelly to the remodeled area, and then request that the patient reinsert the finished product.

Step 8.   If the lift is too long or wide after the adjustment, such results will be readily apparent as the lift will be impossible to insert because of tissue resistance, faulty dental hook retention, and/or patient discomfort. Small gradations in size, accomplished by additional sanding, carving, and retrofitting of the lift throughout the session, should ultimately lead to the best fit possible.

Step 9.   Finally, conduct various speech perceptual and aerodynamic measurements to determine the possible airflow, air pressure, and articulation effects of the adjustment. It should be possible to meet the overall objectives of the session within a 50-minute time frame. *Note:* Many patients complain that the smooth, glass-like hard palate surface of the lift minimizes lingua-alveolar kinesthetic feedback during speech efforts. To help relieve this problem, pseudo-rugae may be constructed with the repair material on the alveolar border of the lift for tongue contact and feedback.

For the patient illustrated here, we had to create an appliance that would serve both to elevate the palate to the level where velopharyngeal valving would normally occur and at the same time to obstruct nasal airflow as much as possible. To do this the posterolateral borders of the lift were built up to facilitate lateral pharyngeal wall contraction and thus effect velopharyngeal closure. Figure 4–4 is a schematic illustration of the velopharyngeal valving effect provided by the palatal-lift appliance. We proceeded with behavioral management exercises with hopes that degrees of improvement would accrue with time and practice.

During the 6 months following the final fitting of his palatal-lift prosthesis, the patient underwent an intensive (5 hours per week) behavioral management program, which included nonspeech and speech exercises designed to induce greater velopharyngeal valving activity. These particular therapeutic efforts

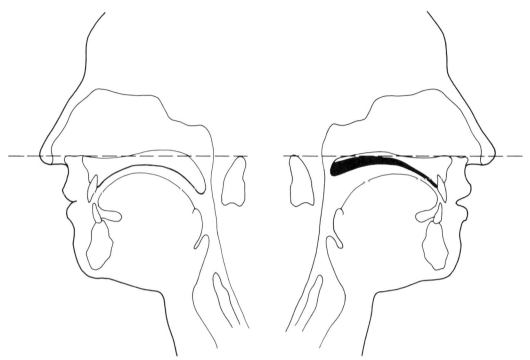

Figure 4–4. Schematic illustrations of the velum assisted by insertion of a palatal-lift appliance. Note the extent to which the prosthesis elevates the velum toward the posterior pharyngeal wall at the level of the palatal plane.

were virtually in vain, as the patient made no demonstrable gains in either related articulatory proficiency or speech aerodynamic features. Notwithstanding the palatal-lift appliance and the exercise program, his severe hypernasality, nasal air emissions, difficulty with pressure consonant productions, and reduction of vocal power persisted, owing in large measure to intractable nasal air wastage through the incompetent velopharyngeal port. As a last ditch effort at rehabilitation, a surgical team was consulted for their opinion about the patient's suitability for surgical intervention. A multiview videofluorographic study was conducted to help decipher whether surgery might prove helpful. The results showed rather surprisingly moderate degrees of both velar and lateral pharyngeal wall movement, which was corroborated upon later review of the videotape. The team vividly recalled that 6 months earlier, immediately following the fitting of the palatal-lift appliance, the videofluorographic studies conducted at that time revealed no movement of the entire valving mechanism. It was hypothesized that wearing of the lift may have stimulated dormant velopharyngeal motor units as well as possibly revived severely damaged ones to degrees that unexplainably were not evident during the peroral examination but were observable with radiologic study. More important, the patient was now judged to be a good candidate for pharyngeal flap surgery, which was performed 4 weeks later. Surgery was a success from a technical standpoint, in that the patient tolerated the procedure without complications and postoperative recovery was unremarkable. However, the speech articulation and aerodynamic effects were equivocal as late as 2 months after the operation, despite continuation of the intensive behavioral management program during this period of time. To date, much better postsurgical results abound in the research literature on neurogenic velopharyngeal incompetency.

Surgical Intervention

Considerations and Objectives

Whereas some dysarthric patients may be sent to the operating table soon after neurologic, speech, and radiologic examinations illustrate significant velopharyngeal valving incompetency, most patients are not considered for this route until they have previously undergone extensive behavioral management treatments with less than optimal results as well as relatively unsuccessful experiences wearing palatal-lift appliances. When surgical intervention seems indicated for the dysarthric patient, regardless of the procedure of choice, the overall goal is to facilitate the anatomically intact velopharyngeal mechanism with hopes of improving its function. The permanence of surgical intervention is attractive to many patients, particularly those who consider the wearing of a lift to be socially stigmatizing, uncomfortable, and rather inconvenient.

Perhaps the best candidate for surgical intervention is the patient who possesses less than severe pre-surgical paralysis of the velopharyngeal mechanism. Those dysarthric patients who suffer from severe involvement prompt guarded prognoses for successful surgical results and may be discouraged from considering surgery as the treatment of choice.

Procedure Options

As mentioned earlier in this chapter, over the years we have seen reports in the medical literature on various surgical approaches to neurogenic velopharyngeal incompetence. On the muscle augmentation side of the spectrum, conflicting evidence exists as to the feasibility of increasing the anatomical bulk of the posterior pharyngeal wall, using material such as Teflon, silicone rubber, silastic pillows, fascia, bone, and cartilage, with the objective of creating a prominence against which the velum can make closure contact to improve speech aerodynamics. Patients for whom such treatments have been successfully reported have been those with only minimal pre-surgical paresis of the velar musculature.

In the past few years, convincing evidence has emerged that the superiorly based posterior pharyngeal flap procedure is the best surgical approach for correction of neurogenic velopharyngeal incompetence. Here we find that the best outcomes with this technique are observed in those patients for whom flaps were constructed with relatively small lateral portals for nasal airflow. Additionally, the good candidate for such intervention is the patient who presents pre-surgically with at least a fair degree of mobility of the lateral pharyngeal walls, which can work in concert with the flap for tight valving during speech motor activities.

Behavioral Management Techniques

Up-Front Considerations

As has been mentioned earlier and shown in Table 4–1, if a patient presents with significant signs and symptoms of velopharyngeal incompetency, it is a good bet that the speech diagnosis rendered will be flaccid, spastic, or a mixed form of dysarthria. Although these patients all will suffer from varying degrees of hypernasality, nasal emissions, and articulatory imprecision as direct consequences of such incompetency, they will differ with respect to the pathophysiology underlying these motor speech disturbances. Because these differences may be rather significant, behavioral management techniques should be sensitive not only to the speech symptoms themselves but also to their cause. A closer examination of the pathologic similarities and the salient differences between these patients should help support this claim. Referring back to Table 4–1, note that, generally speaking, the resonation subsystem signs and symptoms exhibited by flaccid and spastic dysarthric patients are quite similar. The characteristic pathologic differences involve the tonal and reflex activity status of the velopharyngeal musculature as well as the factor of consistency of dysfunction. With respect to this latter point, patients with flaccid dysarthia generally exhibit continuous incompetency, whereas spastic dysarthric patients suffer more from variable degrees of dysfunction. As shown in the table, the flaccid dysarthric patient is plagued by underlying hypotonicity, and the spastic patient by hypertonicity, which in each case contributes to the widespread weakness and paralysis of the velopharyngeal mechanism. The diminished pharyngeal reflex in the flaccid dysarthric patient is of clinical importance if and when a palatal-lift appliance is indicated in the treatment sequence. Reduction or absence of this response fosters fitting of the lift inasmuch as the patient does not usually require a very lengthy adaptation period. The hyperactive gag reflex of the spastic dysarthric patient is likewise of clinical importance, but for different reasons. If a palatal lift is being considered for this type of patient, its fitting may initially be quite a problem in that the inherent stiffness of the velar musculature compounded by a highly sensitive pharyngeal response serves collectively to resist the upward torque of the lift. If the patient is to benefit from this prescription, a behavioral management program like the one described subsequently should be initiated first to try to reduce these antagonistic conditions. Success along these clinical lines may ultimately facilitate the objectives of prosthetic treatment.

When the degree of velopharyngeal incompetence is moderate to severe, behavioral management treatments do not usually yield results clinically significant enough to circumvent the need for alternative prosthetic or surgical intervention. Notwithstanding the likelihood of such a disappointing outcome with these types of patients, it is still clinically most responsible to begin the treatment plan, if only for a prescribed experimental period of time, with the behavioral management approach. For various reasons, the aforementioned case example did not receive such treatments at first, to the chagrin of the treatment team. This clinician usually allows at least 10 hours of concentrated treatment, with signs of little or no improvement, before exploring alternative strategies of management. On the other hand, when the underlying pathophysiologic condition is mild, the prognosis is generally better for improving velopharyngeal functioning and speech resonance balance through clinical exercises. Certainly, such treatments should be the approach of choice initially, leaving prosthetic and surgical methods to much later explorations, if necessary.

Within the context of the aforementioned treatment considerations, when patients are scheduled for behavioral intervention, they may be exposed to speech as well as nonspeech exercises designed specifically to increase velopharyngeal competency so as to improve intraoral air pressure–generating capability and to facilitate resonance balance and articulatory proficiency. Of course, these treatments must be tailored around the differential diagnostic findings as well as the patient's age, overall medical status, and capabilities. Before reviewing the recommended methods of intervention, certain factors that might have an impact on the outcome of therapy are worth brief attention.

First, as mentioned earlier, the success of the behavioral management program is inversely proportional to the extent of the velopharyngeal paralysis; that is, the greater the incompetency of valving, the poorer the prognosis for improvement with exercise. Second, early intervention may improve the chances for success. When therapy is delayed or pushed to lower levels in the treatment hierarchy, undesirable compensations may emerge as the patient attempts volitionally to counter the abnormal resonation and articulation behaviors that may result from such incompetency. Third, parents, spouses, and/or other appropriate loved ones can prove to be invaluable cheerleaders as the patient moves through the exercise regimen. Not only should these individuals be encouraged to support the patient's efforts, but also they must be kept abreast of the objectives of the exercises employed and the criteria adopted for advancement to other steps in the total intervention program. Informed significant others usually develop realistic expectations for improvement, and they can serve as therapy aides in the home environment. Fourth, if the patient can experience some degree of improvement soon after treatment is initiated, however insignificant this might be relative to the total clinical picture, the gains obtained may reinforce the patient's efforts as well as the importance of the treatments themselves. That is why the sequence of techniques begins with the simplest of exercises and gradually progresses in complexity. Fifth, general speech sound and nasality auditory discrimination skills must be evaluated to determine whether or not the patient is capable of differentiating and monitoring acceptable and unacceptable resonation and articulation patterns. Naturally, if such skills are impaired, they too may become the focus of treatment. Sixth, some of the nonspeech exercises are not designed to invigorate velopharyngeal muscle contractions or associated valving activity but rather to direct and facilitate intraoral airflow. Others are in fact designed to try to induce increased muscle function and the extent of velopharyngeal closure; albeit the prognosis for this outcome is generally quite guarded. Last, the speech motor exercises that are found in this treatment package are not designed to train articulatory precision, per se. Such is the purpose of the treatment plan described in the chapter on articulation subsystem disturbances. Here the speech resonation exercises primarily aim to reduce the amount of abnormal air that is forcefully driven through the nasal cavity so as to improve oral-nasal resonance balance during connected speech efforts. Any gains achieved with these techniques, even if they are not completely successful, may at least lay the groundwork for good results with subsequent subsystem treatments.

The first subsection of behavioral techniques is designed exclusively for those dysarthric patients who may require and benefit from treatments to reduce hypertonicity and/or hyperactive reflexes of the velopharyngeal mechanism. All subsequent subsections, however, are designed without regard for particular types of dysarthria. They may be attempted sequentially with any patient who exhibits neurogenic velopharyngeal incompetency.

Treatment Materials

The clinician will need to assemble the following materials in order to employ exercises recommended in this chapter:

1. See-Scape device,
2. Noseclip,
3. Drinking straws,
4. Box of paper clips (28-mm),
5. Box of facial tissues,
6. Finger cots and disposable vinyl examination gloves,
7. Tongue depressors,
8. Tape recorder,
9. Speech Characteristics Chart (see Figure 2–2), and
10. Resonation Subsystem Behavioral Treatment Chart (see Figure 4–5).

Reduction of Pharyngeal Reflex Hyperactivity and Velar Hypertonicity

The exercises in this subsection are designed with two primary objectives: (1) to reduce stiffness (hypertonicity) of the velum, which may facilitate the effects of subsequent velopharyngeal valving exercises, and (2) to decrease the pharyngeal (gag) reflex, which may improve the prognosis for successful fitting of a palatal-lift appliance.

Exercise No. 1

Normally light pressure applied to the first half or two-thirds of the dorsum of the tongue should not evoke a strong pharyngeal response. There are some dysarthric patients who exhibit very strong gag reflexes, even upon tongue-tip contact. Others may show varying degrees of hyperactivity that also can benefit from clinical attention. To lessen such sensitivity in these patients, and potentially to reduce underlying hypertonicity of the velar musculature, the technique of maintained touch or pressure may be helpful. Theorizing that orofacial pressure stimuli are afferent to the principal sensory trigeminal nuclei, which in turn communicate neuroanatomically with the dorsal vagal motor nuclei, neurorehabilitation practitioners employ this technique globally to reduce body part disregard, to normalize touch thresholds, to calm hypersensitivity, and to decrease hypertonicity of involved tissue. The following steps are recommended for the aforementioned purposes, with two important caveats: (1) the degree of pressure and the amount of time it is applied per trial should vary in accordance with the individual patient's response curve, and (2) it is not the overall goal of this particular treatment to convert a hypersensitive and hypertonic mechanism into one that is nonresponsive. Rather, when the patient demonstrates that the velopharyngeal mechanism can tolerate and yield to pressure stimuli, prerequisites that are vital to success with subsequent prosthetic and/or physiologic exercises, those treatments indicated next should be introduced.

Step 1. Familiarize the patient with the overall objectives of the forthcoming techniques without going into more detail than is necessary to defuse any existing apprehension.

Step 2. While seated facing the patient, instruct him or her to open the mouth as wide as possible. Then gently lay a wooden tongue depressor on the midline of the tongue making certain that the distal end of the stick rests approximately 1 inch from the tongue tip.

Step 3. Using a moderate degree of maintained force, press down on the tongue with the stick for 5 seconds, counting aloud so that the patient can strive to achieve the time limit. On a notepad, record the number of seconds the patient was able to tolerate this pressure application without signs of gagging, a biting reflex, or head retraction. Repeat this procedure three times to establish a baseline score. On the Resonation Subsystem Behavioral Treatment Chart (Figure 4–5), enter the date at the top of Column no. 1, and in the respectively labeled cells at the bottom of this column list the number of trials (3), the activity (BH$_1$—symbolizing baseline hyper-reflexia–hypertonicity, Exercise no. 1), and the measurement unit (# seconds). Then put an "X" mark on the grid corresponding to the mean baseline score. If the patient has no difficulty with this stimulus, skip Step 4 and go on to Exercise no. 2.

Step 4. Continue with the same procedure, allowing 15 seconds of rest between trials, until the patient demonstrates such tolerance for the full 5-second application over 10 consecutive trials. Using a separate column, after each set of 10 trials enter on the y-axis grid the mean number of seconds achieved, making certain to list the date, the number of trials (10), the activity (H$_1$), the measurement unit (# seconds), and the target criterion (5 seconds). Once an "X" mark is placed at level 5 on the y-axis, following this recording method, the patient has met the criterion for advancement to the next exercise.

RESONATION SUBSYSTEM BEHAVIORAL TREATMENT CHART

Patient's name: _____

Birthdate: _____ Sex: _____

Speech diagnosis: _____

Medical diagnosis: _____

_____

Clinician: _____

Facility: _____

Address: _____

Comments: _____

ACTIVITY KEY

Feature: | **MEASUREMENT UNIT**
1. Reduction of velar hyperreflexia and hypertonicity (H) | No. of seconds, or 7 point interval scale (1 = normal; 7 = most deviant)
2. Intraoral air pressure generation (nonspeech) (P) | No. of seconds, or Yes = 1/ No = 0
3. Vowel prolongations (V) | No. of seconds, or Yes = 1/ No = 0
4. Intraoral air pressure generation (speech) (A) | Yes = 1/ No = 0
5. Isolated word productions (W) | Yes = 1/ No = 0
6. Sentence productions (S) | Yes = 1/ No = 0
7. Connected speech (C) | Yes = 1/ No = 0

Baseline (pre-treatment): B + activity symbol

Dates:

Average Score: 10 9 8 7 6 5 4 3 2 1 0

No. of trials

Activity symbol

Unit of measure

Target criterion

SESSIONS

Figure 4–5. Virgin chart to be used to record patient responses to resonation subsystem behavioral treatments.

105

Exercise No. 2

With the same objectives as those specified in the preceding exercise, proceed with the following steps:

Step 1. Follow the exact same method as in Exercise no. 1, except that for this exercise position the distal end of the tongue depressor on the halfway mark between the tip and the back of the patient's tongue. If the patient has no difficulty with this stimulus, skip the next step and proceed with Exercise no. 3.

Step 2. Once the patient demonstrates the ability to tolerate the maintained pressure for the full 5-second application over 10 consecutive trials, move on to the next exercise, making certain that data entries on the treatment chart are awarded to separate columns and are categorized in the activity cells as BH_2 and H_2 for baseline and treatment responses, respectively.

Exercise No. 3

The following technique is likewise designed according to the objectives and methods discussed in Exercise no. 1.

Step 1. The exception for this exercise is that the distal end of the tongue depressor is now positioned on the dorsum of the tongue approximately two-thirds of the way back from the tip. If the patient has no difficulty with this stimulus, skip the next step and proceed with Exercise no. 4.

Step 2. After the patient achieves the criterion previously established, the next exercise is indicated. Again the clinician should be certain that data entries are made in columns of the treatment chart separate from those used for the preceding exercises, and that they are categorized as BH_3 and H_3, accordingly, in the activity cells.

Exercise No. 4

Step 1. Encase an index finger in a finger cot or put on a vinyl examination glove.

Step 2. While seated facing the patient, instruct him or her to open the mouth as wide as possible. With the tip of the covered index finger, apply a moderate degree of constant upward force against the alveolar ridge for 5 seconds, counting aloud to alert the patient as to the amount of time elapsed. As in the preceding exercises, establish a baseline level first, and record the result on the treatment chart in a separate column under the activity BH_4. If the patient has no difficulty with this stimulus, skip the next step and proceed with Exercise no. 5.

Step 3. Continue with the exercise procedure using a notepad to record the number of seconds the patient was able to tolerate this maintained finger pressure without signs of gagging, a biting reflex, or head retraction. Repeat this procedure, with 15 seconds of rest between trials, until the patient demonstrates such tolerance for the full 5-second application over 10 consecutive trials. Using a separate column, after each set of 10 trials enter on the y-axis grid the mean number of seconds achieved, making certain to list the date of the session, the number of trials (10), the activity (H_4), the unit of measure (# seconds), and the target criterion (5 seconds). When the patient achieves an "X" mark at level 5 on the grid, the criterion for advancement to the next exercise has been met.

Exercise No. 5

Step 1. Follow the exact same method as in the preceding exercise, except that for this exercise, position and press the fingertip on the midline of the hard palate at the location of the posterior nasal spine.

Step 2. Using the same criterion adopted in Exercise no. 4, once the patient achieves this objective proceed with the following exercise, making certain that data entries on the treatment chart are assigned to separate columns and are categorized in the activity cells as BH_5 and H_5 for baseline and treatment responses, respectively.

Exercise No. 6

Step 1. The patient is once again positioned with an open mouth posture. Using the tip of the covered index finger, with a moderate degree of constant upward force, press upon the alveolar ridge for 2 seconds. Then slowly glide the fingertip posteriorly along the midline of the hard palate to the level of the posterior nasal spine, and keep it at that location for 2 seconds. Then slowly retrace the midline path back to the alveolar ridge, maintaining the same degree of finger pressure along the way, and keep it at that location for 2 seconds. The entire movement, from alveolar ridge to posterior nasal spine to alveolar ridge, should take approximately 10 seconds: 2 seconds at each of the three stops, and 2 seconds to complete each of the two journeys between these stops. Counting aloud will cue the patient about progress as well as the time remaining per trial. On a notepad, record the number of seconds the patient was able to tolerate this mobile pressure without signs of gagging, a biting reflex, or head retraction. Repeat this procedure three times for baseline information, and enter the mean result on the treatment chart, in a separate column listing the date, number of trials (3), activity (BH_6), and measurement unit (# seconds) accordingly. If the patient has no difficulty with this technique, skip Step 2 and move on to Exercise no. 7.

Step 2. Continue with the same exercise, recording the number of seconds the patient tolerated the pressure application, as previously defined. Repeat the procedure with a rest period of 15 seconds between trials, until the patient demonstrates such tolerance for the full 10-second application over 10 consecutive trials. Using a separate column, after each set of 10 trials, enter on the y-axis grid the mean number of seconds achieved, making certain to list in the respective cells the number of trials (10), the activity (H_6), the measurement unit (# seconds), and the target criterion (10 seconds). When the patient achieves an "X" mark at level 10 on the y-axis, the criterion for advancement to the following exercise has been met.

Exercise No. 7

Step 1. With the patient's mouth wide open, place a covered index fingertip on the anteriormost segment of the soft palate, and apply a moderate degree of constant upward force for 5 seconds. Count aloud so that the patient is aware of how much time is left before the end of the trial. Record the number of seconds the patient was able to tolerate this maintained pressure application without signs of gagging, a biting reflex, or head retraction. Repeat this technique three times for baseline reference. If the patient has no difficulty with this stimulus, skip the next step and move on to Exercise no. 8.

Step 2. Continue with the same exercise, allowing 15 seconds of rest between trials, until the patient demonstrates such tolerance for the full 5-second application over 10 consecutive trials. After each set of 10 trials, enter on the y-axis grid the mean number of seconds achieved, listing accordingly the appropriate date, number of trials (10), activity (H_7), measurement unit (# seconds), and the target criterion (5 seconds). An "X" mark at level 5 on the grid symbolizes that the criterion has been met for advancement to Exercise no. 8.

Exercise No. 8

Step 1. Follow the exact same method as in the preceding exercise, except that for this one a tongue depressor is used instead of the fingertip, and the site of pressure application is different. Here the distal end of the stick is pressed upwards, with a moderate degree of constant force, against the middle third of the soft palate for 5 seconds. Again, count aloud to cue the patient as to the time frame.

Step 2. Once the patient achieves the criterion established in Exercise no. 7, proceed to the following exercise, making certain that data entries on the chart are listed as BH_8 and H_8 for baseline and treatment responses, respectively. If baseline scores reveal no difficulty, the exercise itself is skipped, and Exercise no. 9 is introduced at once.

Exercise No. 9

Step 1. Roll a finger cot over the end of a tongue depressor. Request that the patient open the mouth as wide as possible. Using the covered end of the stick, with a moderate degree of constant upward force, press against the anterior third of the soft palate for 2 seconds. Then slowly glide the stick posteriorly along the midline to the middle third of the soft palate, and keep it at that location for 2 seconds. Then slowly retrace the midline path back to the anterior third of the soft palate, maintaining the same degree of upward force along the way, and keep it at that location for an additional 2 seconds. This movement, from the anterior to the middle third and back, should take approximately 10 seconds: 2 seconds at each of the three stops, and 2 seconds to complete each of the two journeys between these stops. Counting aloud will cue the patient, at different points along the route, about the time left in the trial. Record the number of seconds the patient was able to tolerate this mobile pressure without signs of gagging, a biting reflex, or head retraction. Repeat the procedure three times to establish a baseline (BH_9). If no difficulty is determined, skip Step 2 and proceed with Exercise no. 10.

Step 2. Continue with the same exercise, allowing 15 seconds of rest between trials, until the patient demonstrates tolerance for the full 10-second application over 10 consecutive trials. Again, after each set of 10 trials, enter on the y-axis grid the mean number of seconds achieved, listing the date, number of trials (10), activity (H_9), measurement unit (# seconds) and the target criterion (10 seconds). An "X" mark at level 10 on the y-axis reveals that the criterion for advancement to the next exercise has been achieved.

Exercise No. 10

Step 1. The covered tongue depressor is used again for this exercise. With a moderate degree of constant upward force, press the end of the stick against the anterior third of the soft palate for 2 seconds. Then slowly glide the stick posteriorly to the middle third, but along the way smoothly move the stick from the midline position to the right and left lateral borders of the soft palate, making certain to maintain upward pressure throughout the transition. Once the middle third of the soft palate is reached, keep the stick there for 2 seconds, and retrace the lateral stimulation path back to the anterior third, where a final 2 seconds of constant pressure is applied.

Step 2. The same scoring and criterion procedures described in the preceding exercise should be used here as well. Achievement of the criterion for advancement enables the patient to tackle the next and last exercise in this series. Make certain that these activities are classified as BH_{10} and H_{10}, symbolizing baseline and treatment responses, respectively. Again, if baseline performance is unaffected, proceed directly to the next exercise.

Exercise No. 11

Step 1. Connect the plastic nasal olive to the rubber hose of the See-Scape device. Position the olive in the patient's most patent nostril, and tape it in place so that it need not be held during the exercise. Arbitrarily mark with a black felt-tip pen the tube of the device in seven equal increments, classifying the bottom of the tube as no. 1, the middle of the tube as no. 4, the top of the tube as no. 7, and so on in between these levels.

Step 2. Request that the patient prolong the vowel /a/ as long and steadily as possible, and note the level (1 to 7) of the tube to which the Styrofoam float ascends, quantifying the degree of nasal air escape. Repeat this procedure for the /u/ and /i/ vowels until each one is attempted five times. These results will serve as baseline data. Additionally, using a seven-point equal-appearing interval scale, in which 7 represents the greatest deviation from normal (1), rate the perceived degree of hypernasal resonance during each of these baseline trials. In separate columns on the Resonation Subsystem Behavioral Treatment Chart, enter these baseline results using BH_{11a} and BH_{11b} as activity symbols for the nasal airflow and speech perception data, respectively. If these results are within normal limits, skip the next steps and go directly to the next subsection of exercises.

Step 3. Instruct the patient to open the mouth wide. Using a tongue depressor covered with a finger cot, simulate the effect of a palatal-lift appliance by applying a constant and moderate amount of upward and backward force against the body of the soft palate until tissue resistance impedes further displacement. When maximum mechanical lift is obtained, request the patient to prolong the /a/ vowel for at least 5 seconds, counting aloud to encourage the performance effort. The vowel /i/ should be used as an alternative stimulus every other trial.

Step 4. On a notepad, record the level of the tube (1 to 7) to which the float ascends under this condition. Also, render a perceptual rating of hypernasality using the seven-point interval scale. Repeat this procedure, with a rest period of 15 seconds between trials, until the degrees of nasal airflow and the perceptual ratings are at least 3 scale valves improved over the baseline score or "1," if the baseline was "2," "3," or "4," over 10 consecutive trials. After each set of 10 trials, enter the mean nasal flow (H_{11a}) and perceptual rating (H_{11b}) data in separate columns on the y-axis grid, accordingly, making certain to list the appropriate date of the session, number of trials (10), activity symbol (H_{11a} or H_{11b}), measurement unit (1 to 7), and target criterion (?). Once the patient achieves criteria, for this exercise the next subsection of treatments may be introduced.

It is important to note before we review the next series of exercises that most patients who undergo this exercise regimen should show some improvement. Usually, positive results are evident within four to five sessions. However, some patients may take a bit longer, but they too may be expected to make very good gains in the final analysis. This anticipated outcome promotes the opportunity for success with the eventual fitting of a palatal-lift appliance, which may be indicated later in the treatment program. There will be some patients who fail to respond to this first series of exercises, however. The full program should be administered nonetheless, even if the criteria for advancement from one exercise to the next have not been achieved. Experimentation with less strict criteria, at the clinician's discretion, is recommended. Failures at this level of the treatment hierarchy, however, do not bode well for subsequent treatment indications. Notwithstanding this forecast for such patients, the next series of exercises should still be introduced with hopes of better results. Before proceeding with the following exercise regimen, reassess the patient's resonation subsystem under various isolated and contextual speech conditions, and use the Speech Characteristics Chart (see Figure 4–1) to record the perceptual rating (1 to 7). Note whether the exercises just completed have influenced resonance balance by comparing this rating with the baseline judgment previously recorded on the same chart. However, it is highly improbable that such treatments will yield speech resonance effects significant enough to preempt subsequent treatment indications, since they are not designed to accomplish these results.

Nonspeech Intraoral Air Pressure Generation

Velopharyngeal incompetency causes both primary and secondary disturbances. Nasal air emissions, reduced intraoral air pressure–generating capability, and dampened acoustic energy are among the most debilitating of the primary conditions. These result in or contribute to hypernasality, articulatory imprecision, and reduced phonatory energy or volume, respectively. If the patient attempts to compensate for or alter these side effects by abnormally posturing the tongue or hyperadducting the vocal folds, secondary, compounding articulatory and phonatory disturbances may occur. The objective of this subsection is to introduce exercises for increasing intraoral air pressure–generating capability and improving velopharyngeal valving. If the patient can make significant gains under this exercise regimen, the prognosis for successful treatment of the primary and secondary speech disturbances is improved.

The following sequence of exercises is indicated for all dysarthric patients who exhibit velopharyngeal incompetency. Those with underlying velar hypertonicity and hyperactive pharyngeal reflexes will undergo this regimen after completing, whether successfully or not, the exercise program in the preceding subsection. Those patients for whom that program is not indicated will begin their resonation subsystem treatment with this exercise regimen.

Note that many patients, particularly those with moderate to severe incompetency, will not be able to achieve the criteria recommended for advancement within the exercise regimen that follows. If after 30 trials of a given exercise there is little or no evidence to support that continuation of the exercise will yield further improvement, it may be most prudent to discontinue that exercise. Notwithstanding the poor prognosis for gains on the sequentially more difficult exercises that follow, each one in the series should be attempted using the same 30-trial experimental guideline before proceeding with the next one and so on until all the exercises are given a fair trial. If the patient has lip seal difficulty, allow him or her to compensate by using the fingers for assistance during the forthcoming exercises. Note, however, that such compensations should be recorded in the comments section of the treatment chart. Responses to the following exercises may be augmented if the clinician demonstrates task objectives whenever possible, and if the patient is given some opportunity for experimental practice before performances are scored and charted. Finally, periodic reassessment of the speech resonation profile, using the Speech Characteristics (seven-point rating) Chart to measure ongoing treatment effects, is recommended.

Exercise No. 1

Step 1. Briefly familiarize the patient with the overall purpose of the exercise. When necessary, demonstrate the task objective for the patient.

Step 2. Place the See-Scape device upon the tabletop in front of the patient. Instead of the plastic nasal olive, connect a 2-inch piece of drinking straw to the rubber hose. Punch a bleed hole (about the size of a dull pencil point) in one wall of the straw about halfway between the mouth of the hose and the free end of the straw.

Step 3. Instruct the patient to take a deep breath and then blow steadily into the straw with the objective of raising the float to the top of the tube and maintaining it there for a count of 5 seconds. Repeat this procedure three times to establish a baseline, and enter the mean number of seconds achieved on the Resonation Subsystem Behavioral Treatment Chart in a separate column, making certain to record the date, number of trials (3), activity symbol (BP_1), and measurement unit (# seconds) in the appropriate cells of the column. If the patient has no difficulty with this task, skip Step 4 and go on to Exercise no. 2.

Step 4. Repeat the same procedure with 15 seconds of rest between trials until the patient demonstrates the ability to raise the float to the top of the tube for 5 full seconds over 10 consecutive trials. After each set of 10 trials, enter on the y-axis grid of the treatment chart the mean number of seconds achieved, listing the date, number of trials (10), activity symbol (P_1), measurement unit (# seconds), and target criterion (5 seconds). In the respective cells of the column chosen for these data. An "X" mark at level 5 on the y-axis would indicate that the criterion for advancement to Exercise no. 2 has been achieved. Note here that condensation may form in the tube periodically during this exercise, which will retard float dynamics. Occasional cleaning of the interior by threading a facial tissue through one end and out the other should be helpful.

Exercise No. 2

Step 1. This exercise operates with the exact same objective and methodology that were adopted in Exercise no. 1, except that here we drop a single 28-mm paper clip into the tube on top of the float, which makes the task a little harder to perform. Data entries on the treatment chart should, of course, be listed under the symbols BP_2 and P_2 for baseline and treatment results, respectively. Note once again that if the patient has no difficulty with this task on baseline measures, move directly to Exercise no. 3.

Step 2. Once the criterion for advancement to the next treatment has been achieved, Exercise no. 3 is initiated.

Exercise No. 3

Step 1. This exercise also follows the exact same procedures as those detailed in Exercise no. 1, except that here two paper clips are dropped into the tube to resist float dynamics. Note that if the patient has no difficulty with baseline measures the exercise is skipped and Exercise no. 4 is introduced.

Step 2. Once the criterion for advancement has been achieved with treatment, proceed to the next exercise. Be certain to tag the baseline and treatment data on the chart with the symbols BP_3 and P_3, respectively.

Exercise No. 4

Step 1. Look to Exercise no. 1 again for details about the objectives and methods of operation for this exercise. The only difference here is that three paper clips are dropped into the tube prior to the intraoral air pressure–generating measurements. Use the symbols BP_4 and P_4, respectively, for the baseline and treatment data chart recordings. If the patient exhibits no difficulty during the baseline measures, skip the treatment component and move on to Exercise no. 5.

Step 2.   Once the criterion for advancement has been achieved with treatment, proceed to the next exercise.

Exercise No. 5
   Step 1.   This exercise also follows identically the course of Exercise no. 1, except that here four paper clips are dropped into the tube. As discussed in the previous chapter, the resistance achieved with four paper clips roughly simulates a 5 cm H_2O displacement task as may be measured with a water manometer. Be certain to use the activity symbols BP_5 and P_5 when recording on the chart the baseline and treatment data collected, respectively. Again, if the patient performs the baseline measures without difficulty, skip the treatment phase and proceed to Exercise no. 6.
   Step 2.   Following achievement of the criterion for advancement, move on to the next exercise.

Exercise No. 6
   Step 1.   The rules of Exercise no. 1 apply here too. However, for this exercise, drop a total of five paper clips into the tube. Be certain to record baseline (BP_6) and treatment (P_6) responses accordingly on the score chart in the chosen columns for these data. When no signs of difficulty occur during baseline measures, skip the treatments and move on to the next exercise.
   Step 2.   Advance to Exercise no. 7 when the criterion for improvement has been achieved.

Exercise No. 7
   Step 1.   For this exercise the same set-up used in Exercise no. 6 applies, except that six 28-mm paper clips are dropped into the See-Scape tube, and the straw with bleed hole is substituted for the plastic nasal olive.
   Step 2.   Request that the patient take a deep breath and then blow as hard and forcefully as possible into the straw with the objective of causing the paper clips to wedge and remain within the hole of the rubber cap that sits atop the tube as the float descends to the bottom with the cessation of air pressure. Repeat this task three times to gather baseline information. Use a dichotomous yes/no rating system to record the result on the treatment chart, in which Yes = 1 and No = 0. Enter the mean result on the y-axis grid in a separate column chosen for these data, making certain to list the date, number of trials (3), activity symbol (BP_7), and measurement unit (Y/N) in the respective cells of the column. Unless the patient achieves a perfect score during baseline measures, do not skip the next step.
   Step 3.   Continue with the same exercise, allowing 15 seconds of rest between trials, until the patient demonstrates the ability to achieve the aforementioned objective on five consecutive trials. After each set of five trials, enter on the y-axis grid the mean score achieved, and list the date, number of trials (5), activity (P_7), measurement unit (Y/N), and target criterion (5) in the respective cells of the separate column chosen for these data entries. An "X" mark at level 5

on the grid reveals that the criterion for advancement to the next exercise has been met.

Exercise No. 8

Step 1.   Request that the patient try to blow up a small balloon. Repeat the attempt three times using the Yes = 1/No = 0 scoring system, and record the baseline mean on the treatment chart in a column chosen for this information, making certain to list the activity as BP_8 in the appropriate cell. If the patient can perform the task without error, skip the next step and proceed to the next exercise.

Step 2.   Continue with the same exercise, with 15 seconds of rest between trials, until the patient demonstrates the ability to blow up the balloon on five consecutive trials. After each set of five trials, enter on the y-axis grid the mean score achieved, and list the date, number of trials (5), activity (P_8), measurement unit (Y/N), and target criterion (5) in the respective cells of the column chosen for these data. An "X" mark at level 5 on the grid reveals that the criterion has been met for advancement to the next exercise subsection.

Intermittently, a noseclip might be used to demonstrate whether failures to achieve the objectives of these exercises are attributable to velopharyngeal incompetency, respiration subsystem disturbances, or both. Those patients with adequate respiration subsystem controls should be able to perform the intraoral air pressure tasks when the nose is clipped.

Vowel Prolongations

The overall objective of the exercises in this subsection is to improve velopharyngeal closure when the mechanism is stressed with the inherent demands of simple, steady-state non-nasal speech stimuli. We begin with vowels, which are within the phonetic repertoire of most dysarthric patients. It should be noted before getting started here that whereas those patients who failed the preceding exercise preparations will probably suffer disappointments with this regimen as well, others who experienced better success up to this point may continue the trend with these important speech exercises. Irrespective of the patient's track record with previous treatments, this exercise regimen should be administered. The criteria for advancement within the regimen are recommendations that are not etched in stone. Clinicians may wish to adopt more or less stringent criteria, according to their own philosophies and/or the individual patient's prognosis for improvement. As in the preceding subsection, here it is also recommended that if after 30 trials of a given exercise the patient fails to demonstrate improvement over the baseline level significant enough to justify continuation with that exercise, it should be discontinued. Regardless of the poor prognosis for the more difficult exercises that follow in the sequence, each one in the series should be respectively attempted, using the same 30-trial experimental guideline before terminating the exercise and proceeding with the next one. Even if the patient fails to achieve the criteria of the entire regimen, the next subsection of exercises should be attempted.

Exercise No. 1

Step 1.   The standard set-up with the See-Scape device is used for the exercise. Place the nasal olive in the patient's nostril that emits good nasal airflow, and tape it in position to preclude having to hold it during the exercise regimen. With a magic marking pen, draw a line on the tube about 1 inch up from the bottom.

Step 2.   Familiarize the patient with the objective of this exercise, which is to try to minimize nasal airflow during production of the speech stimuli so that the Styrofoam float does not rise beyond the line drawn on the tube.

Step 3.   Instruct the patient to take a deep breath and then prolong the vowel /a:/ for a count of 7 seconds. Disregard the first and last seconds, and note how many of the middle 5 seconds the float remained at or below the line. Repeat this procedure again, but this time use the vowel /u/. For the last of these baseline measures, use the vowel /i/. Calculate the mean number of successful seconds, and enter the result on the treatment chart in a separate column, making certain to list the appropriate date, number of trials (3), activity symbol (BV_1), and measurement unit (# seconds) in the respective cells of this column. If the patient does not demonstrate any difficulty with these trials, skip the next step and move on to Exercise no. 2. As a general rule of thumb, the tape recorder should be periodically used for auditory biofeedback during the exercise.

Step 4.   Continue with this procedure, alternating the vowel used for each trial in concert with the patient's articulatory capability. Use the same scoring method suggested in Step 3 earlier. After each set of 10 trials, compute from the notepad data the mean number of seconds the patient was successful in keeping the float below the target line, and enter this result in a separate column on the y-axis grid, making certain to list the corresponding date, number of trials (10), activity symbol (V_1), and measurement unit (# seconds) in the respective cells of the column. When the patient can produce 10 consecutive trials without the float rising above the target line, the criterion for advancement to the next exercise has been achieved. Be certain to list this target in the criterion cell on the chart.

Exercise No. 2

Step 1.   The same See-Scape set-up and treatment objective established in the preceding exercise will be incorporated into this one.

Step 2.   After familiarizing the patient with the objective, request that he or she take a deep breath and then produce the vowel train /i-u-a/, allowing 2 seconds per vowel. The transition from vowel to vowel should be smooth, occurring on one breath without significant pauses between the shifts. If the float rises above the line drawn on the tube, the trial is graded a "0" (no). If the float remains below the line throughout the trial, the patient is awarded a "1" (yes). Repeat the task two more times, changing the train of vowels as so desired. Add up these three baseline scores and enter the result on the treatment chart in a separate column, making certain to list the date, number of trials (3), activity symbol (BV$_2$), and measurement unit (Y/N) in the appropriate cells of the column. If the patient has no difficulty with this task, skip the next step and proceed with the exercises in the next subsection.

Step 3. Continue with this procedure, alternating the anatomy of the vowel train with respect to the patient's articulatory capability. Using the same dichotomous scoring system as that suggested in the previous step, after each set of 10 trials, tally from a notepad the number of successful trials achieved by the patient, and enter this total in a separate column on the y-axis grid, making certain to list the date, number of trials (10), activity symbol (V$_2$), and measurement unit (Y/N) in the appropriate cells of the column. When the patient can produce 10 consecutive trials without the float rising above the target line, the criterion for advancement to the next subsection of exercises has been achieved. Be certain to list this target criterion in the respective cell at the bottom of the treatment data column.

Speech Intraoral Air Pressure Generation

In the previous exercise regimen the speech tasks were directed at facilitating control of excess nasal airflow, a primary sequela to velopharyngeal incompetency. The treatment techniques in this subsection are aimed at improving intraoral air pressure–generating capability, another problem area associated with such incompetency.

The same guideline for movement within and between the exercises in this regimen as that recommended in the preceding program will be used here. That is, if the patient achieves the criterion suggested for a given exercise, advancement to the exercise that follows in the sequence is indicated. On the other hand, if after 30 trials the patient cannot demonstrate improvement over the baseline level significant enough to warrant continuation with the exercise, it should be discontinued. Irrespective of the poor prognosis for further improvements on the subsequent, generally more difficult exercises, the sequential series should still be administered using the same 30-trial (experimental) guideline before terminating an exercise and proceeding to the next one.

Exercise No. 1

Step 1. Use the See-Scape device. Instead of the plastic nasal olive, connect a 3-inch piece of drinking straw (without bleed hole) to the rubber hose.

Step 2. Familiarize the patient with the objective of the exercise, which is to improve intraoral air pressure control during speech efforts. Such gains should benefit, at least partially, articulatory proficiency; and that is the ultimate goal. The Styrofoam float will serve as visual feedback of oral pressure during the various exercises in this subsection, simulating qualitatively the quantitative effects that may be accomplished in the speech physiology laboratory when a pressure transducer interfaced with an oscilloscope provides visual feedback to the patient regarding intraoral air pressures during contrived bilabial speech sound tasks.

Step 3. Place the straw in the corner of the patient's mouth in such a fashion that it runs parallel to the lips, and the open (free) end rests immediately behind the upper central incisor teeth in the vicinity of, but not touching, the maxillary alveolar ridge. Have prepared a list of nonsense and real words that contain the /p/ sound, such as /po; pai; pi; pa:; pe; pau; a:pa:; i:pi:; e:pe:; ep; pipi; pep ; pupu;/. Request the patient to take a breath and attempt to produce one of these words. Starting off with a consonant-vowel (CV) stimulus and progressing from there in complexity may be the best sequence. Note upon the attempted production of the /p/ consonant whether, as would normally occur, the float rises abruptly to the top of the tube and then reverses its course when the vowel is phased in. This is precisely the type of float action that we set as the objective for this exercise program. If this goal is achieved, the performance is rated a "1." If not, the trial receives a score of "0." Repeat the task three times, alternating the complexity of the stimulus word during each trial to derive a baseline level of ability. If the patient demonstrates no difficulty on these measures, skip the next step and proceed to Exercise no. 2. Be certain to enter the baseline data on the treatment chart under the symbol (BA_1), accordingly. Use of the tape recorder for auditory biofeedback may be facilitative.

Step 4. Using the same stimuli as in Step 3, begin the treatment component with the CV words. Select any of these words, and once again instruct the patient that the objective is to force the float to the top of the tube upon production of the /p/ sound in the stimulus word by building up air pressure within the oral cavity and then suddenly releasing it to create the plosive quality of this sound. Use the dichotomous Yes/No scoring system to rate the performance, as in Step 3 earlier. Continue this procedure, with freedom to select any word in the list as the stimulus for practice until the patient achieves the objective on 10 consecutive word productions. After each set of 10 trials, tally the patient's total score, and enter the result in a separate column on the y-axis grid of the treatment chart, making certain to record the date, number of trials (10), activity symbol (A_1), measurement unit (Y/N), and target criterion (10) in the respective cells of the column. An "X" mark at level 10 on the chart will indicate that the patient has achieved the criterion for advancement to Exercise no. 2.

Exercise No. 2

Step 1. The same exact See-Scape set-up procedure and scoring system used in the preceding exercise will be used here, except that one paper clip (28-mm) is to be dropped into the tube for this exercise.

Step 2. After collecting and recording data on the baseline ability under this weighted float condition, proceed with the treatment regimen if so indicated for the patient.

Step 3. Continue the exercise until the patient achieves the aforementioned objective and criterion, listing the activity symbol (A_2) when entering the data collected on the treatment chart. Once the criterion for advancement is achieved, move on to the next exercise.

Exercise No. 3
Step 1.   This is the exact same exercise as Exercise no. 2 above, except that here two paper clips are dropped into the tube. The procedural methods are identical, but the scoring symbol is "A_3."

Exercise No. 4
Step 1.   Again, the same exercise as Exercise no. 2, except that three paper clips are used. The symbol is "A_4" for data entry. The next exercise is the last one in this subsection.

Exercise No. 5
Step 1.   Finally, follow the same method as that in Exercise no. 2, except that here four paper clips are used, and the symbol is "A_5" for the record.

Isolated Word Productions

Words consisting of pressure consonants serve as the source of stimuli for velopharyngeal closure in this exercise regimen. Depending upon the severity of the patient's articulation subsystem disturbances, these words may vary in composition from simple to complex. The more pressure consonants that can be incorporated into the program, the better, relative to preparing the velopharyngeal mechanism for the demands of connected speech behavior. Before proceeding with the recommended exercises that follow, it will be of help to consult the methodology suggestions that were discussed in the headlines of the preceding subsection, inasmuch as those guidelines apply here as well.

Exercise No. 1
Step 1.   The standard See-Scape set-up is used in this program. Place the nasal olive in the patient's nostril, and tape it in position so that it will not need to be held during the exercise. Draw a line on the tube of the See-Scape about 1 inch up from the bottom, using the marking pen.
Step 2.   Familiarize the patient with the objective of this exercise, which is to try to minimize abnormal nasal air emissions, as will be evidenced by limited (below the target line) or no activity of the Styrofoam float during the word stimuli productions.
Step 3.   Have ready for use several index cards that contain CV, VC, CVC, and CVCV real and nonsense word stimuli that are within the articulatory reach of the patient, making certain that words constructed possess any of the following sounds (p, b, t, d, k, g, s, z, f, ʃ, tʃ, dʒ) but are free of nasals. Request that the patient produce one word at a time, noting the degree of float movement with each utterance. The word list may be ordered by groups from least to most complex, relative to length and phonetic makeup. Starting with the easiest word

group may be the best approach. To establish a baseline, first have the patient attempt at least one word from each of the groups constructed. Score the trial successful (Yes = 1) if the float remains below the target line throughout the production. Add up the positive baseline scores, and enter the result on the treatment chart in a separate column, making certain to list the date, number of trials (?), activity symbol (BW_1), and measurement unit (Y/N) in the respective cells of the column. If these data indicate no difficulty with excess nasal airflow, skip the next step and proceed to the next subsection of exercises. Again, the tape recorder may provide useful auditory biofeedback during the exercise.

Step 4. Continue with this procedure, alternating with each new stimulus the group from which the word is chosen, and use a notepad to keep track of the performance scores. The criterion for advancement to the next subsection is 10 consecutive word productions without excess nasal air emissions, as previously defined. After each set of 10 trials, tally the number of successful trials achieved by the patient, and enter the total in a separate column on the y-axis grid, making certain to list the date, number of trials (10), activity symbol (W_1), measurement unit (Y/N), and target criterion (10) in the respective cells of the column. An "X" mark at level 10 on the grid reveals that the criterion for advancement has been achieved.

Sentence Productions

For this exercise regimen, sentences loaded with pressure consonants and free of nasal sounds serve as the stimuli for velopharyngeal valving. Not unlike the rules governing construction of the isolated words in the preceding subsection, the words chosen for the sentences here should be commensurate with the articulatory capability of the patient. Some patients will be unable to practice this exercise in full, owing to severe articulatory imprecision. Simple sentences consisting of two or three words may promote a modicum of success. They should be attempted, even in the face of a very poor prognosis. The rules governing how to proceed if the patient fails to respond positively to the exercise regimen will be the same as those previously outlined in the headlines of the Vowel Prolongations subsection.

Exercise No. 1

Step 1. Use the exact same See-Scape set-up here as was suggested in the preceding exercise for isolated word productions. The overall objective during the attempts at sentence stimuli production is to keep nasal airflow low enough to prevent the float from rising above the target line on the See-Scape tube. Sentences such as "Pet the puppy," "Two plus two is four," "She baked cookies," "It was a sure shot," "She washed the dishes," and "Watch out for cars" are examples of the types of sentence stimuli that may be employed for this exercise.

Step 2. After familiarizing the patient with the objective of the regimen, have ready index cards that contain the sentences constructed for use with the individual patient. Request that the patient read aloud three of these sentences selected at random, and note the degree of float action that occurs during each trial. If the float rises above the target line at any time during word productions, the performance is rated a "0"; little or no float movement is scored a "1." At the completion of these three baseline trials, enter the total score in a separate column of the treatment chart, using the activity symbol "BS" as the reference for the entry. If the patient scores a "3," skip the next step and proceed to the following subsection. Whenever possible, use the tape recorder for auditory biofeedback of performances.

Step 3. Continue with the exercise, using a different sentence whenever desired, and use a notepad to keep track of the performance scores. The criterion for advancement to the next subsection is 10 consecutive sentence productions without excess nasal airflow, as defined. After each set of 10 trials, tally the number of successful trials achieved, and enter the total in a separate column on the y-axis grid, indicating the date, number of trials (10), activity symbol (S_1), measurement unit (Y/N), and target criterion (10) in the respective cells of the column. An "X" mark at level 10 on the grid is evidence that the criterion for advancement to the next subsection has been met.

Connected Speech

In this exercise we use a paragraph that does not contain nasal sounds. The ultimate objective is to try to train the patient through visual biofeedback to decrease abnormal nasal airflow during connected speech so as to improve resonation balance. Nasal sounds are deliberately omitted from this exercise, so the velopharyngeal mechanism is stressed with consistent demands for closure. Success with this procedure may ready the patient for the more difficult physiologic challenge of connected discourse, which is normally laced with both non-nasal and nasal sounds.

Should the patient fail to achieve the advancement criterion set for this exercise, the aforementioned method in the headlines of the Vowel Prolongations treatment subsection should be followed here as well.

Exercise No. 1

Step 1. The same exact See-Scape set-up used in the earlier Isolated Word Productions treatment subsection will be incorporated into this exercise.

Step 2. The objective is to train the patient to reduce abnormal nasal air emissions, using the visual biofeedback of float activity to facilitate such improvement. Unwanted movements of the float above the target line during production of the words in the stimulus paragraph should be penalized as follows: If more than 80 percent of the words are driven with excess nasal air emissions, the trial is rated a "0." If nasal airflow is kept to a minimum, 20 percent or less, a score of "1" is rendered for the trial. Allow three trials to establish a baseline record, and enter the result in a column separate from previously recorded treatment data, making certain to list the date, number of trials (3), activity symbol (BC_1), and unit of measure (Y/N) as usual in the appropriate cells. If the patient scores a "3" on the baseline measurement, skip Step 3 that follows. Again, the tape recorder may come in handy to highlight the patient's performances.

Step 3. The following paragraph is recommended as the stimulus for this exercise:

> This exercise was developed for people who wish to better their oral airflow ability for speech purposes. As these words are said out loud, if the float rises above the threshold target, that is bad. But if the float stays still, that is good because it shows that all the airflow for these oral speech tasks passed through the oral cavity.

Note that the focus here is not on articulatory proficiency, but rather on the nasal airflow factor and any associated resonance imbalance. Most dysarthric patients who undergo this treatment will not be able to sail through the reading without significant struggle, owing to widespread coexistent speech subsystem disturbances. Notwithstanding this anticipated result, the clinician should encourage the patient to try his or her best to get through the paragraph, which can be presented on an index card for easy visualization. Use the same scoring system here as the one suggested earlier for the baseline measure. Repeat the procedure until the patient achieves the airflow objective discussed in Step 2 on three consecutive trials. After each set of three trials, tally the score awarded (0 to 3), and enter the result on the y-axis grid in a separate column of the treatment chart, listing as usual the date, number of trials (3), activity symbol (C_1), measurement unit (Y/N), and target criterion (3) in the respective cells of the column. An "X" mark at level "3" on the grid will indicate that the patient has met the criterion for completion of the behavioral management program. If the patient does well with this exercise, experimentation with extemporaneous speech activities may prove interesting and valuable.

CONCLUSION

Many patients, however motivated they are, will not make gains in the behavioral management program significant enough to ward off the need for a prosthetic appliance, surgical intervention, or both. Exposure to the exercises in this program will nonetheless prove valuable because it is probable that they will have to be readministered to facilitate the objectives of either one or both of these alternative treatments. Having practiced the various exercises, the patient should experience little difficulty in appreciating their purposes and methods if and when they are reintroduced. Moreover, the effects of such treatments in virtually all cases may not be fully realized or developed until later in the rehabilitation program. The patient must be cautioned that direct treatments of the resonation subsystem rarely by themselves promote the desired levels of speech improvement, irrespective of their technical degree of success. Coexisting articulation and phonation subsystem disturbances, in particular, usually interfere with optimal results until these influential conditions are also successfully treated. However, good results here in the resonation subsystem treatment paradigm do indeed set the stage for the possibility of further gains along these lines.

Figure 4–6 provides a synopsis of the behavioral management program, the sequential exercise regimen, the basic methods and objectives of each application, and the criterion for advancement within the program.

The following case sample may facilitate closure of this chapter.

Illustrative Case No. 2

This 36-year-old school teacher with an otherwise unremarkable medical history experienced over a period of 3 months (prior to the speech-language examination) transient episodes of dizziness, mild clumsiness, indistinct speech, and neck pain. Her family physician suggested that she was much too worried about her job and her failing marriage and treated her symptoms as psychosomatic. Two months later these symptoms progressed to the degree that they became quite debilitating. She complained that her speech was getting worse, that walking was more difficult, and that her neck hurt so much that she could hardly face her job daily.

Upon examination the patient was alert, interactive, and rather cooperative and was equipped with good language and pragmatic skills. She insisted that until very recently many days, even weeks, could go by without significant symptoms. This, she reported, "drove me crazy." She was certain that her doctor's diagnosis was correct. Testing revealed the following significant findings: (1) relatively unsteady, wide-based gait, with a tendency to imbalance with load stress; (2) moderately exaggerated stretch reflexes of the limbs accompanied by similar degrees of hypertonicity and weakness; (3) bilateral Babinski signs; (4) slow and irregular alternate motion rates of the limbs; (5) moderate degrees of hypertonicity and weakness of the tongue, velum, and facial musculature, bilaterally, accompanied by exaggerated reflexes; (6) slow and irregular alternate motion rates of the tongue and lips; (7) articulatory imprecision; (8) harsh voice; (9) periodic loudness outbursts and uncontrollable pitch changes, especially upon vowel prolongations; and (10) moderate degree of hypernasality and excess nasal air emissions. Laboratory studies revealed abnormally high gamma globulin levels, but computed tomography scanning, magnetic resonance imaging, and cerebral blood flow results proved normal.

The speech diagnosis rendered was mixed spastic-ataxic dysarthria, caused by early signs of (suspected) demyelinating disease, possibly multiple sclerosis (MS). In this patient, the wide-based gait suggested cerebellar (ataxic) impairment, as did the prosodic abnormalities and irregular alternate motion rates. Her exaggerated reflexes, Babinski signs, and limb and speech musculature hypertonicity, weakness, and paresis implicated fully the pyramidal system, bilaterally. The diagnosis of MS usually relies on specific findings including (1) multiple white matter lesions; (2) relapsing and remitting symptomatic course; (3) slow, but stepwise deterioration until the illness becomes protracted with time; and (4) onset between the ages of 20 and 50 years. These features result from diffuse and progressive demyelinization of axon sheaths, with a predilection for specific areas

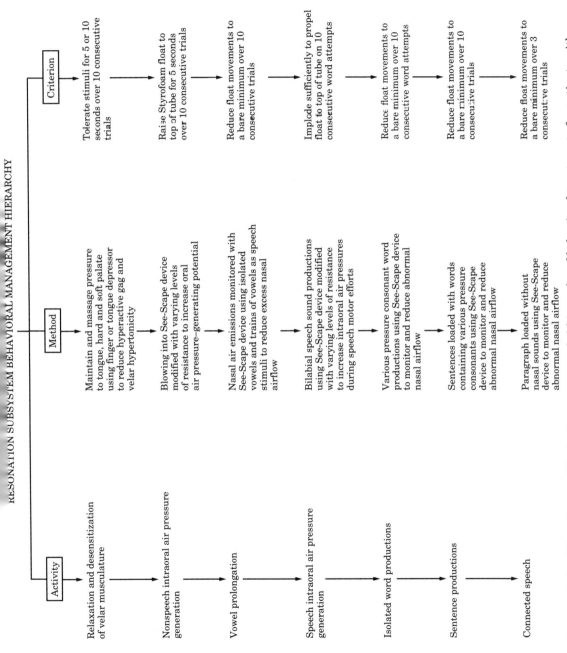

Figure 4–6. Flow diagram illustrating recommended hierarchy of behavioral treatments for patients with resonation subsystem disturbances.

in the central nervous system. These include the (1) optic nerves; (2) brainstem, particularly the medial longitudinal fasciculus and corticobulbar tracts of the pyramidal system; (3) cerebellum; and (4) posterior columns and corticospinal tracts within the spinal cord. However, there is considerable variation as to the loci of lesions and the disease itself. Because the average length of survival following definitive diagnosis is approximately 25 years, this patient's prognosis is uncertain. She was admitted for speech therapy that would occur three times a week, for a 1-hour session each visit. The initial therapeutic focus was on her resonation subsystem disturbances. The overall clinical approach followed in this regard is presented below.

Following the pretreatment protocol of Figure 4–2, we proceeded with baseline testing of the resonation subsystem to establish a framework against which the effects of any treatments administered could be measured. Perceptual ratings of her hypernasality and nasal air emission features were provided by three certified clinicians who listened, on two separate occasions, to various high-quality audio tape recordings made while the patient spoke extemporaneously, and recited words, sentences, and paragraphs. The results yielded a highly reliable inter-rater mean score of 5.7, using the seven-point equal-appearing interval scale, wherein "1" represents normal resonance, and "7" indicates the most deviant degree of hypernasality possible. This baseline result was recorded on the Speech Characteristics Chart for later comparisons.

The oral mechanism examination corroborated the aforementioned diagnostic findings relative to the abnormal velopharyngeal signs and symptoms. The mechanism was rated moderately hypertonic and hyper-reflexive (+3), and moderately paretic (−3), bilaterally. The resultant hypernasality was accompanied by excess nasal airflow, which collectively compounded the coexisting articulation, phonation, and prosody subsystem disturbances.

Speech aerodynamics testing was conducted first using clinical tool adaptations, and second, for quantitative substantiation, with differential airflow and pressure transducers coupled to a computer work station for high-speed analyses of the data. Results of the latter studies revealed (1) abnormal nasal airflow velocities that consistently exceeded 1000 cc/second during attempted productions of various pressure consonants, and (2) intraoral air pressure values that consistently fell below 4 cm H_2O on these same productions. Use of a noseclip to reevaluate these latter values without the nasal air escape factor resulted in greatly improved intraoral pressure recordings. Nearly normal levels were achieved under this testing condition, and the power spectrum of the audio signal was dramatically enhanced as well. These preliminary observations yielded a good prognosis for overall speech improvement if better velopharyngeal closure could be therapeutically accomplished. For comparisons with the laboratory data collected from the patient in this example, See-Scape data were also collected. Those results follow.

1. *Abnormal nasal airflow:* During productions of various non-nasal speech stimuli, the Styrofoam float rose to the top of the tube, indicating nasal

emissions both when there was no paper clip and when one paper clip was used. When two paper clips anchored the float, it rose consistently to the three-quarter mark on the tube during production of the same speech stimuli. The three–paper clip condition retarded float movements to the halfway mark on the tube. With four paper clips, the float was consistently down below the one-quarter mark.

2. *Maximum intraoral air pressure–generating capability (without noseclip):* During vigorous blowing efforts, the float rose to the top of the tube and remained there, indicating oral air pressure emissions, for a total of 3 seconds both when there was no paper clip and when one paper clip was used. With two paper clips weighing down the float, it rose to and remained at the top for no more than 2 seconds. When three paper clips were present, the patient could not raise the float to the top of the tube for more than 1 second. The simulated 5 cm H_2O/5 second intraoral air pressure generation task, achieved with four paper clips within the tube, was very difficult for the patient. She was unable to force the float to the top of the tube for any length of time.

3. *Speech intraoral air pressure values (without noseclip):* During the production of various non-nasal speech stimuli, the Styrofoam float rose to the top of the tube upon the pressure consonant productions, indicating air implosion, both when there was no paper clip and when one paper clip was used. When two paper clips anchored the float, the patient could not generate sufficient intraoral air pressure to propel the float to the top of the tube.

4. *Speech intraoral air pressure values (with noseclip):* When the nose was clipped to prevent nasal airflow wastage during the intraoral air pressure speech tasks, the patient was able to generate sufficient pressure to propel consistently five paper clips and the float to the top of the tube.

Collectively, these measurements led to referral for multiview videofluoroscopic studies of the velopharyngeal mechanism. Results of these appraisals substantiated the speech clinical and laboratory findings regarding the moderate degree of neuromuscular valving incompetency, attributable both to faulty velar and lateral pharyngeal wall activities. Treatment of the resonation subsystem was initiated immediately thereafter. It was the first order of business in the anticipated speech motor control intervention program.

Resonation Subsystem Treatment Hierarchy

The treatment program began with the full-course behavioral management exercise regimen detailed in the preceding subsection. With the first series of exercises, which are designed to desensitize and relax hypertonic and hyper-reflexive velar musculature, the patient made significant improvements. All subsequent exercises, however, yielded results that fell substantially short of the stated objectives and criteria for advancement. The patient made virtually no improvements in velopharyngeal valving capability, practicing neither the non-speech intraoral air pressure–generating exercises nor the speech airflow and pressure stimuli, as determined by speech aerodynamic and perceptual rating re-calculations. After five (experimental) treatment sessions, the behavioral management program was discontinued. Referral to Prosthodontics was made for the fitting of a palatal-lift appliance, which the patient was willing to try. We will first review her successful responses to the velar desensitization and relaxation exercises within the context of the behavioral management program, followed by discussion of the method employed to fit the patient with a lift, and the final outcome.

Behavioral Management Effect

Figure 4–7, *A* through *C* illustrates the patient's responses to the first treatment activity—Reduction of Velar Hyper-reflexia and Hypertonicity. Note that this program began on 2/8/85, with the baseline measurement of tongue-tip pressure tolerance (BH_1), which is the first exercise in this treatment subsection. The "X" mark at level 5 on the grid, in column 1 of Figure 4–7, *A*, was high-lighted above with an asterisk (*), signifying that the criterion was met for that stimulus. Because the patient achieved the objective at the baseline measurement, the exercise itself was skipped, and we proceeded with the next exercise, tolerance of maintained pressure applied to the middle of the tongue.

Baseline measurement (BH_2) shown in column 2 of Figure 4–7, *A* was also collected on 2/8/85, the results of which fell short of the target criterion (5 seconds level). Treatment (H_2) was immediately initiated, and only 30 trials later the patient achieved the criterion for advancement, as indicated by the "X" mark with an asterisk. It took 50 trials for her to meet the criterion set for the next exercise (H_3), which involved pressure stimuli to the back of the tongue, but on 2/10/85 she was able to move on to the fourth baseline measurement (BH_4). No difficulties were exhibited on this or the next two baseline examinations (BH_5 and BH_6), all of which involved hard-palate pressure stimuli. This success enabled us to move on to the seventh exercise, in which baseline scores (BH_7) fell short of the target criterion, as shown on Figure 4–7, *A* in one of the columns dated 2/15/85. This exercise involved pressure stimulation to the anterior velum. It took 90 trials before the patient achieved the criterion set for advancement, but the progress along the way suggested that perseverance might yield good results. Figure 4–7, *B* illustrates that indeed we reached the arbitrary goal on 2/17/85. However, even if we had failed to do so, the improvement made over the baseline score was evidence enough that exercise activity was of value.

We moved on to the eighth exercise, which involved middle velar stimulation requiring treatment. At the end of the 2/20/85 session, the patient achieved the criterion for advancement after 50 treatment trials. Note that in Figure 4–7, *B* on 2/22/85 the ninth exercise, which amounted to mobile pressure stimulation along the midline from the anterior nasal spine to the middle of the velum, yielded poor results. This treatment was discontinued owing to a poor prognosis

RESONATION SUBSYSTEM BEHAVIORAL TREATMENT CHART

Patient's name: S.B.

Birthdate: 10/20/49 Sex: Fe

Speech diagnosis: Mixed Spastic-Ataxic Dysarthria

Medical diagnosis: (Suspected) Early Multiple Sclerosis

Clinician: Dworkin

Facility: Private Practice

Address: Anywhere, USA

ACTIVITY KEY

Feature:
1. Reduction of velar hyperreflexia and hypertonicity (H)
2. Intraoral air pressure generation (nonspeech) (P)
3. Vowel prolongations (V)
4. Intraoral air pressure generation (speech) (A)
5. Isolated word productions (W)
6. Sentence productions (S)
7. Connected speech (C)

Baseline (pre-treatment): B + activity symbol

MEASUREMENT UNIT
No. of seconds, or
7 point interval scale
(1 = normal; 7 = most deviant)
No. of seconds, or
Yes = 1/ No = 0
No. of seconds, or
Yes = 1/ No = 0
Yes = 1/ No = 0

Yes = 1/ No = 0
Yes = 1/ No = 0
Yes = 1/ No = 0

Comments: On occasion the patient found it helpful to use her hand to assist the lip seal during the intraoral air pressure generating exercises.

Dates: 2/8/85 ... 2/10 ... 2/15 ... 2/17

| Activity symbol | BH₁ | BH₂ | BH₃ | H₂ | H₂ | H₃ | H₃ | H₃ | H₃ | H₃ | BH₄ | BH₅ | BH₆ | BH₇ | H₇ | H₇ | H₇ |

No. of trials / Average Score / Unit of measure / Target criterion as plotted on the chart.

SESSIONS

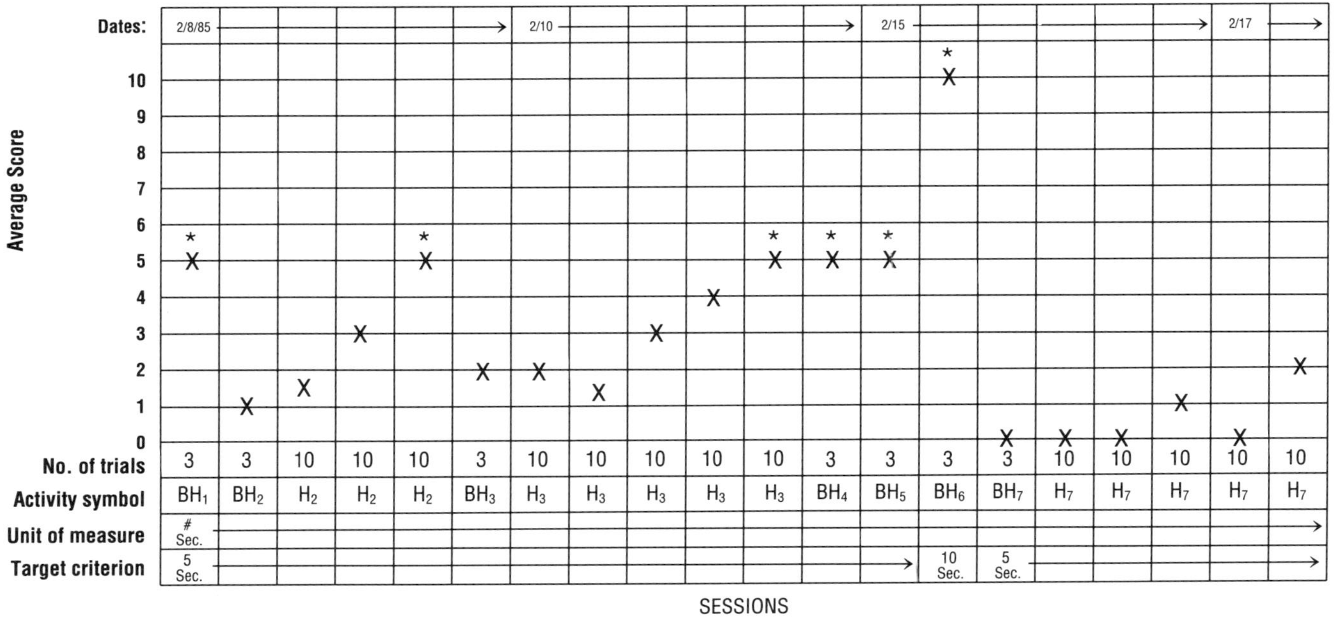

Figure 4–7. A to C, Treatment charts copied from file of patient with mixed dysarthria and significant velopharyngeal valving incompetency. Cells with asterisks (*) represent successful achievement of the criterion chosen for advancement to the next treatment step.

Figure continues on following page.

127

RESONATION SUBSYSTEM BEHAVIORAL TREATMENT CHART

Patient's name: S.B. (continued)

Birthdate: Sex:

Speech diagnosis:

Medical diagnosis:

Clinician:

Facility:

Address:

ACTIVITY KEY

Feature:	MEASUREMENT UNIT
1. Reduction of velar hyperreflexia and hypertonicity (H)	No. of seconds, or 7 point interval scale (1 = normal; 7 = most deviant)
2. Intraoral air pressure generation (nonspeech) (P)	No. of seconds, or Yes = 1/ No = 0
3. Vowel prolongations (V)	No. of seconds, or Yes = 1/ No = 0
4. Intraoral air pressure generation (speech) (A)	Yes = 1/ No = 0
5. Isolated word productions (W)	Yes = 1/ No = 0
6. Sentence productions (S)	Yes = 1/ No = 0
7. Connected speech (C)	Yes = 1/ No = 0

Baseline (pre-treatment): B + activity symbol

Comments:

Dates: 2/17/85   2/20   2/22   2/26

Average Score (0–10)

No. of trials	10	10	10	3	10	10	10	3	10	10	10	3	10	10	10
Activity symbol	H_7	H_7	H_7	BH_8	H_8	H_8	H_8	BH_9	H_9	H_9	H_9	BH_{10}	H_{10}	H_{10}	H_{10}
Unit of measure	# Sec.														
Target criterion	5 Sec.									10 Sec.					

SESSIONS

Figure 4–7. *Continued.*

RESONATION SUBSYSTEM BEHAVIORAL TREATMENT CHART

Patient's name: S.B. (continued)

Birthdate: Sex:

Speech diagnosis: _____

Medical diagnosis: _____

Clinician: _____

Facility: _____

Address: _____

Comments: _____

ACTIVITY KEY

Feature: **MEASUREMENT UNIT**

1. Reduction of velar hyperreflexia   No. of seconds, or
   and hypertonicity (H)   7 point interval scale
      (1 = normal; 7 = most deviant)
2. Intraoral air pressure generation   No. of seconds, or
   (nonspeech) (P)   Yes = 1/ No = 0
3. Vowel prolongations (V)   No. of seconds, or
     Yes = 1/ No = 0
4. Intraoral air pressure generation   Yes = 1/ No = 0
   (speech) (A)
5. Isolated word productions (W)   Yes = 1/ No = 0
6. Sentence productions (S)   Yes = 1/ No = 0
7. Connected speech (C)   Yes = 1/ No = 0

Baseline (pre-treatment): B + activity symbol

Average Score (C)

Dates:	2/26/85						3/2			3/5				
10		*												
9	X	X												
8														
7														
6				X		X	$X_{a,b}$		$X_{a,b}$			$X_{a,b}$		
5					X	X_a X_b	X_b X_a	X_b X_a	X_a X_b	X_b X_a				
4														
3														
2														
1														
0														
No. of trials	10	10	10	3	3	10	10	10	10	10	10			
Activity symbol	H_{10}	H_{10}	BH_{11a}	BH_{11b}	$H_{11a,b}$									
Unit of measure	# Sec.	# Sec.	1–7											
Target criterion	10 Sec.	1	1		a 3.5 / b 2.5									

SESSIONS

Figure 4–7. *Continued.*

129

for further gains. Not particularly hopeful, we proceeded to the tenth exercise, which also involved mobile stimulation of the velum, but in both anteroposterior and lateromedial directions. The need for treatment was revealed by the baseline score (BH_{10}) recorded on 2/22/85 (Figure 4–7, B). Such treatments began on 2/26/85 and continued for 60 trials. At the end of the 2/26/85 session (Figure 4–7, C), she had achieved the criterion for advancement to the last exercise in the subsection.

As can be seen from Figure 4–7, C, she was not as successful with this final stimulation approach. On 3/2/85, the baseline measures were collected. The tasks involved a vowel prolongation as abnormal nasal airflow emission was measured and rated both with the See-Scape apparatus (BH_{11a}) and through perceptual judgments of associated hypernasal resonance (BH_{11b}). As shown, on 3/2/85 the baseline scores were 6.66 and 5.66, respectively. Treatments were begun, during which a tongue depressor was used to simulate the effects of a palatal-lift appliance as vowel prolongations were rehearsed. The patient failed to achieve the target criteria after 70 trials, when the program was terminated.

Because of these and the aforementioned disappointing results with the subsequent regimen, we pursued prosthetic intervention as the next alternative. Results of that approach are presented as follows.

Prosthetic Intervention Effect

Over the course of 3 weeks, the patient was successfully fitted with a palatal-lift appliance. Three adjustments in the length, upper torque, and width were made, with a 5-day adaptation period between each modification. These adjustments were governed by the results of clinical speech aerodynamic and perceptual re-evaluations, which revealed whether additional alterations were needed to effect a tighter velopharyngeal fit. That the final fitting neither completely eliminated excess nasal airflow nor normalized intraoral air pressurization for speech purposes was not an unexpected result in view of the underlying moderate degree of neuromuscular involvement. However, the clinical result was considered to be very good. On all post-treatment measurements, the patient demonstrated at least 75 percent improvement over baseline speech aerodynamic scores. Follow-up videofluorographic analyses revealed that the prosthetic fit anteroposteriorly was anatomically as tight as possible. The residual degrees of abnormal nasal airflow and reduced intraoral air pressure were attributed to the sphincteric incompetency of the lateral pharyngeal walls, which failed in their mesial movements to compress the borders of the elevated palate for sufficient velopharyngeal closure.

Attempts to create a better lateral fit were met with continuous failure. The patient ultimately began to show intolerance as each width adjustment caused more physical discomfort than the preceding unsuccessful one. We settled for the less than ideal result, looking back to the exercise regimen with anticipation that those behavioral treatments might now prove more fruitful than when they were originally administered.

It is important to note here that the patient complained of excess salivation when wearing the lift. Coupled with her faulty tongue control for swallowing, this side effect caused a mild drooling problem. At that time, the patient was merely instructed to try to swallow as often as possible, especially when consciously she perceived a build-up of saliva in her mouth that was about to cause an episode of drooling. She was assured, however erroneous the information was, that once we began to focus on improving her tongue and lip control, the drooling would probably become less of a problem. Also calming was the advice that this side effect is quite common, and that after an adaptation period of a month or so the palatal glands would accommodate to the presence of the lift by secreting less saliva.

It was unfortunate that these predictions did not prove accurate for the patient. She struggled with the drooling problem throughout the intervention program despite the moderate degree of success later achieved with tongue and lip treatments. What to do about this stigmatizing and potentially unhygienic problem was unclear to this clinician at the time. Such ignorance was ultimately at the great expense of the patient. Although she continued to wear the lift, because it facilitated speech improvement, it was evident that she did so reluctantly and with discomfort. Today the approach to this problem would be quite different. The patient would be familiarized with clinical options to reduce the drooling. These would include various surgical procedures that aim at rerouting or interfering with salivary gland secretions, and pharmaceutical prescriptions that produce a "dry-mouth" effect. These procedures, if successful, can wholly influence the primary treatment outcomes, making the therapeutic experience that much more rewarding and long lasting.

The patient was readministered the Behavioral Management treatment paradigm, beginning with the second activity, nonspeech intraoral air pressure generation exercises, and continuing through the entire sequence of activities. Although she did not achieve the criterion set for any one of the activities, the presence of the lift dramatically improved all baseline performances, and moderate degrees of additional improvement were yet accomplished throughout the experimental exercise programs. Her speech resonation perceptual ratings at the completion of this set of treatments averaged 2.6 on the 1 to 7 interval scale, which proved to be more than a 50 percent improvement over original baseline measures. It was hoped that this mild degree of hypernasality and the associated nasal airflow and intraoral air pressure difficulties that remained would improve further when the coexistent articulation subsystem disturbances became the focus of treatment. Of course, the extent to which the patient's progressive disability may eventually overtake the results achieved with such treatments is impossible to know in advance.

The suggested reading list provides sources to which clinicians can turn for additional information on the resonation subsystem.

SUGGESTED READINGS

Dworkin, J. P., & Johns, D. F. (1980). Management of velopharyngeal incompetence in dysarthria: A historical review. *Clinical Otolaryngology, 5,* 61–74.

Dworkin, J. P., & Nadal, J. C. (1991). Nonsurgical treatment of drooling in a patient with closed head injury and severe dysarthria. *Dysphagia, 6,* 40–49.

Gonzales, J. B., & Aronson, A. E. (1970). Palatal lift prosthesis for treatment of anatomic and neurological palatopharyngeal insufficiency. *Cleft Palate Journal, 7,* 91–104.

Johns, D. F. (1985). Surgical and prosthetic management of velopharyngeal incompetency in dysarthria. In D. F. Johns (Ed.), *Clinical management of neurogenic communicative disorders* (pp. 153–177). San Diego, CA: College-Hill Press.

Netsell, R., & Daniel, B. (1979). Dysarthria in adults: Physiologic approach to rehabilitation. *Archives of Physical Medicine and Rehabilitation, 60,* 502–508.

Schweiger, J., Netsell, R., & Sommerfield, R. (1970). Prosthetic management and speech improvement in individuals with dysarthria of the palate. *Journal of The American Dental Association, 80,* 1348–1353.

Shprintzen, R. J., McCall, G. N., & Skolnick, M. L. (1975). A new therapeutic technique for the treatment of velopharyngeal incompetency. *Journal of Speech and Hearing Disorders, 40,* 69–83.

Chapter 5

Treatment of the Phonation Subsystem

POTENTIAL PATIENTS

Voice motor control difficulty is exhibited by most dysarthric and some apractic patients and usually coexists with an assortment of respiration, resonation, articulation, and/or prosody subsystem disturbances. There are, however, as many different types of disordered voice as there are dysarthric and apractic patients who may present with such difficulty. Generally speaking, these types may be clustered into two primary groups: (1) those that are characterized largely by relatively consistent and predictable perceptual/acoustic abnormalities and (2) those with variable, fluctuating, and unpredictable features. Within the former group we may discover spastic, flaccid, and hypokinetic dysarthric patients. The latter group is usually composed of ataxic and hyperkinetic dysarthric patients but may occasionally include those with apraxia of speech. Although it is convenient to group these populations relative to the general types of voice difficulties they may present, even among those patients within the same group there are many symptomatic differences that warrant brief reviews prior to delving into specific treatment recommendations.

Group 1 Patients

Those with spastic dysarthria typically have a strained-strangled voice quality, periodic arrests of phonation, short phrases, and monoloud and monopitch characteristics, owing to hyperadduction, weakness, and paresis of the vocal folds, bilaterally. These features rarely occur in isolation; that is, without coexistent speech subsystem disorders.

Flaccid dysarthric patients will have significant voice problems if the tenth (Vagus) cranial nerve is damaged at any point along its pathway from the origin in the brain stem to the laryngeal musculature. The degree of associated voice difficulty will depend upon the lesion site and whether such involvement is unilateral, bilateral, partial, or complete. Bilateral complete lesions cause total paralysis, weakness, and hypoadduction of the vocal folds, which result in whispered phonation. At risk for aspiration pneumonia, the patient with this history may require tracheostomy or vocal fold augmentation. Bilateral incomplete lesions usually result in an extremely breathy-hoarse, wet-gurgly vocal quality with associated reductions in pitch range and loudness contours, and short phrases. When a unilateral tenth nerve lesion occurs, depending upon the severity of involvement, the paralyzed vocal fold tends to yield a mild to moderate degree of hoarseness, occasional diplophonia, and pitch and loudness restrictions. Generally, when lesions of the Vagus nerve(s) occur within or just outside the brain stem, above the separation of its three primary divisions—(1) pharyngeal, (2) superior laryngeal, and (3) recurrent laryngeal—all those muscles supplied by these nerve branches will be weak and paretic: (1) levator veli palatini, important for velopharyngeal closure and oral-nasal resonance balance; (2) cricothyroid, an extrinsic laryngeal component that chiefly regulates pitch variations; and (3) the intrinsic laryngeal group that enable overall voice motor activities. The patient with such a lesion will probably exhibit both resonation and phonation disturbances. An extracranial lesion of the recurrent branch only, which may occur as a consequence of neck trauma or surgery, generally causes weakness and paresis of the vocal folds themselves. Paradoxically, when this type of lesion is bilateral the vocal folds tend to be fixed in a tightly adducted position, owing to the stretching and adducting effects of the preserved cricothyroid musculature. The voice, consequently, may remain within normal limits, but inhalatory stridor may be produced because the airway is compromised by the narrow glottis. A focal, unilateral, recurrent laryngeal nerve lesion, however, results in a mild to moderate hoarse-breathy quality with coincident loudness and pitch variation disturbances. Flaccid dysphonias may also be observed in patients with myasthenia gravis as well as those with muscular dystrophy. Most often patients with flaccid dysarthria suffer from coexisting articulatory, resonatory, phonatory, and prosodic disturbances, owing to multiple cranial nerve lesions.

Hypokinetic (parkinsonian) dysarthric patients most often present with the characteristics of monopitch, monoloudness, reduced loudness, and harsh-breathy vocal quality, owing to laryngeal and respiratory musculature rigidity and limited range and speed of movements. These phonation subsystem features usually occur in concert with a host of articulatory and prosodic abnormalities, which implicate the orofacial musculature in the differential diagnosis.

Group 2 Patients

Those with ataxic dysarthria may present with hoarse-harsh vocal quality, sudden and irregular loudness and pitch outbursts, and coarse vocal tremor, owing largely to clumsy, incoordinated, and tremorous laryngeal musculature contractions. Similar involvement of the respiratory subsystem usually compounds the dysphonia.

There are quick, slow, and tremor forms of hyperkinetic dysarthria, all of which are characterized, in part, by fluctuating voice abnormalities. Under the "quick" rubric we find patients with Huntington's disease (chorea). The voice motor control difficulties of this population include harsh-strained quality, intermittent breathiness, irregular pitch alterations, occasional arrests of phonation, monopitch, excessive loudness variations, and monoloudness, owing to sudden, involuntary, random, and jerky movements of the laryngeal (and respiratory) musculature. Under the "slow" rubric we discover athetoid patients and those with focal oropharyngeal dyskinesia. The latter patient typically exhibits variably strained-strangled, hoarse-breathy vocal quality, periodic arrests of phonation, excessive loudness variations, monopitch, and episodic inhalatory stridor, owing to uncontrollably slow, undulating, twisting, spasmodic, and involuntary abductor-adductor laryngeal (and supraglottal) musculature contractions. The athetoid patient tends to exhibit similar abnormal voice patterns with associated writhing, and interruptive movements of the head, neck, trunk, and limb musculature. Under the "tremor" rubric there exist patients with essential (organic) voice tremor, although some clinical researchers might place these patients in group 1, and those with laryngeal myoclonus. These patients exhibit rhythmic fluctuations or alterations in loudness, ranging from 4 to 13 Hz, with associated quavering of intonational patterns, monopitch, strained-harsh vocal quality, and episodic laryngospasms and arrests of phonation. These vocal characteristics are due to synchronous tremors of the abductory-adductory laryngeal musculature, which are most evident during vowel prolongations and may occur in concert with additional orofacial and/or limb tremors. Most patients with hyperkinetic dysarthria, irrespective of the form, usually present with co-occurring articulation, phonation, prosody, and/or respiration subsystem disturbances that collectively impair speech motor intelligibility.

Apraxia of phonation has not received much attention in the clinical literature, notwithstanding its presence in some apractic patients. Characterized as a fluctuating or variable condition, this type of dysphonia may range from virtual mutism to inconsistent aphonia (whispered speech) to intermittent pitch and loudness outbursts (squeal-like) to relatively good phonation, owing to difficulty with motor planning of laryngeal (and respiratory) musculature activities during volitional speech efforts. Coexisting speech apraxia and oral (nonspeech) apraxia are almost always evident in these patients.

Note that multifocal lesions may cause mixed forms of motor speech disorders. Any resultant dysphonia usually reflects the characteristic neuromuscular and/or motor planning deficits of the specific components involved in the mixture. Recently, a 22-year-old patient emerged from a severe closed head injury with signs and symptoms of spastic dysarthria mixed with apraxias of speech and phonation. The spastic-flaccid dysarthria of amyotrophic lateral sclerosis is another example of a mixture that may be observed in clinical practice. Table 5–1 provides a synopsis of the differential laryngeal-phonatory features associated with motor speech disorders. (See Chapter 1 for a detailed review of all these disorders.)

TABLE 5–1. Differential Laryngeal-Phonatory Features in Patients with Motor Speech Disorders

Disorder	Voice Characteristics	Laryngeal Pathophysiology	Lesion Site(s)
Spastic dysarthria	*Relatively constant and predictable:* Strained-strangled quality, periodic arrests of phonation, short phrases, monoloudness, and monopitch	Hyperadduction, weakness and paresis of vocal folds, bilaterally	Bilateral corticobulbar tracts of pyramidal system
Flaccid dysarthria	*Relatively Stable:* Hoarse-breathy quality, reduced pitch and loudness range, short phrases, diplophonia, and inhalatory stridor	Hypoadduction, weakness and paralysis of vocal folds, unilaterally, bilaterally, incomplete or complete	Tenth cranial nerve (Vagus), unilaterally or bilaterally anywhere along its course from brainstem to musculature
Hypokinetic dysarthria	*Predictable:* Harsh-breathy quality, monopitch, and reduced loudness	Rigidity and hypokinesia of vocal folds	Substantia nigra of extrapyramidal system
Ataxic dysarthria	*Variable:* Hoarse-harsh quality, sudden and irregular loudness and pitch outbursts, and coarse tremor	Incoordination and intention tremors of vocal folds	Bilateral, generalized cerebellar structures
Quick (chorea) hyperkinetic dysarthria	*Random:* Harsh-strained quality, intermittent breathiness, irregular pitch alterations, arrests of phonation, monopitch, excessive loudness variations and monoloudness	Involuntary, uncontrollable, jerky, and hyperkinetic vocal fold behaviors	Basal ganglia of extrapyramidal system
Slow (dystonia, dyskinesia, athetosis) hyperkinetic dysarthria	*Unpredictable:* Strained-strangled, hoarse-breathy quality, aperiodic arrests of phonation, excessive loudness variations, monopitch, and stridor	Involuntary, uncontrollable slow, undulating, twisting, writhing, spasmodic vocal fold behaviors	Disseminated extrapyramidal structures
Tremor (essential, myoclonous) hyperkinetic dysarthria	*Rhythmic fluctuations or alterations:* in loudness, quavering intonation, monopitch, strained-harsh quality, and episodic laryngospasms with arrests of phonation	Synchronous tremors of abductory-adductory vocal fold musculature	Variable extrapyramidal locations, including cerebral pathways, dentate nucleus, red nucleus, inferior olive, restiform body, and striatum
Apraxia of speech (phonation)	*Inconsistent and intermittent:* Mutism, whispered speech, pitch and loudness outbursts (squeals), and periods of good phonation	Faulty motor planning of vocal fold behaviors during volitional speech efforts	Inferolateral posterior frontal lobe (Broca's area) of language dominant (L) cerebral hemisphere

PRIMARY FOCUS AND GENERAL PRINCIPLES OF VOICE THERAPY

This chapter concentrates on strategies of intervention for neurologic voice disorders. Whereas the bulk of our focus will be on behavioral management techniques, those that may be administered in the usual clinical environment, alternative surgical and pharmaceutical treatments for these disorders will also be discussed, but in less detail.

Irrespective of the types of treatments that are ultimately employed, the objectives generally remain the same: To improve voice motor control and output so that the end result meets the realistic overall needs of the patient and facilitates treatments and performances of the other speech subsystems. Rarely should the achievement of normal voice be the treatment goal. Most patients must learn to settle for much less, especially those with severe pretreatment conditions.

In Chapter 2, a recommended sequence of speech subsystem treatments was discussed. Recall that when respiration and resonation subsystem impairments occur, usually in patients with spastic dysarthria, flaccid dysarthria, and mixed dysarthria containing either or both a spastic and a flaccid component, first-order treatment priority was suggested. The second order of treatment was ascribed to disturbances of the phonation subsystem presented by most dysarthric and some apractic patients. The third, and generally last, order of treatment was to be reserved for the articulation and prosody subsystem difficulties that virtually all patients with motor speech disorders exhibit. Because all patients, even those with the same general diagnosis, do not struggle with identical sets or degrees of speech subsystem disturbances, this recommended treatment hierarchy must be modified to meet the individual differences that prevail in the real clinical world.

As reviewed in Chapters 3 and 4 and illustrated in Table 5–2, when the pa-

TABLE 5–2. Recommended Sequence of Treatments for Commonly Co-occurring Speech Subsystem Impairments in Patients with Motor Speech Disorders

Motor Speech Disorder	Degree of Voice Disturbance	Respiration	Resonation	Phonation	Articulation	Prosody
Spastic dysarthria	Mild	First	First	Second	Second	Third
	Moderate-severe	First	First	Second	Third	Fourth
Flaccid dysarthria	Mild	First	First	Second	Second	Third
	Moderate-severe	First	First	Second	Third	Fourth
Hypokinetic dysarthria	Mild	First	N/A	First	Second	Second
	Moderate-severe	First	N/A	Second	Third	Fourth
Ataxic dysarthria	Mild	First	N/A	First	Second	Second
	Moderate-severe	First	N/A	Second	Third	Fourth
Quick and slow hyperkinetic dysarthria	Mild	First	N/A	First	Second	Second
	Moderate-severe	First	N/A	Second	Third	Fourth
Tremor hyperkinetic dysarthria	Mild	N/A	N/A	First	N/A	N/A
	Moderate-severe	N/A	N/A	First	N/A	N/A
Apraxia of speech	Mild	N/A	N/A	First	Second	Second
	Moderate-severe	N/A	N/A	First	Second	Third

tient presents with respiration and resonation subsystem disturbances, this clinician has discovered that it is almost always most efficient and productive to direct treatments first at these subsystems, regardless of the degree of these disturbances or the existence of other speech subsystem difficulties. If phonation subsystem deficits remain after such treatments they are most effectively treated next in sequence. However, if either respiration or resonation treatment is not indicated, as may be true for patients with hypokinetic, ataxic, and quick and slow forms of hyperkinetic dysarthria, and if the voice difficulty is only mild, then voice therapy may be bumped up to the first order of clinical focus, along with treatment of the respiration (or resonation) subsystem. If neither respiration nor resonation subsystem treatments are indicated, as is probable for patients with the tremorous form of hyperkinetic dysarthria and apraxia of phonation, then the existing voice difficulty, whether mild, moderate, or severe, should be treated first. Also note in Table 5–2 that when the voice disorder is only mild but treatment is not administered until the second order following treatments of the respiration and resonation subsystems (as may be indicated for patients with spastic dysarthria, flaccid dysarthria, or both), then articulation subsystem treatments may be introduced simultaneously on the second order of the sequence hierarchy. Finally, with the exceptions of essential (organic) voice tremor patients and those with apraxia of phonation, for whom voice therapy may be ordered first, other patients with moderate to severe degrees of phonation subsystem disturbances will probably benefit most if such therapy is held in abeyance until antecedent respiration and/or resonation treatments have first been administered and terminated.

This general guide to treatment sequencing was developed over the years by this clinician through trial-and-error experiences with many patients. Tampering with this sequence has led to several disappointing clinical results. Retrospective analyses of these outcomes sprouted the theory that success in voice therapy depends not only upon the specific techniques employed and the patient's prognosis and desire for improvement but upon the timing of the intervention as well. Clinical failures are not always consequences of bad therapy or limited patient potential or motivation. Oftentimes, even clinically sound techniques are unsuccessful because they are administered either too early or too late in the sequence of treatments. In other words, these treatments may be instituted at a time either when the patient may not have been physiologically prepared to benefit most from the applications because of yet untreated subsystem disturbances that interfere with the possibility of success, or when the patient's last ounces of motivation and hope have been drained by a series of other unsuccessful treatments, whether they were administered in the proper sequence or not. Whether clinicians choose to follow the step-by-step treatment recommendations suggested below or prefer merely to adopt some of the procedures as adjuncts to a treatment regimen with which they are more comfortable, the exercises that follow should improve the overall results of voice motor control treatment. Additionally, if the administration methodology is similarly adopted, clinicians will have the means by which to measure the effects of the specific techniques they ultimately select to assist their patients.

SURGICAL INTERVENTION

With the exception of specific muscle augmentation, repositioning, and nerve resection procedures, which are prescribed for a very small percentage of dysarthric patients, there are no known effective methods of surgical treatment of neurogenic voice disorders. Most patients are dependent upon direct therapy, prescription drugs, time, or all three for any voice improvements they may achieve. Even those patients for whom surgical options may be available as "elective" treatment procedures should not be rushed to operating rooms without first submitting them to intensive, viable alternative treatments to establish the need for surgery. What constitutes "intensive" and "viable" ought to be left to the discretion of both the clinician and the surgeon, but it will vary from patient to patient, depending upon the severity of the problem and the therapy-response curve. Let's review the surgical treatment options.

Vocal Fold Augmentation

A commonly employed surgical approach to neurogenic voice disorders in which there is incomplete vocal fold adduction is the *injection of Teflon (polytetrafluoroethylene) paste, collagen, or a Teflon-glycerin suspension* into the paretic vocal fold. This technique was first introduced by Arnold in 1962; since then it has become the standard treatment for this condition. These substances increase the bulk of the pathologic vocal fold, which may be fixed in either the abducted or the paramedian position, and thereby augment glottal closure during voice production by making it easier for the unaffected fold to achieve contact near or across the midline. Some patients, however, end up with worse voices postsurgically, either as a consequence of the injected material itself, a result of faulty surgical approaches (such as improper sites or amounts of injection), or because these patients were poor candidates for the operation initially. A recent patient of this clinician illustrates well this last important point.

Illustrative Case No. 1.   At the age of 25 years, VR was involved in a motorcycle accident and received a moderate-severe closed head injury. In addition to multiple limb, chest, and facial bone fractures, which were successfully treated, the patient was left with numerous cognitive, language, perceptual, psychoemotional, and limb, trunk, and speech motor control disturbances. Four years after this incident, he continued with his pursuits of multidisciplinary rehabilitation treatments on an outpatient basis. His speech diagnosis was mixed ataxic-hypokinetic dysarthria, and he exhibited a mild-moderate degree of bowing of the right vocal fold. Articulation and prosody difficulties were predictably characteristic of the abnormal neuromuscular mixture he presented in the speech subsystems, and phonation was hoarse-harsh with intermittent pitch breaks and reduced loudness variations. Despite direct voice therapy, including use of the Visi-Pitch, electroglottograph, and video-strobolaryngoscope for vocal fold and voice activity feedback, VR failed to make observable gains over the course of more than 15 sessions.

Experimentation with manual compression of the right side of his neck in the region of the thyroid lamina as he attempted phonation revealed marked improvements in voice quality, pitch, and loudness controls. Stroboscopic examination of vocal fold activity during manual compression helped explain these improvements, as it was clearly evident that the right vocal fold was artificially displaced toward the midline of the glottis, enabling relatively good contact and myoelastic-aerodynamic relations with the opposing vocal fold. After numerous replications of these effects using the same external compression technique, the treatment team, including an otolaryngologist, decided that he was a good candidate for permanent right vocal fold augmentation surgery using Teflon paste.

The operation was a technical success in that the patient tolerated the procedure without complication, and weekly laryngeal examinations over a 6 week postoperative course revealed excellent anatomical results. It is unfortunate that VR's voice was moderately worse across all characteristic parameters. He continued with thrice-weekly voice therapy sessions, each lasting roughly 1 hour, hoping that routine exercises and the biofeedback techniques that were incorporated earlier in the treatment program might now prove more advantageous than had been the case prior to surgery, but to no avail. After 15 sessions, his voice remained unimproved. The quality was severely hoarse-harsh and was now laced with intermittent periods of strained-strangled phonation; the pitch averaged 90 Hz, which was approximately 30 Hz lower than his presurgical fundamental. However, episodes of pitch breaks to the upside persisted, and no gains in loudness control were evident. Needless to say, the patient was dejected and prepared to forego the articulation and prosody subsystem treatments scheduled next, for fear of yet additional disappointing results. He was persuaded not to extrapolate failure at the phonation subsystem treatment level to the other subsystems, albeit the advice to press on was with the understanding that it was impossible to predict the extent to which we might overcome or compensate for such failure as we moved ahead in the treatment plan. That the prognosis for later improvements had to be down-graded was reluctantly accepted by the patient.

The treatment team hypothesized that the poor surgical effect could be safely attributed to the underlying laryngeal pathophysiologic condition, inasmuch as from an anatomical point of view the surgery was a success. The right vocal fold no longer suffered from significant bowing and consequently was in a much improved glottal position for vibratory synchrony with the left fold. Why then was VR's voice not only unimproved, but worse? Technically, most patients for whom this operation is prescribed possess an uninvolved intact opposing vocal fold, which can work in concert with the newly designed injected fold for good speech aerodynamic results. VR presented with significant glottal insufficiency because of bowing of the right vocal fold, which simulated unilateral paralysis and prompted consideration of the Teflon paste surgical procedure, but the pathophysiology of this condition was not isolated to the right vocal fold. Rather, underlying this condition was widespread bilateral laryngeal incoordination and hypotonia, consistent with his overall cerebellar-ataxic neuromuscular profile, compounded by a coexistent mixture of hypokinetic-rigidity of the phonation subsystem. It seemed reasonable to conclude that the increased mass of the right vocal fold, accomplished with injection of Teflon paste, created an intolerable load effect that actually exacerbated vibratory incoordination. In retrospect, whereas the patient appeared on the surface to be an excellent candidate for the surgery performed, his neurologic status was a potential contraindication that received little or no consideration presurgically. More than 1 year after the procedure, VR continued to struggle with voice motor control.

Thyroplasty. Introduced initially by Isshiki in 1974, this technique involves use of an alloplastic implant in the thyroid cartilage aimed at displacing medially the paralyzed vocal fold to improve contact with the opposing, uninvolved fold for improved voice production. Although difficult and expensive to perform, this surgical procedure has recently been praised to yield even better results than Teflon injection.

Nerve Transfer. Dating back to the mid-1920s, this surgical treatment for vocal fold paralysis recently involved the ansa cervicalis (hypoglossi)–recurrent laryngeal nerve anastomosis approach, which yielded excellent voice results. If necessary, the reinnervated vocal fold can be injected with Teflon, gelfoam, or other substances to augment the voice effect.

Botulinum A Toxin Injection. In the last few years, various forms of spastic (spasmodic) dysphonia, spasmodic torticollis, and dystonia have been experimentally treated using the toxin from *Clostridium botulinum*. When the toxin is injected transcutaneously or intraorally into the laryngeal musculature, it blocks the release of acetylcholine from the surrounding motor nerve end plates, binds to the muscle membrane, and induces focal flaccid paralysis without the apparent complication of systemic toxicity. These effects are sought to decrease laryngeal spasms and improve vocal quality. Still considered to be in the research stage of development, this procedure may need to be repeated every 3 to 6 months or as needed, as spasmodic muscle activity may return. As with other elective surgical techniques, patients should not be encouraged to give serious consideration to this procedure until and unless alternative treatments, including voice and drug therapy applications, have been less than successful.

Nerve Resection

In the mid-1970s, resection of one recurrent laryngeal nerve was developed as a treatment for intractable adductor spastic dysphonia. Theoretically, the surgically induced vocal fold paralysis would relieve or reduce the laryngospasms and strained-strangled voice characteristic of this disorder. Although initial results of this surgical technique are often encouraging, with time a large percentage of such patients experience recurrence of the laryngeal symptoms and signs. In those patients in whom recurrence of laryngospasms has been reported, factors such as partial muscle reinnervation, hyperactivity of supraglottic structures, and exaggerated adductor muscle activity on the nonsurgical side have been suggested as possible causes. With the advent and reported success of botulinum toxin therapy for select patients with spasmodic dysphonia, nerve resection is used less frequently.

PHARMACEUTICAL INTERVENTION

There are no pharmacologic agents prescribed specifically to treat neurologic voice disorders. Many patients with such difficulties, however, are placed on certain drugs to relieve their overall pathophysiologic symptoms, and voice motor control may improve as a secondary effect of such medication. A differential review of the pharmaceutical approaches to the neurologic diseases that frequently cause motor speech disorders may therefore prove interesting and potentially relevant.

Patients with the *hypokinetic signs of parkinsonism* often benefit from medication that acts to restore striatal dopamine deficiency. In the early to middle stages of the disease, levodopa is often combined with carbidopa (Sinemet), which is an inhibitory drug that blocks the conversion of levodopa to dopamine outside of the subcortex. If and when patients do not respond to this treatment approach, subsequent therapy may include adding a dopamine agonist such as bromocriptine (Parlodel), particularly when the symptoms of tremor and bradykinesia become more pronounced. When the response to medication is good, the patient may demonstrate more fluid and controllable motor behaviors, which may include those of the speech mechanism. However, such improvements do not necessarily eliminate the need for physical, occupational, and speech-language intervention. It should be noted that patients with parkinsonism due to multiple infarcts or associated with other progressive symptoms and signs usually do not respond to dopaminergic therapy.

Patients who present with quick *hyperkinetic symptoms, including those of Huntington's disease,* may experience some early relief with drugs that modify the effects of dopamine. These may include agents that (1) inhibit the neuronal uptake and storage of dopamine, such as a combination of lithium (Lithobid) and tetrabenozine (Nitoman); (2) interfere with the activity of dopamine receptors, such as drugs generically classified as phenothiazine neuroleptics, including haloperidol (Haldol) and chlorpromazine (Thorazine); and (3) have a sedating effect on choreiform movements, such as those drugs in the benzodiazepines class, including diazepam (Valium) and clonazepam (Klonopin). These treatments may provide symptomatic support and therefore reduce the degree of hyperkinesis, allowing for concentrated physical and speech therapy exercises with less uncontrollable, interruptive movement phenomena.

The *slow hyperkinesis of dyskinesia and dystonia* is often treated for symptomatic relief with high doses of anticholinergic agents. These include any of the following drugs: (1) trihexyphenidyl (Artane), (2) ethopropazine (Parsidol), and (3) benzotropine (Cogentin). If any one of these medications prove unsuccessful, another class of drugs is usually attempted, including the antispasticity drug baclofen (Lioresal) or one of the aforementioned agents, Sinemet or Valium. Note that those drugs with neuroleptic actions, such as Haldol, may not be indicated because they tend to substitute parkinsonian symptoms and signs or produce dyskinetic states, both of which can be considered tardive and drug induced in nature. Those patients who experience a reduction in these hyperkinetic movements, as a consequence of successful drug action, may realize some improvement in voice motor potential.

The beta-adrenergic (blocker) agent propranolol (Inderal) has received wide acceptance as the drug of choice to relieve limb symptoms of *essential tremor,* but the laryngeal signs and symptoms have not been as responsive to such treatment.

Those patients with *strained-strangled phonation of spastic dysarthria,* due to widespread hypertonicity and weakness of the speech subsystems, may be placed on muscle relaxation or antispasticity medication. There is a paucity of evidence, however, that such drugs significantly influence the performances of these subsystems. Dantrolene sodium (Dantrium) was prescribed (12 mg four times daily) for a former patient with severe spasticity involving virtually the entire musculoskeletal system, including the speech mechanism; this resulted in significant reduction of spasticity. Further, the perceptual degree of strained-strangled vocal quality with drug therapy alone shifted downward from a severe mean rating of 6.5 to a moderate rating of 5.0 on the 1 to 7 interval scale. The relative change considerably enhanced the patient's voice motor profile.

To relieve or decrease the *intensity of intention tremors in patients with ataxia,* the beta-blocker drugs clonazepam (Klonopin) and propranolol (Inderal) have been used with success. The degrees to which ataxic voice symptoms respond to this treatment approach have not been diligently studied. Informal observations of ataxic dysarthric patients have highlighted the positive secondary effects that these drugs can have on the overall performances of the speech subsystems.

The *flaccid dysarthria due to myasthenia gravis* may respond favorably to the anticholinesterase drug pyridostigmine (Mestinon), especially if the patient is in the initial stage of the disease. The long-term effects of this drug on associated dysarthria are not well understood, however. When this medication is effective, the patient may experience voice improvement.

Although there are no pharmacologic agents that can cure neurologic voice disorders, there are medications that may yield positive perhaps secondary effects on the control, coordination, and output of the phonation subsystem. Thus, the use and influence of appropriate medications should be considered in conjunction with a behavioral voice therapy program. Before proceeding with detailed descriptions of voice therapy techniques, note that Table 5–3 summarizes the surgical and pharmacologic approaches that have been found to promote either direct or indirect improvements in voice motor control.

TABLE 5–3. Laryngeal Surgical and Pharmacologic Interventions for Neurogenic Voice Disorders

Types of Voice Disorders (Populations)	Laryngeal Surgical Intervention Techniques			Classes of Pharmacologic Agents Prescribed						
	VOCAL FOLD AUGMENTATION	BOTULINUM TOXIN INJECTION	RECURRENT NERVE RESECTION	DOPAMINERGICS	CHOLINERGICS (DOPAMINE BLOCKERS)	NEUROLEPTICS	SEDATIVES	BETA-BLOCKERS	ANTISPASTICITY AGENTS (MUSCLE-RELAXANTS)	ANTICHOLINERGICS
Flaccid dysphonia										
1. Unilateral adductor paralyses	X									
2. Bilateral adductor paralyses										
3. Myasthenia gravis										X
Spastic dysphonia										
1. Pseudobulbar palsy		X	X						X	
Ataxic dysphonia								X		
Hyperkinetic dysphonia										
1. Huntington's disease					X	X				
2. Dystonia				X		X	X		X	X
3. Essential tremor							X	X		
Hypokinetic dysphonia										
1. Parkinsonism				X						X
Apraxia of phonation										

144

VOICE THERAPY TECHNIQUES

It might be argued that unless the neurogenic voice disorder is disruptive of speech intelligibility, treatment is not indicated. This view is discouraged here. Speech intelligibility should not be the only yardstick used to measure whether or not dysfunctioning of the phonation subsystem merits clinical attention. Many dysarthric and apractic patients with voice disorders have benefited from voice therapy. This includes even those patients who may have experienced some success with the aforementioned surgical and drug treatment options.

Not unlike the resonation subsystem, the phonation subsystem is particularly difficult to manage with behavioral exercises, regardless of the severity of the underlying pathophysiology. Thus, when a patient is judged ready to receive such intervention, the general rule of thumb found useful by this clinician calls for the discontinuation of a given exercise if after 30 consecutive trials the patient fails to demonstrate any observable trend of improvement over the baseline level. Clinicians may find that moving on to the next exercise indicated in the treatment hierarchy may forestall potential frustration, even though the prognosis for improvement on the subsequent, generally more difficult, task is not enhanced by failures at the previous level. As the new treatment is experimentally phased in, however, the same rule and rationale for discontinuation and advancement to the next exercise in the sequence ought to be adopted. When to proceed with the following exercise if the patient is showing improvement over the baseline level but is continuing to fall short of the criterion set for advancement cannot be predetermined. Clinicians must gauge each patient's potential for further gains on an individual basis. Whereas to stay the course with one patient may prove most beneficial, another patient who is similarly struggling may respond more favorably if the focus is shifted to the next exercise.

The charts shown in this subsection function as valuable aids in logging and tracking patient responses to the treatment administered. They also enable the clinician to demonstrate which techniques appear therapeutically effective, and which do not. Moreover, because nowadays most health practitioners operate within rather stringent guidelines relative to demonstrating accountability for services rendered, charts of baseline and treatment performances may prove very helpful. The Speech Characteristics Chart (see Figure 2–2) should be used both prior to (baseline) and intermittently during the voice therapy regimen to rate and record perceptual judgments of the patient's overall voice production. The comments section of the chart can provide useful space to specify liberally the most salient abnormal voice features that contributed to the baseline rating listed on the graph. The periodic ratings collected and charted throughout the exercise program administered enable subjective measurements of treatment efficacy. Of course, the frequency of these re-evaluations may depend upon the nature of the individual patient's voice disorder, his or her response to the exercises, and the methodology adopted to demonstrate treatment effects. The Phonation Subsystem Behavioral Treatment Chart (Figure 5–1) should be used exclusively

PHONATION SUBSYSTEM BEHAVIORAL TREATMENT CHART

Patient's name: _____

Birthdate: _____ Sex: _____

Speech diagnosis: _____

Medical diagnosis: _____

Clinician: _____

Facility: _____

Address: _____

ACTIVITY KEY

Feature:
1. Relaxation of extrinsic laryngeal musculature (R)
2. Yawn-sigh phonation (Y)
3. Vowel prolongations (V)
4. Speech trains (T)
5. Sentences (S)
6. Contextual speech (C)
7. Holding breath (H)

MEASUREMENT UNIT
7-point interval scale (1 = normal; 7 = most deviant)
7-point interval scale
7-point interval scale or % correct
7-point interval scale or % correct
7-point interval scale or % correct
7-point interval scale or % correct
No. of seconds

Feature:
8. Nonspeech vocal fold valving (N)
9. Phonatory vocal fold valving (P)
10. Hard attack phonation (A)
11. Voice motor planning (M)
12. Laryngeal timing and coordination (L)

MEASUREMENT UNIT
No. of seconds

7-point interval scale or no. of seconds
7-point interval scale or no. of seconds
% Correct
% Correct

Employment strategically treatments above (E + above symbol)

Baseline (pre-treatment): B + activity symbol

Comments: _____

Dates: _____

Average Score: 100, 90, 80, 70, 60, 50, 40, 30, 20, 10, 9, 8, 7, 6, 5, 4, 3, 2, 1, 0

No. of trials
Activity symbol
Unit of measure
Target criterion

SESSIONS

Figure 5–1. Phonation subsystem behavioral treatment chart to be used for tracking efficacy of voice exercises.

to track the patient's ongoing responses to illustrate when advancements within the program are indicated.

Note. In keeping with ethical and professional liability principles, it is usually best to consult with the attending physician before commencing with any voice therapy technique, irrespective of the underlying disorder.

Treatment Materials

The clinician will need to assemble the following materials in order to employ all of the exercises recommended in this subsection:

1. See-Scape device, (Figure 3–4),
2. Noseclip,
3. Tape recorder,
4. Metronome,
5. Stopwatch,
6. Transcervical electronic larynx,
7. Stethoscope,
8. Tiny mirror,
9. Cotton neckerchief,
10. Mini-microphone and speakers,
11. Box of facial tissues and drinking straws,
12. Speech Characteristics Chart (Figure 2–2), and
13. Phonation Subsystem Behavioral Treatment Chart (Figure 5–1)

Patterns of Vocal Fold Vibration Abnormalities

Earlier in this chapter, references were made to two primary groups of patients with neurologic voice disorders: (1) those whose voice problems are caused by relatively predictable and consistent patterns of vocal fold vibration abnormalities, and (2) those with vibratory patterns that are rather variable, fluctuating, and unpredictable. Recall that the first group consists of patients with spastic (at least the tremor and dysarthria voice forms), hypokinetic, and flaccid forms of dysphonia. With the latter two types, the underlying pathophysiologic condition produces *hypoadductory* vocal fold movements, which result in the voice symptoms previously described. Patients with adductor spastic dysphonia, on the other hand, exhibit *hyperadductory* vocal fold activities, which contribute largely to their abnormal voice symptoms. The second group of patients is composed of those with the ataxic, hyperkinetic, and apraxic forms of dysphonia. The pathophysiologic condition underlying these disorders generally produces *variable, hypoadductory/hyperadductory* vocal fold movement abnormalities. For the purpose of convenience, let's categorize and review the behavioral treatment packages that follow according to these abnormal vocal fold movement subtypes.

Note. Treatment techniques for loudness and pitch abnormalities will be reserved for the chapter on the prosody subsystem. The exercises laced through-out this chapter address mostly vocal "quality" disturbances.

Treatments of the Hyperadductory Laryngeal Mechanism

It is important to caution at the outset that the strained-strangled voice ex-hibited by many patients with spastic dysarthria, usually symptomatic of excess laryngeal tension and associated hyperadduction of the vocal folds, generally is quite resistant to any kind of treatment. The experiences of this clinician in treating the dysphonia of spastic dysarthria have been disappointing, particu-larly with regard to those patients whose symptoms exceeded mild degrees of in-volvement. Patients with this voice disorder are, however, usually entitled to a trial of voice therapy.

The overall objectives of the exercises in this subsection are to improve the quality of voice and increase the number of syllables produced per breath. These goals may be realized directly through exercises aimed at (1) facilitating relax-ation of any existing influential supralaryngeal muscular tension, (2) reducing vocal fold hyperadduction, and (3) improving voice output control. Because it may also be necessary and beneficial to employ indirect approaches (those compensa-tory phonation strategies that bypass the therapeutically nonresponsive laryn-geal mechanism), they too are included in the hierarchy of treatment alterna-tives presented next. Remember to enter a baseline perceptual rating of the patient's voice on the Speech Characteristics Chart for comparison with subse-quent periodic ratings throughout the exercises that follow.

Relaxation Exercise No. 1

Step 1. To bring about relaxation of hypertonic laryngeal musculature, as-pects of the "rag doll" exercise, prescribed earlier for respiration subsystem relax-ation, may be modified for help here. Prior to initiating this exercise, however, use the Phonation Subsystem Behavioral Treatment Chart (Figure 5–1) to rate the baseline impression of head and neck rigidity, making certain to use the ac-tivity symbol "BR$_1$" at the bottom of the column in which the recording is en-tered. Note that the y-axis should be treated as an equal-appearing interval scale for this rating, in which "7" represents the most severe degree of hypertonicity, and "1" signifies a state of normal tone. If the baseline rating proves to be within an acceptable range of normal, so that the relaxation exercise may be omitted from the treatment regimen, move on to Exercise no. 2.

Step 2. After the baseline rating, proceed in the following manner: First, stand behind the comfortably seated patient, and gently grasp both sides of his or her head. Second, instruct the patient to relax as much as possible so that the head can be passively manipulated into different positions. Third, gently pull the head backwards until the patient's chin is pointing up towards the ceiling, and hold that position to an out-loud count of 10. Fourth, upon completion of this count, smoothly glide the head forward so that the chin points toward the lap, and again count to 10. Fifth, upon completion of this count, pull the patient's head into the normal upright position, and then gradually twist it as far as possible to the right side for a count of 10, then bring it back to the midline and smoothly across to the far left side for another count of 10. Sixth, upon completion of this count, reposition the head in the midline position, and allow a 30-second rest period. On a notepad, use the seven-point scale to rate the overall degree of head and neck musculature hypertonicity perceived during the passive movements. Repeat this procedure until the degree of rigidity is at least three scale valves improved over the baseline rating or "1," if this rating was "2," "3," or "4," over 10 consecutive trials.

Step 3. After each set of 10 trials, enter the mean perceptual rating data in a separate column on the y-axis grid of the Phonation Subsystem Behavioral Treatment Chart, making certain to list the appropriate date of the session, number of trials (10), activity symbol (R_1), measurement unit (1 to 7), and target criterion (?) in the respective cells of the column. Once the patient achieves the criterion for this exercise, move on to Exercise no. 2. Remember that the next exercise should also be introduced if after 30 trials or more the prognosis is poor for accomplishing further gains or the criterion selected.

Relaxation Exercise No. 2

Step 1. Follow the exact same baseline procedure as that in Step 1 of the preceding exercise, using a separate column on the treatment chart for this rating. However, the symbol "BR_2" should be entered in the activity cell of the column, signifying that the rating rendered represents the baseline status of head and neck muscle tone prior to the second relaxation exercise.

Step 2. After administering the baseline rating, follow the exact same procedure as that in Step 2 of the preceding exercise, except that here all head manipulations are conducted to counts of 5, not 10, and they are repeated one full cycle before the 30-second rest period.

Step 3. When charting clusters of data collected, make certain that the activity symbol "R_2" is used in the cell at the bottom of the column in which the mean rating is recorded. Exercise no. 3 is to be introduced upon achievement of the criterion selected or when no further progress is anticipated if the current exercise were continued.

Relaxation Exercise No. 3

Step 1. Follow the exact same baseline procedure as that in Step 1 of Exercise no. 1, again using a separate column on the treatment chart for this rating. In the activity cell, the symbol "BR_3" will highlight that the rating rendered represents the baseline status of head and neck muscle tone prior to the third and final relaxation exercise.

Step 2. After this baseline rating, administer the exact same procedure as that in Step 2 of Exercise no. 1. However, here the aforementioned head manipulations should be conducted to counts of 2 in each position and should be repeated for five full cycles before a 30-second rest period is permitted.

Step 3. As in the previous two exercises, a 1 to 7 rating is rendered on a notepad with respect to the perceived degree of head and neck muscle tone. After each set of 10 trials, the mean perceptual rating is calculated and entered on the y-axis grid of the treatment chart in the column corresponding to the cells signifying the respective date of the session and activity symbol (R_3). The next exercise is indicated upon achievement of the criterion selected or when continuation of this exercise is considered counterproductive.

Yawn-Sigh Exercise No. 1

Step 1. Render a baseline perceptual rating of the patient's voice on the Speech Characteristics Chart for comparison with the previous similar rating(s) entered to date. If the hyperfunctional voice symptoms have not moderated to an acceptable level as a result of treatment administered thus far, advance to the next step.

Step 2. For reduction of vocal hyperadduction and its symptomatic effects on phonation during isolated sound and word productions the "yawn-sigh" approach to phonation is first recommended. This technique of voice intervention may be helpful in reducing vocal hyperfunction because yawning inherently relaxes any existing tension in the pharyngeal and laryngeal musculature. Prior to initiating this exercise use the Phonation Subsystem Behavioral Treatment Chart to rate the patient's overall baseline voice motor control producing all of the following isolated sound and word stimuli: (1) /i/, (2) /u/, (3) /o/, (4) /hi/, (5) /hu/, (6) /ho/, (7) /ʃi/, (8) /ʃu/, (9) /ʃo/, (10) /pi/, (11) /pu/, (12) /po/, (13) /mi/, (14) /mu/, (15) /mo/, (16) /si/, (17) /su/, (18) /so/, (19) /ipi/, (20) /upu/, (21) /opo/, (22) /iʃi/, (23) /uʃu/, (24) /oʃo/, (25) /imi/, (26) /umu/, (27) /omo/, (28) /ihi/, (29) /uhu/, (30) /oho/, (31) /isi/, (32) /usu/, and (33) /oso/. It is important to note that for those patients who are unable to articulate all these stimuli with any degree of precision, a modified or even different list can be constructed for their practice. Most patients, however, should be capable of working with the items recommended. Even moderate to severe articulatory imprecision is acceptable, provided that the patient can be focused therapeutically on phonation. The stimuli may be written on index cards and presented to the patient for recitation and/or they may be verbally demonstrated by the clinician, followed by patient repetition.

Step 3. The overall rating rendered should conform to the rules of the aforementioned seven-point equal-appearing interval scale. In a separate column on the treatment chart, enter the 1 to 7 rating of the degree and characteristic symptoms of vocal hyperfunction on the y-axis grid, making certain to list the appropriate date and activity symbol (BY[1]) in the respective cells of the column. This symbol represents the baseline status of vocal fold hyperadduction prior to the easy onset of phonation exercises. If the baseline rating is within an acceptable range of normal, skip this exercise and advance to the next one.

Step 4. Demonstrate for the patient a slow inspiratory yawn with a wide-open mouth posture, followed by a prolonged expiratory sigh accompanied by soft phonation of the vowel /aː/. Focus the patient on the breathy, relaxed, low-volume voice result. After four or five demonstrations, the yawn component of the exercise is faded out so that each new demonstration consists of a normal inspiration followed by prolonged sigh phonation of the vowel. After several demonstrations of this approach, the sigh is faded and replaced by less breathy phonation that strives to approximate normal quality. The clinician should alternate the vowels used during these demonstrations.

Step 5. A tape recorder should be used so that the patient can listen to the responses intermittently throughout the exercise for auditory feedback. Instruct the patient to attempt the yawn-sigh maneuver beginning with the vowel /i/, prolonging the sound as long as possible and in as steady and breathy a manner as possible on one exhalation. On a notepad, rate the performance using the aforementioned scale of 1 to 7. Have the patient repeat this task, periodically switching the vowel used, until the degree of vocal fold hyperadduction, as characterized mainly by a strained-strangled voice quality and/or intermittent arrests of phonation, is at least three scale values improved over the baseline rating or "1," if this rating was "2," "3," or "4," over 10 consecutive trials.

Step 6. After each set of 10 trials, enter the mean perceptual rating data in a separate column on the y-axis grid of the treatment chart, listing the date, number of trials (10), activity symbol (Y_1), measurement unit (1 to 7), and target criterion (?) in the respective cells of the column. Allow a 30-second rest period, and continue with the same exercise until the patient achieves the criterion or if after 30 trials or more the prognosis is poor for additional gains. Advance to the next exercise accordingly.

Yawn-Sigh Exercise No. 2
Step 1. Altering slightly the procedures of the preceding exercise, the patient is now requested to replace the yawn component during each trial by as normal as possible an inspiratory maneuver followed by the prolonged sigh of the vowel stimulus. As before, rate the performance using the same method for advancement to the next exercise. Remember that for this exercise the symbol "Y_2" will be used when charting the patient's progress. Once again, a tape recorder can prove useful for periodic auditory feedback.

Yawn-Sigh Exercise No. 3
Step 1. For this exercise, both the yawn and the sigh conditions are faded during each trial as the patient is required to try to prolong the vowel stimulus with as nearly normal vocal quality as possible. Again, use exactly the same method for rating and charting the patient's progress as that described in Step 5 of Exercise no. 1. However, the symbol "Y_3" will be used for these data. Note that if the patient fails to achieve the criterion set, experimentation with higher or lower pitch and various loudness levels may yield better results, and is worth trying.

Vowel Prolongation No. 1
Step 1. Randomly select 15 of the stimulus items from Step 2 of Yawn-Sigh Exercise no. 1 above for this baseline measurement. Request that the pa-

tient prolong the production of each item using the very best vocal quality possible. Following the same scoring procedure recommended in that exercise, rate the patient's baseline performance, making certain to use the symbol "BV" on the treatment chart. Additionally, engage the patient in conversational speech, and use the Speech Characteristics Chart to record the perceptual rating of vocal hyperfunction during connected discourse. Compare this rating with the previously recorded baseline score to measure the overall efficacy of the treatments administered thus far. Move on to the next step if so indicated by these baseline data.

Step 2. Place the See-Scape apparatus on the tabletop in front of the patient, and connect a 2-inch piece of drinking straw to the rubber hose in lieu of the plastic nasal olive. With a black marking pen, draw a line on the tube about 1 inch from the top. Have available a tape recorder for periodic feedback of the patient's voice efforts during this exercise. Also use a stopwatch on occasion to illustrate for the patient the length of time of each prolonged vocalization. If the patient can see the seconds tick by during the performance, such visual feedback can be rather motivating and facilitative. If the patient presents with persistent resonation subsystem imbalance, which can dampen the acoustic signal, a nose-clip should be used throughout this regimen except during practice of those stimuli containing nasal consonants.

Step 3. Proceed in the following way: First, demonstrate the overall objective of this exercise by placing the straw between the lips, enabling the end to come into light contact with the central incisor teeth. Then inhale normally, and steadily prolong the vowel /i/ to illustrate that with the generation of good vocal quality the Styrofoam float travels up to and remains fixed at (or within 1 inch from) the top of the tube. Second, also demonstrate that breathy phonation induces similar float activity and may be considered initially as an acceptable compensatory strategy. Third, for illustrative purposes, simulate the effects of vocal hyperfunction by prolonging the vowel using strained-strangled voice quality. Discuss that under this abnormal condition, movements of the float are undesirably erratic, owing to the aerodynamic disturbances precipitated by the hyperadducting vocal folds.

Step 4. Using the same stimuli as those in Step 2 of Yawn-Sign Exercise no. 1, begin by accordingly positioning the straw in the patient's mouth and requesting steady prolongation of the vowel /i/, with the objective of propelling and maintaining the float above the line drawn near the top of the tube for at least 90 percent of the duration of the production. Achieving this goal warrants a *correct* rating, whereas failure to do so is rated *incorrect*. The patient should be informed that breathy-soft phonation will not be acceptable at the outset of this program, and that such productions will be rated incorrect, irrespective of the resultant float activity. Rate the performance using this dichotomous scoring system. Periodically select for practice a different speech stimulus from among the 33 V, CV, and VCV options listed, making certain that the patient understands that the *vowels* are prolonged, not the consonants. Continue this procedure until either the patient achieves at least 80 percent correct over 10 consecutive trials, or 30 trials elapsed without evidence that if the patient is pressed to keep trying this criterion will be realized.

Step 5. After each set of 10 trials, tally the correct percentage score from the notepad, and enter the result in a separate column on the y-axis grid of the treatment chart. Be certain to list the date, number of trials (10), activity symbol (V_1), measurement unit (percentage correct), and target criterion (80 percent) in the respective cells of the column, and allow a 30-second rest period between sets of 10 trials. Note that if the patient fails to achieve the criterion here, he or she should advance to Exercise no. 2. On the other hand, if the patient succeeds with this exercise, the next exercise should be skipped, and he or she should proceed to the Speech Train exercise.

Vowel Prolongation Exercise No. 2

Step 1. Follow exactly the same set-up as that in the preceding exercise. Once again, demonstrate breathy-soft prolongation of the vowel /i/, noting that the float should travel up to and remain fixed at or within an inch of the top of the tube for the duration of the production.

Step 2. Ask the patient to try this compensatory vocal quality technique, and use the dichotomous scoring system to rate the performance. Follow the same methodology as that in Steps 4 and 5 above to direct and measure the patient's progress and eligibility for advancement to the next exercise. However, the symbol "V_2" is used on the treatment chart in logging these data. Note that if the patient fails to achieve the criterion here, the prognosis is poor for success with the more difficult speech stimuli in the subsequent exercises. Nevertheless, these treatments should be attempted on a trial basis in the event that they may trigger an accurate or near accurate physiologic response.

Speech Train Exercise No. 1

Step 1. Use the Speech Characteristics Chart to record a perceptual (1 to 7 point) rating of the voice, as determined through extemporaneous conversation with the patient. Advance to the next step if treatment is still indicated.

Step 2. Prior to initiating this exercise, instruct the patient to take a deep breath, and then prolong a train of any three of the 33 speech stimuli in Step 2 of Yawn-Sigh Exercise no. 1. For example, let's suppose that the following three stimulus items were chosen for this baseline measurement: /i-upu-mi/. Upon completion of inhalation, the patient faces the task of prolonging the /i/, then gliding without voice stoppage into a prolonged /upu/, and completing the exhalation with smooth transition to the /mi/ component of the train. Producing this V-VCV-CV sequence with virtually no cessation of voice activity is the target objective, as roughly equal time is afforded to each stimulus member of the train. Using the seven-point interval scale, rate on a notepad the overall degree of vocal hyperfunction present during the patient's effort to perform this task, remembering that a score of "7" represents marked impairment, and a "1" rating is symbolic of normal functioning. Repeat this same procedure four more times, selecting a different train of speech stimuli each time.

Step 3. Upon completion of these baseline trials, enter the mean perceptual rating in a separate column on the treatment chart, making certain to tag the data with the activity symbol "BT" in the appropriate cell at the bottom of the column. If the baseline score suggests the need for further intervention, move on to the next step.

Step 4. The See-Scape apparatus is used for this exercise in the same fashion as that discussed in Vowel Prolongation Exercise no. 1. Demonstrate the task for the patient by positioning the end of the straw lightly against the central incisor teeth and prolonging a train of three stimulus items chosen from the aforementioned list, making certain that good voice quality is maintained throughout the production, and an equal amount of phonation time is given to each stimulus component, as in the baseline measure of the preceding task. Note that this technique will propel and stabilize the Styrofoam float above the line drawn on the tube, with little or no fluctuation throughout the entire trial. The objective for the patient is to accomplish this target for at least 90 percent of the duration of each speech train production. If the patient achieves this criterion, a *correct* rating is rendered, whereas failure to do so warrants an *incorrect* rating. Breathy phonation is not penalized if indeed it appears to be the only successful method the patient can employ to compensate for or reduce the adverse effects of vocal hyperfunction. Request the patient to produce, as demonstrated, a chosen speech train. Rate the performance using the dichotomous scoring system. Periodically select for the exercise a different train of three stimuli from among the various options. Continue with the procedure until either the patient achieves at least 80 percent correct over 10 consecutive trials, or 30 trials elapse without evidence that continuation is warranted.

Step 5. After each set of 10 trials, tally the correct percentage score from the notepad, and enter the result in a separate column on the y-axis grid of the Phonation Subsystem Behavioral Treatment Chart. The date, number of trials (10), activity symbol (T_1), measurement unit (percentage correct), and target criterion (80 percent) are to be listed in their respective cells in the column. Allow 30 seconds rest between sets of 10 trials. Advance to the next exercise when indicated. As a reminder, the tape recorder can be very useful for occasional feedback and discussion of the patient's performances.

Sentence Production Exercise No. 1
Step 1. From the following list randomly select three sentences of differing lengths, and request that the patient read each one of them out loud. For clarity and ease of presentation, it may be best to have these sentences typewritten on index cards, with no more than two or three sentences per card. Using the seven-point scale again, rate the perceived vocal quality during each sentence production, remembering that overall a score of "7" should be assigned to profound vocal hyperfunction and that normal quality gets a "1" rating. Tally the mean rating, and enter the baseline result on the y-axis grid of the treatment chart, making certain that data relative to the date, number of trials (3), activity symbol (BS), and measurement unit (1 to 7) are recorded in the respective cells of

the chosen column. Follow the same perceptual scoring method with the patient engaged in conversational speech; however, the Speech Characteristics Chart is used to record this impression, as was the case for the previous connected discourse baseline ratings. If all these baseline data support the need for additional treatment of vocal hyperfunction, move on to the next step.

1. Hurry up.
2. Don't cry.
3. Stay put.
4. Pet the puppy.
5. The grass is mowed.
6. Give the baby a kiss.
7. Put on your shoes.
8. May I go to the store?
9. Mary makes beautiful music.
10. Put the cookies in the cabinet.
11. The mechanic said the transmission is bad.
12. Shopping at the grocery is time consuming.
13. Vegetables and potatoes should be included in all meals.
14. Grandfather likes to be modern in his language.
15. The washing machine is broken.
16. The dictionary can help with spelling.
17. Let's serve cheese and crackers at the party.
18. Charlie spoke at the graduation ceremony.
19. Baseball is my favorite sport.
20. This exercise helps me practice better voice control.
21. With each word produced in this sentence, the float should move toward the top of the tube.
22. If the float moves swiftly toward or stays near or at the bottom of the tube as the words in these sentences are produced, this may mean that my voice quality is too strained.
23. It's okay for the float to travel toward the bottom of the tube when I take a breath or pause between words.
24. Certain words contain sounds that make the float move upwards with great force.
25. Other words are produced with less airflow, and the float does not move as much.

Step 2. Use the See-Scape device for this exercise, and substitute the straw for the nasal olive as before. Demonstrate the task for the patient by placing the straw between the lips, with the end in light contact with the central incisor teeth, and reading aloud any one of the longer stimulus sentences. Have the patient note that as the words in the sentence are produced with good vocal quality and aerodynamics, albeit at times with slight articulatory imprecision owing to the presence of the straw, the float moves toward or remains near the top of the tube, except during normal breaths and intersyllabic pauses. That this characteristic float activity is the objective of the exercise should be made clear to the patient. For negative practice purposes, also illustrate the abnormal or undesirable float effects in response to periodic simulated vocal hyperfunction during the production of sentences.

Step 3. Request that the patient perform the task, beginning with one of the simpler sentences. Assure the patient that any coexistent speech subsystem disturbances that may compromise the performances here will not be weighed in the scoring procedure. Remind the patient that the objective is to generate voice during the word productions that is as free of vocal strain as possible, as evidenced by generally upward float activity. Using the dichotomous correct/incorrect scale, rate on a notepad the entire sentence correct if the float is so active for at least 90 percent of the duration of voice output, irrespective of the amount of time it takes the patient to complete the task. An incorrect rating is rendered otherwise. Breathy-soft phonation is not penalized as long as the aforementioned 90 percent criterion is achieved. Periodically select a different sentence stimulus for practice, commensurate with the patient's level of ability, and continue with the procedure until either the patient achieves at least 80 percent correct over 10 consecutive trials or 30 trials elapse without evidence that additional exercise will yield better results.

Step 4. After each set of 10 trials, tally the correct percentage score from the notepad and enter the sum in a separate column on the y-axis grid of the treatment chart. The date, number of trials (10), activity symbol (S_1), measurement unit (percentage correct), and target criterion (80 percent) should be recorded in their respective cells in the column. Allow 30 seconds of rest between sets of 10 trials, and advance to the next exercise when indicated.

Note. Emphasize to the patient the importance of focusing as much as possible on improving voice control regardless of the associated motor speech difficulties. Encourage him or her to vocalize every word in the stimulus sentence, even if the output is unintelligible, inasmuch as the objective is to reduce *vocal* hyperfunction. The clinician should not fall prey to temptations to treat breakdowns of the other speech subsystems during voice therapy. Such an approach may confuse and frustrate the patient as well as minimize progress.

Contextual Speech Exercise No. 1

Step 1. Using the Speech Characteristics Chart and the Phonation Subsystem Behavioral Treatment Chart, render baseline ratings of the patient's voice during extemporaneous speech efforts. If this observation supports the need for continued intervention, proceed to the next step.

Step 2. Use the See-Scape device in exactly the same manner as that in the preceding exercise. Once the straw is effectively positioned between the patient's lips, engage him or her in conversation about a topic of interest. Point out that the objective here is to try to generate voice during contextual speech that is as free as possible of a strained-strangled quality irrespective of the coexistence of residual or untreated speech subsystem disturbances. In addition to the cues that auditory feedback and monitoring may provide, both with and without a tape recorder, relative to the ongoing voice characteristics, the activity of the Styrofoam float should highlight visually the associated acoustic aerodynamics. As stated earlier, if the float clings to or near the bottom of the tube during the majority of phonation time, this result may be attributable to vocal fold hyperadduction and consequent poor translaryngeal and intraoral airflow. An accompanying strained-strangled vocal quality corroborates this explanation perceptually. On the other hand, when the float is more active and hovers near the top of the tube during the majority of phonation time, this response may be accounted for by the result of more relaxed vocal fold vibratory patterns and adequate airflow dynamics. Accompanying voice quality that falls within the breathy to normal range helps substantiate this conclusion. Follow the same scoring format as that recommended in Step 3 of the preceding exercise, except that here the correct/incorrect rating is rendered after the patient generates a full minute of conversational speech. Continue with this exercise until either the patient demonstrates at least 80 percent correct performances over 10 consecutive minutes, or 30 minutes of treatment expire without signs of improvement or promise for additional gains with further exercise.

Step 3. After each 10-minute sample of patient conversational speech, tally the total correct percentage score from the notepad, and enter the result on the treatment chart in the usual way, categorizing this activity with the "C_1" symbol. Note that if the patient fails to achieve the criterion at this level of intervention, and the persistent vocal hyperfunction continues to threaten the prognosis for significant improvements of the yet-untreated speech subsystems, experimentation with compensatory instrumentation techniques may be helpful. Case studies are provided for illustrative purposes.

Illustrative Case No. 2. The patient is a 24-year-old who came to the speech pathology service roughly 3 years after his severe closed head injury with resultant spastic paresis of the limb, trunk, and speech musculature and virtual unintelligibility. Coexistent cognitive, linguistic, and perceptual impairments were rather mild in degree. Full-course respiration subsystem treatment, akin to those recommended in Chapter 3, resulted in minimal improvement: No more than four syllables per breath were possible, and oppositional inhalatory/exhalatory breathing patterns plagued most speech efforts. Similarly disabling was his velopharyngeal incompetency, which rendered every vocalization, however primitive, hypernasal with accompanying excess nasal air emission. Nonresponsive to the resonation subsystem behavioral therapy, the patient was fitted with a palatal-lift appliance, which yielded moderate speech aerodynamic improvement.

With apprehension we next proceeded to treat the symptoms of severe vocal hyperfunction. Phonatory efforts, no matter how brief, literally fatigued the patient. After careful study of these abnormal signs and symptoms, aided by speech aerodynamic, electroglottographic, video-strobolaryngoscopic, and respirometric examinations, it was determined that because vocal fold hyperadduction was so severe during all phases of phonation, the prognosis for improvement with voice therapy was very poor. Notwithstanding this forecast, the patient was administered the entire treatment protocol previously described. Figure 5–2, *A* and *B* il-

PHONATION SUBSYSTEM BEHAVIORAL TREATMENT CHART

Patient's name: P.P.

Birthdate: 5/17/60   Sex: M

Speech diagnosis: Spastic dysarthria

Medical diagnosis: Closed head injury

Clinician: Dworkin

Facility: Private practice

Address: Anywhere, USA

ACTIVITY KEY

Feature:	MEASUREMENT UNIT
1. Relaxation of extrinsic laryngeal musculature (R)	7-point interval scale (1 = normal; 7 = most deviant)
2. Yawn-sigh phonation (Y)	7-point interval scale
3. Vowel prolongations (V)	7-point interval scale or % correct
4. Speech trains (T)	7-point interval scale or % correct
5. Sentences (S)	7-point interval scale or % correct
6. Contextual speech (C)	7-point interval scale or % correct
7. Holding breath (H)	No. of seconds

Feature:	MEASUREMENT UNIT
8. Nonspeech vocal fold valving (N)	No. of seconds
9. Phonatory vocal fold valving (P)	7-point interval scale or no. of seconds
10. Hard attack phonation (A)	7-point interval scale or no. of seconds
11. Voice motor planning (M)	% Correct
12. Laryngeal timing and coordination (L)	% Correct

Employment strategically treatments above (E + above symbol)

Baseline (pre-treatment): B + activity symbol

Comments: Because the patient experiences rapid and severe fatigue during virtually all phonation exercises owing to underlying vocal fold hyper-adduction, many more rest periods than usual are required per treatment session. The severity of the subsystem dysfunction prompted adoption of more lenient criteria for advancement than prescribed in the treatment protocol. All improvements were with breathy quality.

Average Score (y-axis: 0, 5, 10, 20, 30, 40, 50, 60, 70, 80, 90, 100)

Dates:	6/13/89			6/15			6/16				5/20				
Activity symbol	BR₁	R₁	R₁	BR₂	R₂	R₂	BR₃	R₃	R₃	BY₁	Y₁	Y₁	Y₁	Y₂	Y₂	Y₃
Unit of measure	1–7															
Target criterion	3			3			3			4						

SESSIONS

Figure 5–2. **A** and **B**, Treatment charts illustrating a spastic dysarthric patient's response to the vocal fold hyperadduction intervention regimen. The criteria for advancement within the program vary in accordance with the task and the patient's individual baseline scores. For the relaxation exercises the criterion for the patient was a score of "3" on the 7-point interval scale (three scale values improved over baseline [6 − 3 = 3]). For the yawn-sigh exercises the criterion was a score of "4" on the 7-point interval scale (7 − 3 = 4). Scores of 80 percent are the standard criteria for all patients on the vowel prolongation, speech train, sentence, and contextual speech exercises. The absence of asterisks in any of the columns of data

PHONATION SUBSYSTEM BEHAVIORAL TREATMENT CHART

Patient's name: P.P. (continued)

Birthdate: ___ Sex: ___

Speech diagnosis: ___

Medical diagnosis: ___

Clinician: ___

Facility: ___

Address: ___

ACTIVITY KEY

Feature:	MEASUREMENT UNIT
1. Relaxation of extrinsic laryngeal musculature (R)	7-point interval scale (1 = normal; 7 = most deviant)
2. Yawn-sigh phonation (Y)	7-point interval scale
3. Vowel prolongations (V)	7-point interval scale or % correct
4. Speech trains (T)	7-point interval scale or % correct
5. Sentences (S)	7-point interval scale or % correct
6. Contextual speech (C)	7-point interval scale or % correct
7. Holding breath (H)	No. of seconds

Feature:	MEASUREMENT UNIT
8. Nonspeech vocal fold valving (N)	No. of seconds
9. Phonatory vocal fold valving (P)	7-point interval scale or no. of seconds
10. Hard attack phonation (A)	7-point interval scale or no. of seconds
11. Voice motor planning (M)	% Correct
12. Laryngeal timing and coordination (L)	% Correct

Employment strategically treatments above (E = above symbol)

Baseline (pre-treatment): B + activity symbol

Dates: 6/20/89, 6/22, 6/25

No. of trials	5											3	5		5		5	5
Activity symbol	Y_3	BV_1	V_1	V_1	V_2	V_2	V_2	BT	T_1	T_1	T_1	BC	S_1	S_1	S_1	BC	C_1	C_1
Unit of measure	1–7	1	% corr.	% corr.				1–7	% corr.			1–7	% corr.			1–7	% corr.	% corr.
Target criterion	4	1	80%	80%				1	80%			1	80%			1	80%	80%

Average Score

SESSIONS

B

Comments:

Figure 5–2. *Continued.*

159

lustrates his responses to the exercises prescribed. As can be seen from these figures, the patient failed to achieve the criterion targets set for all the exercises. It is important to note, however, that when he compensated by using breathy-soft phonation, his performances were measurably improved over those trials when attempts to normalize vocal quality were required. It is unfortunate that poor breath support compounded the volume difficulty he experienced during breathy phonation, rendering his speech efforts virtually inaudible outside of the quiet clinical environment.

With the palatal lift in position, breathy speech output was only moderately imprecise. This observation prompted consideration of methods by which we might be able to increase the volume of the voice without taxing the respiration or phonation subsystems, which through experience with the patient proved counterproductive on numerous clinical trials. It was hypothesized that if the breathy speech could be mechanically amplified, this result would improve the patient's communication efforts, as well as facilitate forthcoming articulation subsystem treatments. Experimentation with an earpiece microphone connected to a pocket-size amplifier and speaker system was unsuccessful in that the patient could not generate sufficient speech acoustic energy to induce external meatus bone vibration for the microphone response. In lieu of the earpiece microphone, a Radio Shack "Walkie-Talkie Headset," not unlike that used by a telephone operator, was interfaced with the miniature amplifier and speaker. Clipped to the patient's shirt pocket, the speaker projected his whispered-breathy utterances so that he could be heard easily across an average-size room without having to strain at phonation. In addition, not only did use of this augmentative system increase threefold the number of syllables per breath that the patient could sustain during attempts at connected discourse, but also it significantly reduced the symptoms of communication fatigue. However, because he continued to struggle with episodic vocal hyperfunction while using this system, albeit to a much lesser degree than without it, exercises were designed to reduce such occurrences. After five treatment sessions, only small gains were made in this regard. Thus, we moved on to the rehabilitation needs of the articulation subsystem, which will not be discussed here.

Illustrative Case No. 3. MG is a 48-year-old female with a moderate degree of spastic dysarthria. Whereas her articulation subsystem was only mildly dysfunctional at the time of the initial examination, involvements of the phonation and resonation subsystems were much more pronounced. The patient reported that the hypernasality had become noticeably worse in the few weeks immediately prior to the examination, and that when she attempted to speak she got a "squeezed-off, choking feeling in my throat." Perceptual, acoustic, laryngoscopic, video-strobolaryngoscopic, and clinical speech aerodynamic studies confirmed the presence of moderate to severe bilateral paresis of the velopharyngeal valving mechanism and a similar degree of involvement of the laryngeal mechanism, owing to underlying hypertonicity and weakness of the associated musculature. Her voice was characterized by a moderately to severely strained-strangled quality with the usual secondary concomitant acoustic effects. Any voice that was generated without extreme resistance was articulated with a fair degree of precision, but the moderate amount of hypernasal resonance and excess nasal air emission present significantly dampened the intelligibility of such utterances. A tentative diagnosis of progressive supranuclear palsy was made, but it was speculated that if the equivocal lower motor neuron signs and symptoms in her hands definitively progressed, then amyotrophic lateral sclerosis might be a more representative and accurate diagnosis. MG refused to be fitted with a palatal-lift appliance, despite her failure to respond to full-course resonation subsystem behavioral therapy. Because of the progressive nature of her illness, possible surgical intervention was not considered in her case. Thus, her persistent hypernasality plagued articulation efforts. Her responses to the treatment to improve vocal hyperfunction were equally unsuccessful. Over the course of 2 months following the initial examination, in which she was seen for these treatments on a three-times-per-week basis, her voice and resonation symptoms worsened. Curiously, symptom progression was not as evident when the speech and nonspeech functions of the articulation subsystem were separately evaluated. It was decided at that time to explore a compensatory means of vocalization, one that might bypass the phonation and resonation subsystems and yet take advantage of the patient's residual articulatory capabilities.

Reflections on methods of voice rehabilitation for laryngectomy patients highlighted the possible usefulness of the transcervical mechanical instrument for MG. Initially she did not care for the acoustics of this device and found placement against the neck difficult to navigate. Moreover, it took a few sessions to train her to turn off her own voice when articulating the artificial voice source. Once she learned consciously to articulate only and allow the Western Electric device to provide the acoustics, she was able to communicate with relative ease and at length. Still inconsistent and inefficient in her skills of positioning the instrument against the neck, which may have been attributable to progressive weakening of her hands, we considered switching to the Cooper-Rand intraoral electrolarynx. Experimenting with this device we discovered that placement of the plastic tube in the mouth triggered a hyperactive pharyngeal reflex and tended to interfere with her articulatory agility. Unable to adjust to these side effects, she opted to continue to work with the original transcervical instrument. Although the patient was unfortunately lost to long-term follow-up, 3 months after her introduction to this device, she was reported to be using it quite effectively to communicate with her family and friends.

Treatments of the Hypoadductory Laryngeal Mechanism

Most commonly observed in hypokinetic and flaccid dysarthric patients, hypoadduction of the vocal folds results largely in a hoarse-breathy vocal quality and reduced control of pitch and loudness, as shown in Table 5–1. Unlike those patients with hyperadduction of the vocal folds, these patients may have a fair to good prognosis for voice improvement with therapy. Of course, the severity of the disorder and the underlying etiology invariably influences the overall response to such treatment. Patients with Parkinson's disease can make good gains early in their clinical course but may experience setbacks as their condition progresses. Patients with lower motor neuron diseases or injuries may initially respond well to voice therapy, but if their medical conditions are progressive in nature they too may experience later difficulties in maintaining such improvements. Notwithstanding these possibilities all patients, regardless of their prognoses at the outset, should be considered candidates for the treatment program described in this subsection if they present with hypofunctional voice characteristics.

The overall objectives of the following exercises are to improve voice quality and to increase the number of syllables that can be produced per breath. To achieve these goals, the exercises developed here were designed to (1) increase the forces of vocal fold adduction during phonation, and (2) convert these improved forces into better voice motor control during connected discourse.

It is important to remember that for most patients this is administered following treatment of the respiration and/or resonation subsystem. Not infrequently when improvements are realized as a result of these preceding treatments, patients approach voice therapy motivated to continue their successful track record. Moreover, these important physiologic gains provide a supportive background for further treatment success. Patients who have struggled with these previous subsystem treatments may not fare well in voice therapy either, but they should not be discouraged from making legitimate efforts to beat the odds. Also note that if the patient presents with residual velopharyngeal incompetence, which appears to compound the voice disorder about to be treated, discretionary use of a noseclip during the following exercises may prove fruitful.

Holding Breath Exercise No. 1

Step 1. As a precursor to vocal fold valving exercises during phonation efforts, here we try to induce glottal closure by requiring the patient to hold the breath for set periods of time. Prior to initiating the exercise, however, use the Phonation Subsystem Behavioral Treatment Chart to rate the patient's baseline ability by instructing him or her to inhale deeply and then hold the breath for as long as possible with the lips closed. Place a small mirror under the patient's nostrils to detect airflow, and use a stopwatch to record the number of seconds that elapse between the end of inspiration and the beginning of expiration. Repeat this procedure three times, calculate the mean number of seconds achieved, and enter the result on the y-axis grid of the treatment chart in a separate column chosen for this finding. Make certain to tag the recording with the activity symbol "BH" at the bottom of the column. Also render a baseline perceptual rating of the patient's voice on the Speech Characteristics Chart for comparison with subsequent periodic ratings throughout the various exercises in the regimen. If the patient is unable to hold the breath on these baseline measures for at least an average of 15 seconds, proceed with Step 2. Otherwise skip this exercise, and advance to the next exercise in the sequence.

Step 2. Assemble the See-Scape apparatus on the tabletop in front of the patient, and place the plastic nasal olive in either nostril, preferably the one with the least amount of resistance to nasal airflow. Using a marking pen, draw a line on the tube at approximately the halfway mark. Familiarize the patient with the objective of the exercise, which is to take a deep breath and then hold it for as long as possible. Once the patient learns that exhalation will be evident by movement of the float, instruct him or her to close the mouth and lips, inhale deeply through the nose, and then hold the breath. At the moment the patient begins the breath-holding phase, start the stopwatch or note the position of the second hand on a wristwatch. The clock stops when the float moves and remains above the line drawn on the tube for more than 2 consecutive seconds, which signals (transglottal) exhalatory airflow. Record the number of seconds achieved during the breath-holding phase, and repeat the task until the patient (1) demonstrates at least 75 percent improvement over the baseline score or 15 seconds, whichever is less, over 10 consecutive trials, or (2) fails to exhibit an improvement trend that warrants further practice of this exercise. Calculate this target criterion according to the baseline score, and enter the figure in the respective cell at the bottom of the anticipated treatment data column.

Step 3. After each set of 10 trials, tally the mean number of seconds accomplished, give the patient a 30-second break, and enter the result on the y-axis grid of the treatment chart using a separate column for these data. The appropriate date, activity symbol (H_1), number of trials (10), measurement unit (# seconds), and target criterion (?) should also be recorded in the respective cells of the column. Advance to the next exercise if the patient does not achieve the criterion here. If, on the other hand, the criterion has been met, skip the next exercise and proceed with the one following it.

Nonspeech Vocal Fold Valving Exercise No. 1

Step 1. Yet again, request the patient to hold the breath for as long as possible. Following the same method of baseline recording as that recommended in Step 1 of the preceding exercise, enter on the treatment chart the mean number of seconds achieved, using the symbol "BN" to represent these data.

Step 2. Tape the nasal olive of the See-Scape device to the most patent nostril of the patient so that his or her hands are free to participate in this exercise. Depending upon the upper limb strength and coordination of the patient, the following methods to induce vocal fold valving will be attempted to discover which one proves most efficacious: (1) clasp hands together at chest level, with arms bent 90 degrees at the elbow, and squeeze the palms together as hard as possible; (2) grasp the bottom of the seat with both hands, if possible, and pull up as hard as possible, as if to lift off the ground the chair on which one is sitting; and (3) push down on the seat bottom with both hands, as if to cause the chair to collapse. To determine the extent to which any of these methods promote glottal closure, have the patient take a deep breath and then begin a slow exhalation. As soon as the float moves above the halfway mark on the See-Scape tube, signaling the start of the exhalation cycle, perform the first of these valving maneuvers with the objective of assisting a legitimate effort to hold the breath. If and when the float drops below the midline or to the bottom of the tube during this trial, encourage the patient to keep squeezing the hands together so as to maintain for as long as possible the breath-holding phase. Use a stopwatch or wristwatch to time the achievement. As before, the clock stops when the float resumes its upward course beyond the halfway mark for 2 consecutive seconds, indicating expiratory airflow. Repeat this procedure with the remaining two valving techniques, and compare the results to determine the method that is most helpful for the patient. Use that method in the next step, or select the one that may work best with practice if the results of the preliminary trials are equivocal.

Step 3. Request that the patient inhale deeply and then begin exhaling. As soon as the float travels past the halfway mark on the tube, instruct the patient to invoke the chosen valving maneuver in concert with conscious effort to cease exhaling. The clock starts when the float drops below the mark and stops upon exhalation, as previously defined. Record the number of seconds accomplished, and continue the exercise following the exact same procedural criterion and scoring format as that outlined in Steps 2 and 3 of the preceding exercise. Be certain to use the symbol "N_1" to tag the results of this exercise on the treatment chart.

Phonatory Vocal Fold Valving Exercise No. 1

Step 1. Request the patient to take a deep breath and then at a comfortable loudness and pitch level say the vowel /a:/ as long and steadily as possible. Repeat the task three times. On the y-axis grid of the phonation subsystem behavioral treatment chart, enter in a separate column the total mean number of seconds the patient sustained the vowel, making certain to tag this baseline result with the activity symbol "BP_1" at the bottom of the column. Additionally, using the seven-point interval scale, rate the overall voice characteristics during these baseline trials, and enter the mean result on the treatment chart in the column adjacent to the one just used to record the mean length of vowel prolongations. For these data, the symbol "BP_2" is listed in the activity cell at the bottom of the column. As always, Step 2, which follows, is not indicated if the patient performs within normal limits on these baseline measures.

Step 2. Using one of the three aforementioned vocal fold valving maneuvers, as determined either in the preceding exercise or through experimentation prior to this exercise, the patient is instructed to inhale deeply and then prolong the vowel /a:/ while simultaneously employing the maneuver selected to induce vocal fold valving. A tape recorder can prove very helpful for auditory biofeedback. The objectives here are twofold: (1) to prolong the vowel either 75 percent longer than was demonstrated during the baseline measures or a full 20 seconds, whichever is less, and (2) to generate voice that on the seven-point scale is rated at least three scale values improved over the baseline score, or "1" if this score was "2," "3," or "4." On a notepad, list these scores separately and repeat this task, altering the vowel stimulus in concert with the patient's articulatory proficiency, until either these objectives are each met over 10 consecutive trials or the patient fails to exhibit a significant improvement trend to justify continuation of the exercise.

Step 3. After each set of 10 trials, compute both the mean number of seconds achieved and the mean of the perceptual ratings rendered, and enter each of these results in separate columns on the y-axis grid of the treatment chart, respectively tagging these data with the activity symbols "P_1" and "P_2." Make certain that the appropriate date, number of trials (10), measurement unit (# seconds, or 1 to 7), and target criterion (?) data are similarly recorded in the respective cells of the columns. Afford the patient 30-second rest periods between trials. Note that those patients who do not achieve the criteria here should proceed to the next exercise. Those patients who are successful, however, can skip the next exercise and advance to the following one.

Hard-Attack Phonation Exercise No. 1

For those flaccid and hypokinetic dysarthric patients who have failed to improve with the preceding exercises, the hard glottal attack technique may facilitate adduction of the vocal folds during voice production. The purposeful therapeutic use of hard-attack phonation should be considered negative practice, however, and administered with limitations in order to minimize the possibility of abusive side effects.

Step 1. To establish a baseline against which the effects of treatment can be compared, request that the patient perform the following tasks as best as possible: (1) prolong the vowel /a:/; (2) sing up and down an octave scale at comfortable pitch and loudness levels; and (3) answer pertinent background questions so that context voice characteristics can be measured. Use the Phonation Subsystem Behavioral Treatment Chart to record these impressions. For the first task, record the number of seconds of vowel prolongation, making certain to enter this result on the y-axis grid in a separate column and that the activity symbol "BA_1" is used to tag the score. For both the second and the third baseline tasks, the seven-point interval scale should be used for these perceptual ratings. Each score is best logged in a separate column of the treatment chart. The symbols "BA_2" and "BA_3" are used to tag these data on the chart in the respective activity cells. Proceed with the next step if any of these scores fall below the levels set for the patient.

Step 2. Place an open palm on the patient's abdomen. After requesting that he or she inhale deeply and then hold the breath, intermittently yet firmly pump the abdomen to cause air to be exhaled. Instruct the patient to try to resist this external effort by bearing down as hard as possible at the level of the glottis. Strong glottal resistance should trigger audible vocal straining. If this does not result, tell the patient to bear down in a fashion like that required to bench press an inconceivable amount of weight. Imagining the pushing process of natural childbirth or the act of straining during defecation may similarly evoke vocal fold adduction. At the moment of perceptible strangled voice quality, instruct the patient to try to bellow and prolong the vowel /a:/ with the best vocal quality possible. As soon as voice is produced, pumping of the abdomen is terminated. Initially, the patient's challenge is to blend induced vocal straining into more controlled and adequate phonation. Ultimately the former component of this process needs to fade, to reduce laryngeal tension and stress, as volitional glottal resistance for voice purposes is practiced. Once the patient understands the objective here, proceed to Step 3.

Note. Allowing the patient to strain at phonation for protracted periods of time can produce acute laryngeal edema. Therefore, during this exercise, it is most efficient to govern very quick transitions from the artificially strained to the more natural voice outputs. The use of a stethoscope, a tape recorder, or both can be used for feedback to the patient relative to the ongoing status of his or her vocal efforts. Likewise, discussion about the differential perceptual features of the induced strained-strangled voice quality versus normal voice quality can be an added advantage.

Step 3. Follow the procedure in Step 2, but this time use the seven-point scale to rate on a notepad the patient's performance, in which at the extremes a score of "1" represents smooth and quick transition from strained voice quality to normal vocal quality and length of prolongation, and a "7" indicates failure to improve voice output during the trial. Repeat the task until the patient achieves a mean rating that is at least three scale valves improved over the baseline score or "1," if this score was "2," "3," or "4," over 10 consecutive trials.

Step 4. After each set of 10 trials, calculate the mean rating and enter the result in a separate column on the y-axis grid of the treatment chart, making certain to record the date of the session, activity symbol (A_1), number of trials (10), measurement unit (1 to 7), and target criterion (?) in the respective cells of the column. Allow a 30-second rest period between all trials, during which discussions about the performances can take place. As always, if the patient fails to demonstrate a significant improvement trend to justify continuation of the exercise, stop the regimen, as earlier suggested, after 30 consecutive trials of poor performance. If the patient meets the criterion here, move on to the two next steps. Otherwise, skip these steps and proceed to the following exercise. To reduce monotony, the vowel stimulus can be periodically switched.

Step 5. Follow the same procedure as in the preceding steps, except that here abdominal pumping by the clinician is eliminated, as the patient is required to self-generate a hard glottal attack that is blended immediately into prolongation of a vowel. When logging patient performances be sure to tag these data with the activity symbol "A_2." Attempt Step 6 whether or not the patient achieves the aforementioned criterion for advancement.

Step 6. Follow the same procedure as that in the preceding step, but this time the patient is instructed to fade the hard-attack and attempt vowel prolongations without audible grunting. Bearing down to accomplish glottal resistance may still be necessary; however, the approach to phonation must now be imperceptible or demonstrably less strained. The activity symbol "A_3" is used to identify these data on the treatment chart. Advance to the next exercise when so indicated.

Speech Train Exercise No. 1

Step 1. Follow the exact same procedures as that detailed earlier in the Speech Train exercise for patients with vocal fold hyperadduction. Note that the patient is allowed, in fact encouraged, to employ whatever technique desired to generate vocal fold valving. Here we can add to the list of speech stimuli strings of numbers, such as 1 to 10 and 10 to 20, that the patient is instructed to count aloud on one breath. Days of the week and months of the year similarly serve as excellent trains of speech stimuli for this exercise. Remember that the patient is to afford each element of the train roughly equal phonation time during the prolongation sequence, and that here the degree of vocal hypofunction, *not* hyperfunction, is rated during each trial. Advance to the next exercise as indicated.

Sentence Production Exercise No. 1
Step 1. Follow the exact same procedures as that detailed earlier in the treatment exercise subsection of the same name for patients with vocal fold hyperadduction. Again, here vocal hypofunction, *not* hyperfunction, is rated. Advance to the next exercise as indicated, making certain that during these performances the patient is encouraged to employ the vocal fold valving method that may have been learned in the preceding exercises.

Contextual Speech Exercise No. 1
Step 1. Follow the procedures recommended in the treatment subsection described for patients with hyperfunctional voice disorders. Of course, here the effects of vocal fold hypofunction *rather than* hyperadduction are measured. Note that if the patient unsuccessfully moves through all the exercises in this regimen, prior to abandoning in defeat the phonation subsystem, some compensatory techniques might be worth a try. These will be addressed through case illustrations.

Illustrative Case No. 4. PP is a 58-year-old male who presented to the Speech Pathology Service with severe breathy-hoarse phonation 6 months following thyroid gland surgery during which the right recurrent laryngeal nerve had to be sacrificed. Paralyzed and atrophied between the paramedian and abducted position, the right vocal fold caused excess escape of unphonated air during voice efforts. The severity of the glottal chink could not be overcome with the aforementioned treatment regimen, as virtually no improvement was observed throughout the various exercises. Unwilling to consider surgical intervention to correct the problem, the patient felt strongly that if the volume of his voice could be amplified, he would be able to get on with his life with less discomfort. We fitted a lapel microphone and miniature amplifier and speaker system akin to the one described in case no. 2 above, which he wore clipped to his belt. With amplification his breathy voice was easier to hear in most environments and afforded him a personally acceptable means of communication, although the treatment team felt that vocal fold augmentation would probably yield better results. Oftentimes what the patient desires is neglected or "pooh-poohed" by clinicians who, in good faith, believe that they know what treatments will be most effective. However, this particular patient was content with the clinical outcome, which was in part self-directed, and that is *truly* most important.

Illustrative Case No. 5. VK presented with left unilateral vocal fold paralysis due to brainstem injury involving multiple cranial nerves, including the left Vagus nerve. Both routine mirror and stroboscopic laryngeal studies revealed that the affected fold was displaced in the paramedian position without significant signs of atrophy, since only 6 weeks had elapsed since his accident. The resultant flaccid dysphonia was characterized by moderately hoarse vocal quality with associated reduction in the range of pitch and loudness control. After reasonably good success in fitting him with a palatal-lift appliance to compensate for bilateral weakness and paralysis of the velopharyngeal mechanism, the preceding phonation subsystem treatment regimen was administered in full. The results were not encouraging, as the patient continued to struggle with the same pretherapeutic degree of voice difficulty. Exploring the alternatives to this clinical program the patient was not opposed to submitting to the Teflon-glycerin augmentation procedure described earlier.

Not unlike other patients with similar voice disorders, such as case no. 1 above, when VK twisted his head sharply to the right side he could generate moderate improvements in vocal quality, pitch, and loudness. As he adjusted his head posture gradually back toward the midline, these voice parameters commensurately deteriorated. It was hypothesized that this head torque displaced medially the left vocal fold, thereby simulating the valving effects of the anticipated surgical procedure. Experimenting with external compression force applied with two fingers to the left half of the thyroid lamina yielded similar effects. When the force was moderate in degree and applied steadily, the patient could demonstrate reasonably good voice. Withdrawal of the stimulus immediately reversed the effect. The inducing of voice improvement with these compensatory techniques suggested that the results of vocal fold augmentation would prove even more rewarding. With the endorsement of the laryngeal surgeon, who was unable to schedule the patient for another 7 weeks, the efficacy of these compensatory techniques was explored further.

The patient practiced numerous variations of head twisting maneuvers, coupled with phonation activities, in an effort to discover which position, if any, would render the best voice most consistently. As expected, this exercise was frustrating for the patient. Slight modifications in the torque led to noticeable adverse shifts in voice quality, and neck stiffness was an unacceptable side effect. After three treatment sessions we abandoned this approach and experimented with the manual compression technique, as we awaited the date of surgery.

Having little desire to use the hand to compress the larynx, the patient was favorably disposed to wearing a cotton neckerchief. Rolled up and tied firmly, but comfortably around his neck at the level of the thyroid cartilage, the kerchief induced roughly the same improved voice effects that were achieved with the successful head twisting maneuvers. Laryngoscopic examinations revealed that the kerchief displaced medially not only the left paralyzed vocal fold but also the right uninvolved one. It is unfortunate that when it was removed, carryover was not evident. Because the kerchief had a tendency to loosen over a brief period of time, necessitating numerous readjustments to ensure adequate compressive force, a 4-cm-wide elastic band with Velcro tabs was constructed as a successful replacement. This material design lent itself to easy fitting and remained securely in place regardless of the amount of head turning or neck perspiration. The patient wore this band most of the day, apparently unaffected by its presence and pleased with its moderately positive voice effects. He continued to wear it as a quasi-prosthesis until the day of surgery. Concerned about the potential adverse soft tissue and vascular effects of long-term use of the band, the treatment team could not recommend without strong reservation this mechanical therapeutic approach in lieu of surgical intervention. More important, the patient desired the operation and its potential long-lasting, unrestricting benefits. Surgery was indeed performed without complication. Two months later the patient suffered from only mild dysphonia, leading to the general consensus that the operation was quite successful.

Retrospectively, not only did use of the neck band provide the patient with immediate voice gratification, but it also helped motivate him to think positively about the upcoming surgery. However, the extent to which these factors influenced the actual results of the surgical procedure is unclear. Notwithstanding such uncertainty, these results and additional similar findings since then support continued experimentation with this methodology for those patients with flaccid dysphonia who are not responsive to alternative behavioral treatments. For those patients with high risks for CVAs, extreme caution should be exercised when considering this technique. The presence of this device around the neck can prove medically counterproductive if cerebral blood flow is further compromised.

Treatments of the Abnormally Fluctuating Laryngeal Mechanism

Reviewing Table 5–1 once again highlights that patients with ataxic dysarthria, hyperkinetic dysarthria, and apraxia of speech may present with significant voice disorders that result, characteristically, from fluctuating vocal fold movement abnormalities. Because these patients vary considerably with respect to their laryngeal pathophysiologic conditions, the treatment programs will be segregated here into three population subsections. This breakdown, however, does not discriminate against the use of the same treatment methods for patients who exhibit similar voice difficulties but whose overall diagnoses differ. Therefore, when possible and feasible those exercises that lend themselves to cross-population application will be referenced accordingly, but not repeated verbatim.

Apraxia of Phonation

Owing to faulty motor planning of vocal fold adjustments during volitional speech efforts, patients with apraxia of phonation exhibit episodic and variable signs and symptoms including (1) no laryngeal sound, either voiced or voiceless, (2) whispered speech, (3) asynchrony of articulatory and exhalatory movements, (4) arrests of phonation, and (5) strident vocalizations that at times are camouflaged by periods of normal voice production. For some patients the condition is so severe as to render them mute. Notwithstanding the usual coexistence of speech apraxia in these patients, therapy should focus initially on the voice disorder component because gains at this level of intervention ordinarily promote successes with the large-scale articulation and prosody subsystem exercises to follow. Whereas the voice motor planning treatment program introduced here may prematurely tax these other subsystems, such stimulation is deliberately contained by the relatively simple constitution of the various phonation exercises. To avoid overtaxing these related subsystems and inducing unwanted speech praxis interferences, vowels only will serve as the phonetic stimuli. The underlying speech apraxia will be tackled later in the course of the treatment program, permitting virtually all of the focus here to be on phonation subsystem difficulty. The overall objective of these exercises is to achieve greater consistency and precision of voice motor control so that the phonation subsystem is accessible during all volitionally programmed as well as therapeutically manipulated speech efforts. *Note:* When working with the metronome, the Index of Metronomic Levels in Chapter 2 (Table 2–2) will provide helpful information regarding expected performances at different speeds on various tasks. Moreover, all data entries on the treatment chart must reflect real time spent practicing the task. Time-outs automatically stop the clock and do not figure in the scores awarded.

Voice Motor Planning Exercise No. 1 (Isolated Vowel Repetitions at 30 bpm)

Step 1. Begin by rendering a baseline rating of the patient's vocal difficulty during conversational speech. Use the seven-point interval scale, in which at the extremes a score of "7" indicates marked impairment, and a "1" symbolizes normal ability, and enter the result on the y-axis grid of the Speech Characteristics Chart (see Figure 2–2) in a separate column from previously recorded data. Tag this entry with the activity symbol BV, making certain to list the date of data collection. As a final baseline measure, request that the patient repeat the vowel /a/, roughly one repetition every 2 seconds, for at least 30 continuous seconds. Several trials should be permitted. Rate each utterance independently as either *correct* or *incorrect* relative to the absence or presence, respectively, of signs or symptoms of apraxia of phonation. A correct rating is awarded only if there are no (1) perceptible periods of arrests of phonation during the utterance, (2) pitch breaks, (3) loudness outbursts or reductions, and (4) signs of delayed voice onset time. Repeat this task three times, and calculate from the notepad ratings the total percentage of correct productions. Extract the baseline result, and enter the score on the Phonation Subsystem Behavioral Treatment Chart, making certain to list the appropriate date, minutes of testing, activity symbol (BM$_1$), and unit of measure (percentage correct) in the respective cells of the data column. A score of less than 80 percent correct indicates the need for Step 2, which follows. Otherwise, move on to the next exercise. Note that the vowel used can be switched periodically.

Step 2. A standard metronome is used here for external temporal pacing stimuli. Placed on the tabletop in front of the patient, this device is set at 30 beats per minute (bpm). The patient is encouraged but not required to tap the finger or foot to the beat during the exercise, as pairing such motor gestures with speech activities can also be therapeutic. Inform the patient that this exercise program involves repeating vowels to the beat of the metronome. Caution the patient not to become frustrated if and when errors occur. That errors will probably occur should be understood as par for the course, especially in the beginning. Encourage the patient to try to get past the breakdown as quickly as possible and back on beat. Demonstrate for the patient that the primary objectives are to program voice onset and offset, according to the designated metronomic beat, with consistent accuracy relative to the timing of each utterance and the underlying vocal quality, pitch, and loudness controls. As the clinician performs the task the patient's open hand should be taken and pressed lightly against the thyroid cartilage so that laryngeal vibrations can be kinesthetically discerned during the voice components of the exercise. If a stethoscope is available, place the earpieces on the patient and the diaphragm on your thyroid cartilage, and repeat the task so that the patient can hear the differences between the voiced and voiceless segments of the exercise. These feedback techniques may prove helpful throughout all the exercises in this subsection. Of course the patient may feel and listen to his or her own vocal fold vibrations during the treatment program, if so desired and fruitful.

Step 3.   Once the patient is adequately familiarized with the objectives, request that he or she produce the vowel /a/ to the beat of the metronome: One production per beat for 30 continuous seconds. A stopwatch can be used to signal starting and stopping. At 30 bpm for 30 seconds, a maximum of 15 accurate repetitions (one every 2 seconds) can be achieved for the trial for a total score of 100 percent. All patient productions that meet or exceed the performance objectives should be graded correct, whereas those that are plagued by any of the aforementioned salient features of apraxia of phonation are subtracted from the percentage correct. Note that if the patient stops at any time during the trial, because of apractic breakdowns or anything else, penalties accrue and are weighed in the score for the trial. That is, the clock runs for the 30 seconds, and the patient is expected to continue throughout this period without interruption. For the purposes of this regimen, a total mean score of at least 80 percent correct productions over 10 consecutive trials will serve as the criterion for advancement to the next exercise. As with all exercises in this text, the criterion recommended is not etched in stone. Some patients may benefit more from different sets of criteria than those outlined here or in the other treatment subdivisions. Generally speaking, however, if after 30 trials the patient fails to demonstrate an observable improvement trend, discontinue this exercise and proceed with cautious pessimism to the following, more difficult exercise in the treatment sequence. Use of a notepad to record the patient's correct percentage score per trial is recommended.

Step 4.   After each set of 10 trials calculate from the notepad scores the mean percentage of correct productions and enter the result on the y-axis grid of the Phonation Subsystem Behavioral Treatment Chart in a separate column. Tag these data with the "M_1" symbol, making certain to list the appropriate date, number of trials (10), measurement unit (percentage correct), and target criterion (80 percent correct) in the respective cells of the column. To reduce the potential for boredom and adaptation effects, the vowel stimulus can and should be changed periodically. Proceed with the next exercise when indicated.

Voice Motor Planning Exercise No. 2 (Isolated Vowel Repetitions at 60 bpm)
    Step 1. Follow exactly the same baseline method as that recommended in Step 1 of the preceding exercise, except that here the patient is asked to repeat a vowel at a speed of one production every second for at least 30 seconds. Note that the symbol "BM_2" is used on the treatment chart to tag these baseline data.
    Step 2. The procedure detailed in the preceding exercise is adopted, except that here the metronome is set at 60 bpm, and data entries on the treatment chart are identified by the "M_2" activity symbol. Proceed with the next exercise when so indicated.

Voice Motor Planning Exercise No. 3 (Isolated Vowel Repetitions at 90 bpm)
    Step 1. The baseline rules of the preceding exercises apply, except that here the vowel should be repeated at a speed a little faster than one production every second for at least 30 seconds. The symbol "BM_3" represents this finding.
    Step 2. The method employed in Exercise no. 1, Steps 2 to 4 are followed, except that here the metronome is set at 90 bpm, and data entries on the treatment chart are tagged with the "M_3" activity symbol. Advance to the next exercise as usual.

Voice Motor Planning Exercise No. 4 (Isolated Vowel Repetitions at 120 bpm)
    Step 1. The baseline method of Exercise no. 1 above is again adopted, except that here the requested speed of vowel repetition is roughly one production every half second for at least 30 seconds. The symbol "BM_4" is used to tag this baseline impression on the treatment chart.
    Step 2. Again, follow exactly the same method as that in the preceding exercises, except that here the speed of the metronome is set at 120 bpm. Data entries on the treatment chart are identified by the "M_4" activity symbol. Advance in the usual way.

Voice Motor Planning Exercise No. 5 (Two-Vowel Sequence at 30 bpm)
    Step 1. As before, use the Speech Characteristics Chart to render a baseline impression of the patient's voice motor programming skills during connected discourse. Be sure to tag this "BV" update with the appropriate date of data collection. Additionally, establish a baseline of the patient's ability to repeat a sequence of any two different vowels (e.g., /i-u/), producing one and then the other, roughly 2 seconds apart, for at least 30 continuous seconds. Several trials should be permitted. Using the Phonation Subsystem Behavioral Treatment Chart, record the overall percentage of error-free vowel combinations produced, that is, those sequential repetitions without evident features of apraxia of phonation. Enter the result on the y-axis grid, using the symbol "BM_5" to identify the score. Proceed with the next steps as indicated.

Step 2. Set the metronome to a speed of 30 bpm, select any vowel pair (e.g., /i-u/ or /a-i/), and request that the patient repeat the sequence to the beat for 30 continuous seconds. That is, if the /i-u/ pair were the stimulus the /i/ component is produced in concert with the first beat, the /u/ is produced on the second beat, the /i/ is repeated on the third beat, the /u/ is pronounced on the fourth beat, and so on until 30 seconds have elapsed. To reduce potential boredom and possible adaptation effects, periodically alter the composition of the vowel pair. At 30 bpm for 30 seconds, a maximum of seven and a half pairs can be produced error-free for the trial, for a total score of 100 percent correct. Each vowel pair is judged individually. Each pair that meets or exceeds the previous behaviorally defined performance objectives for consistent, accurate voice control should be graded correct. Those vowel pairs that suffer from voice apractic breakdowns are ruled incorrect and detract from the total percentage correct for the trial. A total mean score of at least 80 percent correct productions over 10 consecutive trials is arbitrarily recommended as the criterion for advancement to the next exercise. After each trial, enter on a notepad the patient's correct percentage score.

Step 3. Following each set of 10 trials, calculate the mean score from the notepad, and enter this result on the y-axis grid of the treatment chart in a separate column. The symbol "M_5" is used to tag these data. As usual, list the date of the session, number of trials (10), measurement unit (percentage correct), and target criterion (80 percent correct) in the respective cells of the column. Proceed with the next exercise when the criterion is met or the patient performs with no demonstrable signs to support continuation of the exercise.

Voice Motor Planning Exercise No. 6 (Two-Vowel Sequence at 60 bpm)

Step 1. Follow exactly the same procedures as those outlined in the preceding exercise, except that here the metronome is set at 60 bpm, and the baseline and therapy scores are respectively tagged "BM_6" and "M_6" on the treatment chart. Note that the speed of baseline productions must be increased to approximate 60 bpm. Advance as usual.

Voice Motor Planning Exercise No. 7 (Two-Vowel Sequence at 90 bpm)

Step 1. Again follow exactly the same procedures as those in Exercise no. 5, except that here the metronome is set at 90 bpm, and the baseline and therapy scores are respectively tagged "BM_7" and "M_7" on the treatment chart. Note that the speed of baseline productions must be increased to approximate 90 bpm. Advance as usual.

Voice Motor Planning Exercise No. 8 (Two-Vowel Sequence at 120 bpm)

Step 1. For this exercise, once again the same basic method as that detailed in Exercise no. 5 is followed, except that here the speed of the metronome is 120 bpm, and the baseline and therapy scores are labeled "BM_8" and "M_8" on the treatment chart. Note that the speed of baseline productions must be increased to approximate 120 bpm. Advance as usual.

Voice Motor Planning Exercise No. 9 (Three-Vowel Sequence at 30 bpm)

Step 1. The Speech Characteristics Chart is used again to render a baseline impression of the patient's voice motor programming skills during connected discourse. On the Phonation Subsystem Behavioral Treatment Chart score the ability to repeat sequentially a train of any three different vowels (e.g., /i-u-a/), producing the first one, then the second one, and then the last one roughly 2 seconds apart from one another for at least 30 continuous seconds. Several trials should be permitted. The overall percentage of error-free vowel trains produced is rated, that is, those completed without the aforementioned salient features of apraxia of phonation. Enter the baseline score on the y-axis grid of the chart, using the symbol "BM$_9$" for identification. Proceed to the next step as indicated. As a reminder, less than 80 percent correct baseline productions constitutes the recommended need for treatment.

Step 2. Set the metronome to a speed of 30 bpm, select any train of three vowels, and request that the patient repeat the sequence to the beat for 30 continuous seconds. If the /i-u-a/ sequence is selected as the train with which to begin the exercise, the /i/ component is produced on the first beat, the /u/ on the second beat, the /a/ on the third beat, the /i/, /u/, and /a/, respectively, on the fourth, fifth, and sixth beats, and so forth until 30 seconds have elapsed. To reduce potential boredom and possible order effects, the train composition should be periodically altered. At 30 bpm for 30 seconds, a maximum of five complete trains can be produced error-free for the trial, yielding a total score of 100 percent correct. Because this exercise is more complex, from a motor planning point of view, than the previous exercises, the patient should be permitted to jump in and out of the beat as desired to gain voice control, not unlike the act of jump rope in which the player jumping can opt out when the going gets too rough to handle at the moment. Opting out in this exercise should not be penalized, even if it takes several beats before the patient re-enters the task. However, do not render a score for the trial until 30 seconds of actual performances can be rated. As before, a total mean score of at least 80 percent correct productions over 10 consecutive trials will serve as the criterion for advancement to the next exercise. If after 30 trials the patient fails to demonstrate an observable improvement trend, discontinue this exercise and proceed, nonetheless, with the next exercise. As usual, a notepad works well for the recording of the patient's score per trial.

Step 3. After each set of 10 trials, the mean percentage of correct productions can be calculated from the notepad scores and entered on the y-axis grid of the treatment chart in a separate column. The activity symbol "M$_9$" is used to tag these data, and the appropriate date, number of trials (10), measurement unit (percentage correct), and target criterion (80 percent correct) must be recorded in the respective cells of the column. Proceed with the next exercise when so indicated.

Voice Motor Planning Exercise No. 10 (Three-Vowel Sequence at 60 bpm)

Step 1. Follow exactly the same baseline and treatment methods detailed in the preceding exercise, except that here the speed of the metronome is set at

60 bpm. The symbols "BM_{10}" and "M_{10}" are respectively used on the treatment chart to identify the baseline and therapy data. Note that the speed of baseline (nonmetronomic) productions must be increased to approximate 60 bpm. Advance as usual.

Voice Motor Planning Exercise No. 11 (Three-Vowel Sequence at 90 bpm)
    Step 1.   Again, follow the procedures of Exercise no. 9. However, this time, the speed of the metronome is set at 90 bpm, and the baseline and therapy activities are identified on the treatment chart as "BM_{11}" and "M_{11}," respectively. Note that the speed of baseline productions must approximate 90 bpm. Advance as usual.

Voice Motor Planning Exercise No. 12 (Three-Vowel Sequence at 120 bpm)
    Step 1.   The procedures of Exercise no. 9 are employed yet again, but here the speed of the metronome is set 120 bpm. The baseline and therapy data logged on the treatment chart are identified, respectively, with the symbols "BM_{12}" and "M_{12}." Note that baseline efforts must approximate 120 bpm to be graded as correct productions. Advance as usual.

Voice Motor Planning Exercises Nos. 13 to 16 (Four-Vowel Sequence at 30, 60, 90, and 120 bpm)
    Step 1.   Follow the same routes of Exercises nos. 9 to 12 above; however, for these exercises, the train stimuli will consist of four different vowels in sequence (e.g., /u-a-i-o/). Remember to adjust the baseline and therapeutic speeds of production according to the designated 30, 60, 90, and 120 bpm paradigms. The symbols "BM_{13-16}" and "M_{13-16}" should be used on the treatment chart to tag the data collected.

Voice Motor Planning Exercise No. 17 (Voiced and Voiceless Alternates at 30 bpm)
    Step 1.   Establish baseline ability by requesting that the patient alternate productions of the sequence /a-h-i/ several times, with a 2-second wedge between the sounds. That is, /a/ for 2 seconds, then /h/ for 2 seconds, then /i/ for 2 seconds, then /a/ for 2 seconds, and so forth. Rate the entire train, not its individual parts, following the same rating criteria as those used throughout this regimen. Repeat this procedure three times, altering the composition of the train each time (e.g., /u-h-a/, or /h-i-o/, or /h-æ-h/), and tally from the notepad scores the total number of trains that the patient produced correctly. Record this baseline finding on the treatment chart in the usual way, using the activity symbol "BM_{17}". Adopting the previous criterion for treatment, a score less than 80 percent correct justifies introduction of the next step.
    Step 2.   Set the metronome at 30 bpm, and instruct the patient to repeat the voiced and voiceless alternates train /a-h-i/ to the beat of one sound per beat continuously for 30 seconds. Employ the rating, scoring, charting, and advancement methods adopted earlier. When recording the data on the chart, list the ap-

propriate activity symbol (M_{17}). Note the need to alter the composition of the train periodically throughout the exercise, as suggested in the previous step, to reduce potential boredom and possible order effects.

Voice Motor Planning Exercises Nos. 18 to 20 (Voiced and Voiceless Alternates at 60, 90, and 120 bpm)

These exercises are identical in design to the first one above except that for these three the sequences are produced at metronomic speed equivalents of 60, 90, and 120 bpm, respectively. When charting these data be sure to record the correct activity symbols (M_{18}, M_{19}, or M_{20}). The prefix "B" is used to indicate baseline scores. Faster rates can be practiced with patients who have demonstrated the ability to experiment at such levels.

Note that if at the completion of Exercise no. 20 the patient has achieved the criterion set, experimentation with trains that contain more than four vowels as well as those composed of simple voiceless consonants at different metronomic speeds may prove additionally rewarding. Naturally, failure to meet the criterion at the lesser therapeutic level does not bode well for success in such advanced course work. In such instances, the program should be terminated after Exercise no. 20, and any other subsystem disturbances should be addressed according to the aforementioned recommended treatment sequence.

Ataxic Dysphonia

The hoarse-harsh vocal quality and concomitant loudness and pitch irregularities that chiefly characterize ataxic dysphonia result largely from the underlying incoordination of the vocal folds. Frequently compounding these pathophysiologic signs and symptoms are dysrhythmic respiratory patterns that tend to influence abnormally not only speech breathing activities but also the aerodynamic forces that regulate phonation. The following treatments are designed to improve the timing and coordination of laryngeal activities so as to enhance the physiologic backdrop for control of voice quality. Treatments of the associated phonation prosodic disturbances will be discussed in detail in Chapter 7. Some patients with ataxic dysphonia and coexistent respiration subsystem involvement may have already undergone the full-course speech breathing treatment program described in Chapter 3, which precludes the need to address directly the respiration subsystem during voice therapy. Others with mild degrees of dysphonia, as shown in Table 5–2, may be scheduled for simultaneous respiration and phonation subsystem treatments.

Laryngeal Timing and Coordination Exercise No. 1

Step 1. As usual, begin with a baseline measure of voice motor control during conversational speech. Use the Speech Characteristics Chart to record the subjective impression, remembering that the yardstick here is the seven-point interval scale. Additionally, request the patient to take a deep breath and then repeat the consonant-vowel (CV) syllable /pi/ three times, prolonging the vowel each time for 3 seconds without taking breaths between the productions. Allow the patient numerous trials, grading dichotomously each cluster of three repetitions collectively as either *correct* or *incorrect*. Compute the percentage of correct trials, and enter this baseline result on the y-axis grid of the Phonation Subsystem Behavioral Treatment Chart. The symbol "BL$_1$" should be used to tag these data. A score of less than 80 percent correct warrants continuation with Step 2. Otherwise proceed with Exercise no. 2.

Step 2. The See-Scape device will be used here. Substitute a 2- to 3-inch piece of drinking straw for the plastic nasal olive. If a small leak exists between the body of the straw and the rubber hose, a piece of tape can be used to create a tighter seal. Using a marking pen, divide the test tube into four equal divisions by drawing horizontal lines on the one-fourth, one-half, and three-quarter levels of the tube. Place the straw between the patient's lips so that the end rests lightly against the central incisor teeth. The straw remains in this position for the duration of the exercise, even though it may slightly interfere with production of the /p/.

Step 3. Place a noseclip on the patient and instruct him or her to inhale deeply through the mouth, and then repeat the CV syllable /pi/ three times, prolonging the vowel portion each time for 3 seconds without breathing between the productions. Counting aloud for the patient or placing a stopwatch in full view is recommended. Note the instantaneous ascent of the Styrofoam float to the top of the tube upon the first production. It should remain fixed at the top throughout the 3-second vowel-prolongation phase. At the completion of the first 3 seconds, the patient is required to repeat the CV syllable in the same fashion two more times without taking breaths prior to the productions. Performed correctly these repetitions will be characterized by a float that is firmly fixed at the top of the tube for the duration of the trial. The performance should be graded correct only if this outcome is achieved. If sudden inspiratory activity and/or intermittent vocal fold hyperadduction causes the float to descend to or below the three-quarter mark, the performance is graded incorrect. Each cluster of three repetitions constitutes a single trial. Use a notepad to grade the trial correct or incorrect. The suggested criterion for advancement to the next exercise is a total mean score of at least 80 percent correct productions over 10 consecutive trials. If after 30 trials no improvement trend is discernible, proceed with the next exercise. Rarely at this point is it fruitful to press the patient further with the same exercise.

Step 4. After each set of 10 trials, calculate from the notepad scores the mean percentage of correct trials, and record the result on the y-axis grid of the treatment chart in a separate column, usually the one next to the baseline entry. Tag these data with the "L$_1$" activity symbol, making certain to list the date, number of trials (10), measurement unit (percentage correct), and target criterion (80 percent correct) in the respective cells of the column. To reduce the potential for boredom and adaptation effects, the following stimuli may also be used throughout the exercise: /pu; ti; tu; ki; ku; ʃi; ʃu; si; su; fi; and fu/. Also note that here no attempts are made to improve the quality of the voice output. Advance to the next exercise when indicated.

Laryngeal Timing and Coordination Exercise No. 2

Step 1. Enter on the Speech Characteristics Chart another baseline perceptual rating (1 to 7) of voice motor control during connected discourse. Any score from 2 to 7 may justify the need for this exercise. As a precursor to this exercise, establish a baseline score of the patient's ability to repeat any of the aforementioned CV syllables three times, prolonging the vowel each time for 3 seconds with a breath-holding pause of 1 second between productions. Permit several trials, grading dichotomously each cluster of three repetitions collectively as either *correct* or *incorrect*. Compute the percentage of correct trials, and enter the score on the treatment chart in the usual way, using the symbol "BL$_2$" to represent the baseline data. Again, with a score of less than 80 percent correct, proceed to Step 2. Otherwise skip this step, and move on to Exercise no. 3.

Step 2. Use the same exact See-Scape set-up as that in the preceding exercise. Once the straw and noseclip are in position, request that the patient inhale deeply through the mouth and then repeat the CV syllable /pi/ three times, prolonging the vowel each time for 3 seconds with a breath-holding pause of 1 second duration between repetitions. Educate the patient that upon the first /pi/ production, the Styrofoam float should ascend rapidly to and remain fixed at the top of the tube as the vowel is prolonged. Immediately following this first production, the breath must be held for 1 second, as will be evidenced by the slow descent of the float: If the patient inhales, the float will rapidly fall to the bottom of the tube, which disqualifies the trial as incorrect. After completion of this pause, the patient is required to repeat the CV syllable in the same fashion, followed by another pause and so on for the third production. If the trial is performed correctly, it will be characterized by a float that remains firmly fixed at the top of the tube during all the /pi/ productions and descends slowly between them as the patient holds his or her breath each time for about 1 second. Rapid descent of the float, caused by unwanted inspiratory activity, and faulty rise characteristics due to poor voice motor control are abnormal performance features that individually or in tandem yield a rating of incorrect. Each cluster of three repetitions constitutes a single trial.

Step 3. Follow the same scoring and charting method as that detailed in Step 2 of the preceding exercise, except that here the data entries on the treatment chart are tagged with the "L$_2$" activity symbol. Note that the alternate CV syllables previously introduced can and should be incorporated into this exercise as well. As with the preceding exercise, the focus here is not on control of voice quality but rather on the timing and coordination of the phonation and respiration subsystems. Advance to the next exercise when so indicated.

Laryngeal Timing and Coordination Exercise No. 3

Step 1. In the usual way, rate overall voice motor control on the Speech Characteristics Chart. As an additional baseline measure, request that the patient take a deep breath and produce the following vowel train on that breath, prolonging in sequence each vowel roughly 2 seconds: /u-a-i-ɛ-o-ɪ/. The transition from one vowel to the next must be smooth, without significant voice offset time, variations in the length of each prolongation, or signs of inspiration. Allow the patient several trials, and grade the total percentage of correct performances. Enter this result on the phonation subsystem behavioral treatment chart with the activity symbol "BL$_3$" to identify the data. If the patient has a perceptual rating above "1" and a score of less than 80 percent correct performances on these baseline measures, he or she should move on to the next step. Otherwise skip this step and proceed with Exercise no. 4.

Step 2. Use the See-Scape device again. After fastening a noseclip on the patient and positioning the straw as described in the preceding exercises, have the patient inhale deeply through the mouth and then produce the following vowel train on that one breath, prolonging in sequence each vowel roughly 2 seconds: /u-a-i-ɛ-o-I/. A *correct* performance must meet these objectives: (1) upon the /u/ production the float travels swiftly to the top of the tube and remains fixed in that position, (2) the smooth transition, without another breath, to the /a/ causes the float to descend slowly to the bottom of the tube, (3) next, shifting to the /i/, again on the same initial breath, propels the float back up to the top of the tube, and it remains there throughout the prolongation, (4) phasing in the /ɛ/, as with the preceding /a/, results in another slow descent of the float to the bottom of the tube, (5) when the /o/ is produced next, again on the same initial breath, the float returns to the top of the tube, and it remains there until, (6) the final vowel in the train, the /I/, is produced, and the float descends slowly to the bottom of the tube to complete the trial.

If the patient significantly pauses between the vowels, varies the length of each production, or inhales during the trial, as would be evident by rapid descent of the float, the performance is rated incorrect. The criterion for advancement to the next exercise is a total mean score of at least 80 percent correct productions over 10 consecutive trials.

Step 3. As usual, a notepad can be effectively used to rate each performance correct or incorrect, and after each set of 10 trials, the mean correct percentage can be calculated and transferred to the y-axis grid of the treatment chart in a separate column. The activity symbol "L$_3$" is used here to tag these data, and the usual information relative to the date, number of trials (10), measurement unit (percentage correct), and target criterion (80 percent correct) should be listed in the respective cells of the column. The same discontinuation plan should be invoked here as that suggested in the preceding exercises. The following vowel trains are examples of effective alternatives to the original train throughout this regimen: (1) /i-a-o-ɛ-u-I/, (2) /o-ɛ-i-I-u-a/, (3) /u-ɛ-o-I-i-a/, (4) /I-u-a-i-ɛ-o/, and so on. When designing other substitutions make certain that the train is composed of these vowels and that the anatomy of adjacent pairs consists of a tense (i-u-o) and lax (a-ɛ-I) vowel, irrespective of which form is ordered first. Advance to the next exercise when so indicated.

Laryngeal Timing and Coordination Exercise No. 4

Step 1. Render a perceptual rating of the patient's voice on the Speech Characteristics Chart as usual. Also seek baseline information on the patient's ability to perform variations of the task in the preceding exercise. That is to say, request that he or she take a deep breath and produce a vowel train on that breath, prolonging in sequence the vowels for different lengths of time; however, none should exceed 3 seconds. The same grading and advancement criteria as those suggested in Step 1 of the preceding exercise are recommended here. The symbol "BL$_4$" is used to tag these baseline data.

Step 2. Follow the exact same See-Scape method as that in the preceding exercise, except that here the vowel train segments are prolonged not for uniform lengths of time but for variable time intervals on one breath. For the /u-a-i-ɛ-o-ɪ/ train, we begin the /u/ prolongation for 3 seconds, followed by the /a/ for 1 second, the /i/ for 2 seconds, the /ɛ/ for 3 seconds, the /o/ for 1 second, and finally the/ ɪ/ for 2 seconds. A stopwatch and the verbal cue "switch" should be used to prompt the patient from one segment of the train to the next.

Step 3. The criteria for grading the performances either correct or incorrect and for advancing within the program are adopted precisely from the preceding exercise, as are the recommended vowel train alternatives to reduce potential boredom and possible order effects. Note that the length of time assigned to each of the vowels in the train can be adjusted in any way desirable, provided that adjacent components differ in length and form (tense/lax) and that the patient can generate sufficient lung-thorax support to prolong the entire train on one breath.

Laryngeal Timing and Coordination Exercise No. 5

Step 1. As usual, offer a perceptual rating of voice motor control on the Speech Characteristics Chart. Establish a baseline regarding the patient's ability to produce sequentially on one breath the train of words that follow, prolonging the final sound of each word for a length of time different from that of the preceding word and varying the amount of pause time between the words on the train. Do not, however, exceed 3 seconds on any of the prolongations or pauses so as not to exhaust breath support for the entire train: *paper-cookie-fee-show-sue.* The same grading and advancement criteria outlined in Step 1 of Exercise no. 3 should be used, but the symbol "BL$_5$" is listed on the treatment chart to tag these baseline data. Alternative word stimuli may include the following options: *pea, puppy, tea, tie, key, tee-pee, she, see, bee, bye-bye, and baby.*

Step 2. Prepare the patient with the exact same See-Scape set-up as that used in the preceding exercises. Request that the patient produce sequentially on one deep breath the aforementioned word train in the following way. First, the patient produces the word "paper" and prolongs the final sound for 2 seconds, noting that the Styrofoam float should be fixed at the *top* of the tube during this production. Second, immediately following this production, the patient pauses, by holding the breath, until the float descends to the *halfway mark* on the tube, and then produces the word "cookie," which should propel the float back up to the *top* as the final vowel is prolonged for 3 seconds. Third, following this production, the patient pauses again until the float descends to the *three-quarter mark* and then produces the word "fee" to raise the float to the *top* as the word is prolonged for 1 second. Fourth, following this production, the patient pauses again until the float descends to the *one-quarter mark* and then produces the word "show" to raise the float to the *top* as the word is prolonged for 2 seconds. Finally, following this production, the patient pauses one last time until the float descends to the *bottom* of the tube and then produces the word "sue," noting the float's ascent to the *top* of the tube as this word is prolonged for a terminal 3 seconds. Use of a stopwatch and/or a verbal cue, such as "switch," to signal the patient when to shift from one word to the next in the train, is recommended and will forestall possible debate concerning the timing of the performances.

Step 3. Follow the same rating and advancement criteria as those detailed in the preceding exercises; however, here use "L_5" as the activity symbol on the treatment chart when logging the data collected. Note that the word stimuli chosen for the train may include any combination of those listed in Step 1 earlier. Furthermore, the prolongation and pause times can be made to vary in any way desirable as long as the patient can readily muster the breath support to complete the train without the need to inhale because of depletion of the original air supply.

Laryngeal Timing and Coordination Exercise No. 6
Step 1. By now there may be signs of improved voice motor control, owing to possible successes experienced with the previous exercises. Render a baseline perceptual rating of such control during connected discourse, and enter the result on the Speech Characteristics Chart in the usual way. Proceed with Step 2 if the voice disorder is still of clinical significance. Otherwise, move on to the next subsystem requiring therapy, as indicated in the sequence of treatments individually designed for the patient.

Step 2. To improve residual vocal quality disturbances borrow from the earlier subsection on treatments of the hypoadductory laryngeal mechanism the Speech Train, Sentence, and Contextual Speech exercises, and officially administer them as may be indicated for practice with the present patient.

Hyperkinetic Dysphonias

Table 5–1 summarizes different types of hyperkinetic disorders and the abnormal voice characteristics that they typically cause. For the *quick and slow hyperkinetic populations,* the voice therapy programs may best be designed using some of the exercises described earlier for other types of patients that may also be applicable to these patients because of overlapping characteristic voice difficulties. To improve the strained-strangled feature, we can employ strategically any or all of the exercises in the earlier subsection on treatment of the hyperadductory laryngeal mechanism. To combat the aperiodic hoarse-breathy feature that may plague patients, administration of any or all of the exercises from the earlier subsection on treatment of the hypoadduction laryngeal mechanism may prove facilitative. Even the immediately preceding laryngeal timing and coordination exercise regimen designed specifically for the ataxic dysphonic patient may be adapted successfully for use with some of these patients. If the voice is severely involved but the articulation subsystem is impaired to a lesser degree, which occurs on occasion, the compensatory technique used successfully with Case no. 3 above may be worth a shot if alternative treatments have proved fruitless.

Note: When entering the results of such adapted exercises on the Phonation Subsystem Behavioral Treatment Chart, use the activity symbol "E + the symbol of the exercise selected for therapy." For example, the symbol "ET" would be used on the chart to tag the results of the employment (E) of the Speech Train (T) exercises. One important caveat is warranted here: The voice disorders of these patients are often resistant to improvements despite the integrity of the treatments prescribed. Notwithstanding this probable shortcoming, as well as the oftentimes degenerative nature of their medical diagnoses, voice therapy in concert with applicable pharmaceutical intervention should be administered with cautious optimism and guarded prognoses.

For patients with *organic voice tremor,* voice therapy generally leads to disappointing results. Patients with myoclonus, on the other hand, do not tend to suffer in this respect, in that their voice tremors are less perceptible. However, when the adventitious movements involve other components of the speech mechanism (e.g., soft palate, face, and tongue), speech production can be affected. Pharmacologic therapy has been disappointing. However, clinicians may wish to communicate with neurologists about the feasibility of prescription drugs for these types of patients.

Figure 5–3 is a flow diagram that illustrates the overall sequence of voice therapy techniques, segregated according to possible neurogenic patterns of vocal fold vibration abnormalities, as listed and reviewed in this chapter. Before we close, another case sample is presented next.

Illustrative Case No. 6. NR is a 22-year-old male who experienced a severe closed head injury in an automobile accident at the age of 21 years, which resulted in bi-frontal lobe lesions, confirmed by multiple computed tomography scans. At the time of this accident, he was enrolled in a junior college. Whereas he exhibited mild cognitive and linguistic deficits following this incident, his primary difficulties were with motor speech control. Language testing, including examinations for aphasia, yielded equivocal findings. Differential evaluations for the presence of motor speech disorders resulted in unequivocal signs and symptoms of severe apraxia of speech, marked predominantly by a phonatory component, and co-occuring unilateral upper motor neuron dysarthria of milder dimensions. The classic apraxia features of highly variable sound and word transpositions and associated struggle phenomena were evident in NR's articulatory efforts. Most pronounced was his phonatory apraxia, characterized by inconsistent failures to program (volitionally) voice onset time or appropriate pitch and loudness controls. Intermittent periods of aphonia, followed by sudden and unpredictable bursts of high-pitched, squeal-like vocalizations, were quite common throughout attempts at communication. Video-stroboscopic and routine flexible fiberoptic laryngeal examinations revealed a healthy-appearing larynx; vocal fold movements, however, to command were slow but complete in their adductory-abductory cycles whenever phonation was produced.

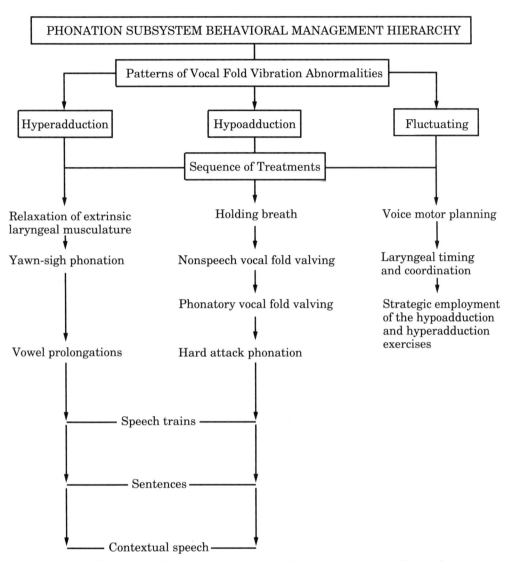

Figure 5–3. Phonation subsystem voice therapy hierarchy segregated by underlying vocal fold vibration abnormalities: hyperadduction, hypoadduction, and fluctuation.

Prior to registering for the present rehabilitation program, NR withdrew from 6 months of intensive therapy during which routine voice and articulation exercises were unsuccessful.

The treatment team, consisting of four speech pathologists, determined that the initial focus of intervention should be on the apraxia of phonation disturbances. As such, the voice motor planning exercise regimen detailed earlier for apraxia of phonation was administered. In the interests of time and space, only the overall results of these treatments will be presented here for demonstration purposes.

At the outset of the program, a baseline score of "7" was rendered on the speech characteristics chart, indicating marked impairment of voice motor planning skills. The severity of this disorder had a camouflaging effect on the degree of his concomitant speech motor difficulties. The voice exercises were initiated in early March, scheduled for five 1-hour sessions per week. He zipped through the first four exercises to criteria after just nine sessions. Exercises nos. 5 through 8, however, were quite a bit more grueling for NR, taking him 19 sessions ultimately to achieve criteria. Even Exercise no. 5, which required the sequential repetition of two vowels at a speed (30 bpm) that separated the two into essentially isolated sounds, not unlike the task of Exercise no. 1, required six sessions to meet the objective. Maintenance testing at this time revealed preservation of the learned behaviors to date. Exercises 9 through 12 required NR to sequence three different vowels at different metronomic speeds. Notwithstanding his easy mastery of the task at 30 bpm, he struggled for 23 sessions, with subtle signs of improvement, before achieving the criteria set. On the most difficult exercises, nos. 13 through 16, NR demonstrated good voice motor control by attaining all objectives relatively quickly—in just five sessions. At that time, we reserved further work on praxis until the articulation subsystem treatments, which were scheduled next in sequence. NR progressed from an original baseline voice motor control score of "7" to a therapeutically induced score of "3" during conversational speech. The treatment team attributed this significant improvement to both the intensive exercise program and NR's dogged determination to whip this problem.

It should be noted in all fairness, however, that about halfway into these treatments NR began to overcompensate by voicing even normally voiceless sounds. Because intensive therapeutic work on speech praxis was forthcoming, this phenomenon was not formally addressed directly during voice therapy. (The suggested readings provide additional information on neurogenic voice disorders and their management.)

SUGGESTED READINGS

Arnold, G. E. (1962). Vocal rehabilitation of paralytic dysphonia. Technique of intracordal injection. *Archives of Otolaryngology, 76,* 358–368.

Aronson, A. E. (1990). *Clinical voice disorders: An interdisciplinary approach* (3rd ed.). New York: Thieme-Stratton, Inc.

Boone, D. R. (1990). *The voice and voice therapy* (2nd ed.). Englewood Cliffs, NJ: Prentice-Hall, Inc.

Crumley, R. L. (1990). Teflon versus thyroplasty versus nerve transfer: A comparison. *Annals of Otology, Rhinology, Laryngology, 99,* 759–763.

Dedo, H. H. (1976). Recurrent laryngeal nerve section for spastic dysphonia. *Annals of Otology, Rhinology and Laryngology, 85,* 451–459.

Finitzo, T., & Freeman, F. (1989). Spasmodic dysphonia, whether and where: Results of seven years of research. *Journal of Speech and Hearing Research, 32,* 541–555.

Ford, C., & Bless, D. (1986). Clinical experience with injectable collagen in vocal fold augmentation. *Laryngoscope, 96,* 863–883.

Froeschels, E. (1952). *Dysarthric speech: Speech in cerebral palsy.* Magnolia, MA: Expression Co.

Froeschels, E., Kastein, S., & Weiss, D. (1955). A method of therapy for paralytic conditions of the mechanisms of phonation, respiration, and glutination. *Journal of Speech and Hearing Disorders, 20,* 365–370.

Hartman, D. E. (1984). Neurogenic dysphonia. *Annals of Otolaryngology, Rhinology, Laryngology, 93,* 57–64.

Isshiki, N , Morita, H., Okamura, H., & Hiramoto, M. (1974). Thyroplasty as a new phonosurgical technique. *Acta Otolaryngologica, 78,* 451–457.

Ludlow, C., Naunton, M., Sedory, M., Schulz, M., & Hallett, M. (1988). Effects of botulinum toxin injections on speech in adductor spasmodic dysphonia. *Neurology, 38,* 1220–1225.

Miller, R., Woodson, M., & Jankovic, J. (1987). Botulinum toxin injection of the vocal fold for spasmodic dysphonia. *Archives of Otolaryngology, Head and Neck Surgery, 113,* 602–605.

Moncur, J., & Brackett, I. (1974). *Modifying vocal behavior.* New York: Harper & Row.

Ramig, L., Harada-Fazoli, K., Scherer, R., & Bonatati, C. (1990). Changes in phonation of Parkinson's disease patients following voice therapy. Presented to the *Clinical Dysarthria Conference,* San Antonio, TX.

Stemple, J. C. (1984). *Clinical voice pathology: Theory and management.* Columbus, OH: Charles E. Merrill, Publishers.

Chapter 6

Treatment of the Articulation Subsystem

WHEN TO BEGIN

A good percentage of clinical time is spent treating the articulation sub-system in patients with motor speech disorders. Speech clinicians realize, how-ever, that disturbances of the articulation subsystem rarely occur in isolation. Coexisting respiration, resonation, phonation, and/or prosody subsystem break-downs are not uncommon, as reviewed in detail in the preceding chapters. That neuromuscular and motor planning deficits involving any one or more of the as-sociated speech subsystems may adversely influence the performance of the artic-ulation subsystem is well documented. So to, as proposed here, is the understand-ing that because these subsystems are functionally interdependent, their coexisting disturbances should be treated sequentially, according to the natural order of their physiologic relationship and degree of impairment. Earlier, ration-ales were presented for treating sequentially respiration, resonation, and phona-tion problems before administering articulation subsystem treatments. Despite the severity of the articulation difficulty and the temptation to render first-order treatment priority to this problem, experienced clinicians recognize up front the need to delay such full-scale intervention until efforts can be made to improve the underlying physiologic support for speech through the treatment of other sub-systems, when needed. Primed in this way for intensive therapy, the articulation subsystem may prove most responsive. Skirting these preparatory steps with ea-gerness to stimulate immediate improvements in articulatory proficiency, so that patients may possess a ready means of more intelligible communication, this cli-nician has failed on numerous occasions in the past. Rather than achieving the stated objectives, many patients exposed to such mismanagement dropped out of therapy frustrated, with little to show for *their* honest efforts.

CHARACTERISTIC DIFFERENCES BETWEEN PATIENTS

The pathophysiology underlying articulatory imprecision in patients with motor speech disorders is not usually uniform, either within or between patient subgroups. The neuromuscular or motor planning deficit often varies in degree from patient to patient, as does the resultant articulation disorder. Even patients with virtually the same etiology and medical and speech diagnoses may differ with respect to both their overall disabilities and their ultimate responses to identical treatments. When patients do present with similar articulation subsystem symptoms, their diagnoses do not always coincide; they may indeed belong to different population subgroups, possess dissimilar etiologies, and struggle with incongruous movement abnormalities. This complex matrix was also realized and addressed in earlier chapters when attention was focused on other speech subsystems.

The following sections describe the disturbances of the articulation subsystem that patients with motor speech disorders are likely to exhibit.

Spastic Dysarthria. Generalized hypertonicity, weakness, immobility, abnormal force physiology, and exaggerated reflexes of virtually all muscles of the speech mechanism produce obvious dysfunction of the articulation subsystem. Speech is slow-labored and imprecise articulatory efforts, compounded by disturbances of respiration; resonation, and phonation often render speech unintelligible.

The following sequence of treatments is generally recommended for the spastic dysarthric patient:

1. Lingual, labial, and mandibular musculature tone reduction.
2. Lingual, labial, and mandibular musculature strengthening.
3. Lingual, labial, and mandibular force physiology training.
4. Phonetic stimulation in various contexts.

Hypokinetic Dysarthria. Widespread rigidity and associated paresis of virtually all muscles of the speech mechanism justify treatments to improve respiration, phonation, articulation, and indeed prosody. The sequence of articulation subsystem exercises recommended above for patients with spastic dysarthria is generally followed for those with hypokinetic dysarthria. Variations of the force physiology and phonetic training programs are necessary, however, to address the pathophysiologic differences between these populations. In addition, weakness of the tongue, lip, and/or jaw musculature may not prove salient for all patients with hypokinetic dysarthria.

Hyperkinetic Dysarthria. Movement abnormalities in patients with this motor speech disorder are either (1) characteristically quick, unsustained, and jerky, as observed in those with Huntington's disease; (2) predominantly slow, sustained, and writhing, as seen in individuals with dystonia and athetosis; or (3) tremorous, as occur in essential tremor and myoclonus. These involuntary disturbances may adversely affect functioning of the entire speech mechanism. Depending on the severity of their problem, many such patients are best scheduled for treatment of the respiration and phonation subsystems before the initiation of therapy for coexistent difficulties with articulation and prosody. Because these individuals may possess diverse pathologic conditions, they cannot be treated according to a uniform sequence of exercises. Instead, their presenting signs and symptoms should dictate whether specific exercises are indicated. Whereas this caveat applies to all other dysarthric populations as well, its employment here is especially predominant and noteworthy. With this precaution in mind, the following sequence of articulation subsystem exercises is *generally* recommended for patients with hyperkinetic dysarthria:

1. Lingual, labial, and mandibular force physiology training.
2. Phonetic stimulation in various contexts.

Note. If the patient exhibits significant, consistent disturbances in muscle tone and strength, treatments aimed at these conditions should be employed in sequence, as recommended earlier for spastic and hypokinetic dysarthric patients.

Ataxic Dysarthria. Widespread incoordination in timing, speed, range, and force of muscular activities throughout the speech mechanism is characteristic of this motor speech disorder. However, not unlike hypokinetic and hyperkinetic dysarthric patients, whose lesion sites are generally within the extrapyramidal system, those with ataxic dysarthria usually do not exhibit significant breakdown of the resonation subsystem. After indicated treatments of the respiration and phonation subsystems, these patients are primed for articulation exercises according to the sequence below:

1. Lingual, labial, and mandibular force physiology training.
2. Phonetic stimulation in various contexts.

Note. If the patient presents with significant degrees of hypotonia and/or muscle weakness, specific strengthening exercises may be indicated in sequence before the above named therapies. Also, the nature of the force physiology program for these patients will vary somewhat from that designed for other dysarthric patients whose mechanism difficulties are not caused primarily by faulty timing and coordination.

Flaccid Dysarthria. Focal or multiple speech subsystem difficulties, depending on the extent and number of cranial nerve lesions, generally cause commensurate hypotonicity, weakness, paralysis, abnormal force physiology, and diminished reflexes of involved musculature. When indicated, respiration, resonation, and phonation subsystem impairments may be treated in this order, depending on the severity of involvements, prior to treatments of the articulation subsystem. Specific articulation exercises should vary in concert with the muscle groups that are disturbed and the degree of their involvement. The following sequence of articulation subsystem treatments is recommended:

1. Lingual, labial, and/or mandibular musculature strengthening.
2. Lingual, labial, and/or mandibular force physiology training.
3. Phonetic stimulation in various contexts.

Mixed Dysarthria. In mixed motor speech disorders, the treatment program should address first the component of the mixture that is most severe, although on occasion discrepancies occur in component levels of involvement.

Whereas, for example, the articulation subsystem may suffer predominantly from the flaccid pathophysiology associated with advancing amyotrophic lateral sclerosis (ALS), in the same patient the phonation subsystem may be suffering from apparently intractable spasticity and vocal hyperfunction. Therapeutic focus would shift with respect to the initial treatments indicated per subsystem. The exercises designed for vocal fold hyperadduction might effectively be administered first, followed by the aforementioned intervention package for the flaccid articulatory component. Any coexisting respiration or resonation disturbances would respectively be treated before these other conditions. More complex mixtures than this example create even greater challenges regarding the appropriate types and sequences of treatments. Irrespective of the presenting condition, however, clinicians should resist swerving from the suggested hierarchy of subsystem treatments: Respiration first, followed sequentially by the resonation, phonation, articulation, and prosody subsystems. Adjustments are made not in the sequence, but rather in the specific subsystem exercise protocols that clinically are judged most indicated on the basis of the severity and coincident pathophysiology. At times, the employment of more than one treatment regimen may prove fruitful. For example, exercises for both the hyperadducting and hypoadducting vocal fold mechanism may be indicated for the mixed spastic-flaccid dysphonic (dysarthric) patient. The regimen administered first, in this case, may be contingent upon which of the two debilitating conditions is considered most predominant.

Apraxia of Speech. Disturbances of the articulation and prosody subsystems receive primary attention in the treatment program for this disorder. The sequence of exercises includes:

1. Nonspeech oral motor planning activities.
2. Simple phonetic motor planning stimulation.
3. Complex phonetic motor planning stimulation.

TABLE 6–1. Overall Sequence (Left to Right) of Articulation Subsystem Exercises Segregated According to Type of Motor Speech Disorder

	EXERCISES				
Disorder	Tone Reduction	Strengthening	Force Physiology Training	Phonetic Stimulation	Motor Planning Activities
Spastic dysarthria	X	X	X	X	
Hypokinetic dysarthria	X		X	X	
Hyperkinetic dysarthria			X	X	
Ataxic dysarthria			X	X	
Flaccid dysarthria		X	X	X	
Apraxia of speech				X	X

For mixed disorders, assume the logical sequence of treatments prescribed for the respective components. The absence of an "X" mark in a given column indicates that the exercise above is generally not administered to patients with the disorder listed in the corresponding row of the table. Exceptions are not uncommon, however.

Note. Once the patient completes this program, the prosody exercise regimen is introduced wherein factors such as loudness, pitch, rate, pause time, and stress are addressed.

Table 6–1 summarizes the overall sequence of articulation subsystem exercises recommended differentially for patients with motor speech disorders. Generally speaking, when the degree of articulation imprecision is moderate or severe, such exercises should be exclusively administered after necessary treatments of the respiration, resonation, and phonation subsystems, but before those indicated to improve prosody. On the other hand, mild disturbances of articulation may not require such therapeutic segregation; instead, dual subsystem treatments may prove successful if logically ordered and scheduled. Focus on the articulation and prosody subsystems, for example, is a natural combination for simultaneous treatment.

METHOD TO FOLLOW WHEN EMPLOYING THE ARTICULATION SUBSYSTEM EXERCISES

Whereas drug therapy may enhance the sensorimotor potential of a given patient, improvements in articulation proficiency are usually not evidenced without intensive behavioral therapy. Surgical procedures to restore articulatory skills, such as anastomoses of cranial nerves, have been implemented, but are by no means prescribed routinely for the treatment of motor speech disorders.

Table 6-1 provides a general synopsis of probable exercise requirements for dysarthric and apractic patients. Patients may present, however, with signs and symptoms that require a different set and sequence of articulation subsystem treatments from those recommended in Table 6–1. Hyperkinetic and ataxic dysarthric patients, for example, may exhibit significant abnormalities in orofacial muscle tone and/or strength that demand clinical attention before force physiology training. The patient with parkinsonian (hypokinetic) dysarthria may suffer from associated orofacial muscle weakness that may best be scheduled for treatment between the tonal and force physiology exercise programs. Regardless of the modifications that need to be made in the number and types of treatments administered to a given patient, adherence to the left to right exercise sequence recommended in Table 6–1 is advised.

Ordered according to this sequence, each of the treatment subsections below takes into account the types of patients for whom the exercises are most indicated. This approach tends to reduce redundancy, thus preserving space for salient treatment information. For patients who present with hypertonicity of the articulation musculature, irrespective of their speech diagnosis, the *tone reduction* therapy program is prescribed first. When orofacial muscle strength is compromised, the *strengthening exercises* are introduced before force physiology training, but after indicated treatments of coexistent hypertonicity of the same musculature. All dysarthric patients undergo an intensive *force physiology regimen,* designed specifically to improve the underlying articulation subsystem pathophysiology, after any necessary tone and/or strengthening exercises have been administered to the same musculature. *Phonetic stimulation* is a core treatment component for all patients. It is scheduled, however, when the articulators have been physiologically prepared, i.e., through the preceding exercise hierarchy. The *speech motor planning* activities, reserved primarily for apractic patients, are phased in along with or subsequent to phonetic practice.

It is not unlikely that the sequence of treatments will vary from one involved muscle group to the next. That is to say, at any given point in the program, the tongue may be undergoing one particular form of treatment, the lips another, and the jaw yet another, as indicated by their different difficulties and responses. In any case, it is usually most prudent to delay the phonetic practice segments until the patient has completed (to criteria if possible) the prescribed physiologic exercises for all the articulators. Advancement within the program is generally contingent on the achievement of criteria set for all exercises. As with all previously administered speech subsystem treatments, however, movements from one exercise to the next may be dictated not only by such success but also by the patient's failure to demonstrate any observable trend of improvement after several consecutive trials. Here we will maintain the general rule of thumb advocated earlier calling for discontinuation of a given exercise if after 30 consecutive trials no such trend is evident. Although the succeeding exercise may be no easier for the patient, it is phased in with cautious optimism according to the same advancement or discontinuation guidelines. The most difficult decision the clinician faces is when the patient illustrates some gains but continues to fall short of criteria levels despite concentrated efforts to go the distance. Should the exercise in question be administered further, or would it be best to move on in the interests of time, cost, and patient motivation? Perhaps modifications of the same technique will make a discernible difference in the ultimate outcome. Because each patient's capabilities and stamina must be judged individually, universal answers to these and other similar questions are neither useful nor possible. Stopping short of a patient's inherent potential can be counterproductive, but pushing too hard can be disastrous. Establishing a balanced approach is not easy: It taps the clinical intuition skills of us all.

TREATMENT MATERIALS

The clinician needs to assemble the following materials in order to employ all the exercises recommended in this chapter:

1. See-Scape Device* (see Chapter 3 references),
2. Mirror,
3. Tape recorder,
4. Metronome,
5. Stopwatch or wristwatch with second hand,

*Pro-Ed, 8700 Shoal Creek Blvd; Austin, Tx 78758.

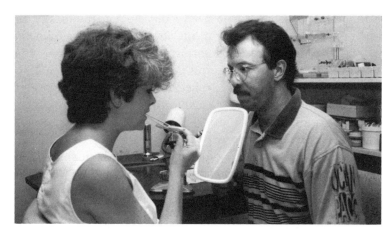

Figure 6–1.   Recommended seating arrangement for most articulation subsystem treatments. Note the mirror positioned for visual biofeedback to the patient, yet unobtrusive from the clinician's point of view. This arrangement affords the clinician the best direct view of the patient's mouth, while the patient is able not only to see her own performances but also to glance up easily at the clinician for any necessary prompts during an exercise.

6. Stethoscope,
7. Bite blocks (plastic)*, or putty material†,
8. Tongue depressors,
9. Roll of ½ inch Scotch tape,
10. Cotton-tipped applicators,
11. Vinyl examination gloves and finger cots,
12. Drinking straws and facial tissues,
13. Button (size of nickel) and string or dental floss,
14. Gauze pads, and
15. Treatment charts.

Before the exercises are introduced, it may be worth noting Figure 6–1, which illustrates the recommended physical set-up for all treatment sessions. A mirror supported by a small table vise permits the patient easy visual feedback of all articulator activities, while at the same time enabling the clinician to view and manipulate these structures. Use of examination gloves and finger cots is recommended for sanitary purposes when conducting most of these exercises.

TREATMENT OF HYPERTONICITY

Tone refers to the inherent elasticity of muscle tissue, and can be measured by the amount of resistance detected by an examiner as a body part is moved

*Edgewood Press, Inc., Box 811, Nicholasville, KY 40356.
† Citricon Base and Universal Accelerator; Sybron/Kerr, Romulus, MI 48174 (or from most local dental supply companies).

through its range of motion with no active muscle contraction by the patient. Normally, such resistance is very slight but not too relaxed, soft, or flabby, as in the hypotonus of flaccid paralysis. Treatment for this condition is usually approached through a muscle-strengthening program. Increased tone, on the other hand, occurs in two primary forms: (1) spasticity, as observed in patients with pyramidal system (upper motor neuron) lesions; and (2) rigidity, as evidenced in patients with extrapyramidal system lesions. Spastic hypertonus does not typically involve all muscles to the same degree. This is especially true of those within the speech mechanism. The condition is often most dramatic during only the initial part of a given movement, not throughout the full excursion. When lessening of resistance is felt as the muscle continues to be passively stretched, this effect is known as the "clasp-knife" phenomenon, seen often in the joints of hypertonic limbs. A similar effect may be observed in such measures of the tongue and jaw musculature of spastic dysarthric patients. The hypertonus of rigidity, characteristic of parkinsonism, usually affects the full range of motion, resulting in perceived stiffness for the entire measurement. "Lead pipe" or "plastic" hypertonicity are terms frequently used to describe the severity of this condition. In patients with the hypokinesia of Parkinson's disease and parkinsonism, the underlying rigidity of virtually all the muscles of the body is compounded by superimposed rhythmic contractions of certain muscle groups. This perceived phenomenon is termed "cogwheel" rigidity, but its existence is generally limited to joints of the limbs and neck. Whether of the spastic or rigid type, hypertonia of muscle tissue imposes strict limitations on volitional movement control. Exercises to reduce or normalize tone are almost always indicated for patients with these conditions. The regimen below is designed for such purposes and is subdivided into three articulator categories: Tongue, lips, and jaw. Note that tone measurements depend largely on examiner perceptions and are therefore subject to inconsistency and error. The greater the experience in conducting such evaluations, in both pathologic and normal populations, the more accurate and reliable the examiner's judgments tend to be. In the beginning especially, measures of inter- and intrajudge reliability will prove valuable by ensuring that the data collected are as accurate as possible.

Tongue Hypertonicity Exercise No. 1

Step 1. As shown in Figure 6–2, request the patient to stick out the tongue so that it can be gently grasped with a gauze pad. Once the tongue is positioned and secured in this fashion, instruct the patient to relax as much as possible to allow the tongue to be (passively) pulled slowly forward and laterally to measure its inherent tissue elasticity. Maintain the tongue in each manipulated direction for at least 3 seconds. Repeat this technique three times before rendering a baseline rating of overall muscle tone on the Tone Improvement Chart (Figure 6–3), which is based on a popularly used scale ranging from +4 to −4. To record these baseline data, enter on the y-axis grid the perceived degree of muscle tone, making certain to list the date of data collection, the number of trials

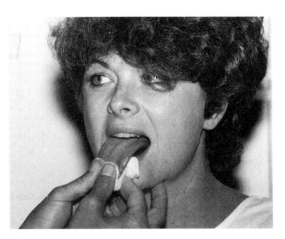

Figure 6–2.
Forward pull of the tongue as required in the tone reduction therapy regimen. Note that the thumbs and index fingers do the pulling as the remaining fingers of each hand are positioned gently against the undersurface of the patient's chin for leverage and head balance control.

(3), the musculature tested ("T" for tongue), and the activity (BF_1, BR/L_1), indicating forward and lateral tone baselines. A score of "+1.5" or higher generally warrants a prescription for the following tone reduction steps. If the patient achieves a score closer to "0" (normal tone) or in fact is rated as having a hypotonic (−1 to −4) tongue, this exercise is not indicated.

Step 2. Employ the same technique as in the preceding step, except that here the tongue is stretched in the forward direction only, withdrawn from the patient's mouth to the level of natural anatomical resistance (Figure 6–2), and held steady in this final position to an out-loud count of 10 seconds. In the early stages of this exercise the patient may protest in mild discomfort. Encourage the patient to bear with the exercise with the understanding that this side effect usually lessens as the hypertonicity is reduced.

Step 3. On a notepad record the perceived degree of hypertonicity as the tongue was maintained in this fully extended position, making certain to use the −4 to +4 scale. Repeat this procedure until the patient achieves a mean tone rating that is at least 3 scale values improved over the baseline ratings, or "0" if the baseline score was a 2 or 3, over 10 consecutive trials, allowing a 10-second rest period after each measurement.

Step 4. After each set of 10 trials, enter the mean rating in a separate column on the y-axis grid of the Tone Improvement Chart, listing the date, number of trials (10), musculature treated (T), activity symbol (F_1), and calculated target criterion (?) in the respective cells of the column. As always, if the patient fails to demonstrate a discernible trend of improvement after 30 consecutive trials, it may be best to discontinue and proceed with the next exercise.

Note. Avoid pulling the tongue too far out of the patient's mouth, which can cause the lingual frenum to tear and bleed. One overzealous patient decided to speed this treatment process by pulling his own tongue while at home. It took 10 days for his frenum to heal. Another common and counterproductive problem during this exercise is the exertion of too much finger pressure on the tongue, causing pain. Pulling the tongue too forcefully and quickly forward may also

TONE IMPROVEMENT CHART

Patient's name:

Birthdate: _____ **Sex:** _____

Speech diagnosis:

Medical diagnosis:

Clinician:

Facility:

Address:

Comments:

ACTIVITY KEY

1. Musculature: Tongue (T); Lip (L); Velum (V); Jaw (J)

2. Activity: Forward tongue pull (F); Lateral tongue pull (R/L); Up/Down lip pull (U/D); Open/Close Jaw excursions (O/C); Velar Massage (A/P)

Baseline (pre-treatment): B + feature symbol

TREATMENT RESPONSES

Dates:

Subjective Rating	
Very Increased	+ 4
	+ 3
	+ 2
	+ 1
Normal	0
	– 1
	– 2
Very Decreased	– 3
	– 4

No. of trials

Musculature

Activity symbol

Target criterion

SESSIONS

Figure 6–3. Blank Tone Improvement Chart to be used for articulator tone reduction therapy.

cause pain. The best approach is gentle grasping accompanied by slow, gradual, and steady pulling to complete extension.

Tongue Hypertonicity Exercise No. 2

Step 1. Derive a baseline score for right/left lateral muscle tone by gently pulling the extended tongue to one corner of the mouth, holding it there for roughly 3 seconds, and then smoothly gliding it over to the opposite corner for another 3-second holding phase. Following basically the scoring procedure outlined in the preceding exercise, enter this baseline result on the tone chart in the usual way, making certain that the entry is tagged with the "BR/L$_2$" activity symbol. Proceed as directed in Step 1 above.

Step 2. Request the patient to protrude the tongue so that it can be grasped gently. Next, pull it forward as completely as possible, noting that if the criterion set in Exercise no. 1 has been met, extending the tongue in this fashion should be possible without difficulty. Once fully withdrawn the tongue is slowly pulled to the right corner of the mouth, held there for an out-loud count of 10 seconds, and then smoothly moved across the midline to the left corner for another count of 10 seconds to complete the trial. Although the degree of hypertonicity present will probably produce resistance to these adjustments, maintaining the lateral pulling forces along the way usually proves fruitful after 10 or 15 trials with most patients.

Step 3. Follow the same scoring and advancement procedures detailed in the preceding exercise, Steps 3 and 4, making certain that on the Tone Improvement Chart these data are tagged with the activity symbol "R/L$_1$."

Tongue Hypertonicity Exercise No. 3

Step 1. Take another baseline score following the exact same method detailed in Exercise no. 1, Step 1. Proceed with this exercise if this finding suggests the need for additional treatment. If not, move on to the next indicated exercise subcategory for the patient. *Note:* Tag these baseline data with the activity symbol "BF$_2$, BR/L$_3$."

Step 2. After requesting the patient to protrude the tongue, grasp and pull it gently forward until it is fully withdrawn. Upon completion of an out-loud count of 10 seconds, immediately but smoothly glide the tongue to the right corner of the mouth, maintaining the gentle pulling force along the way and during a 10-second count in this position. Finish the trial by slowly pulling the tongue across the midline to the left corner of the mouth and holding it there for a final count of 10 seconds. Remember the importance of stretching or extending the tongue throughout the entire trial, even if the patient objects initially and the stiffness factor seems invincible. Eventually, these obstacles should fade as the hypertonicity lessens.

Step 3. Record in the usual way the perceptual score for the whole trial. Follow the scoring and advancement criteria detailed in Exercise no. 1, but make certain that on the tone improvement chart the data collected during this exercise are tagged with the activity symbol "F,R/L$_1$."

Note. These three exercises are generally sufficient to reduce significantly hypertonicity of the tongue musculature, regardless of the type or etiology. In most cases, results are evident within a few treatment sessions. In the beginning it may appear that the degree of stiffness is so great as to be impossible to overcome with any kind of exercise. As mentioned earlier, the patient may also feel helpless as pain and tenderness are evoked with each tug on the tongue. Patience and perseverance are truly virtuous here. Affording the patient ongoing views of the treatment chart as results of the exercises are logged may provide additional motivation to persevere, especially if the scores are improving. Periodic examinations of the lingual frenum are advised, as on rare occasions this connective tissue may avulse, requiring rest from treatment.

Lip Hypertonicity Exercise No. 1

Step 1. With the patient's mouth at rest, gently grasp the lower lip with a gauze pad and pull it slightly outward and then downward toward the chin, exposing the lower teeth and gingival tissue. Hold the lip firmly and steadily in this position for a count of 3 seconds. Repeat the procedure three times. Next, grasp the upper lip and pull it outward and then upward toward the nose, exposing the upper teeth and gum line. Hold the lip in this position for a count of 3, and repeat the procedure three times. Render a mean baseline rating of overall lip tone on the y-axis grid of the Tone Improvement Chart, making certain to record the date, number of trials (three), musculature ("L" for lips), and activity symbol (BU/D$_1$). Proceed with the next step if the mean rating is equal to or exceeds "+1.5"; otherwise this exercise regimen is not indicated.

Step 2. Here the focus is on the lower lip only. Proceeding as in Step 1 above, instruct the patient to relax as much as possible so that the lip can be passively pulled toward the chin. Once the lip is in the fully lowered position, count aloud for 10 seconds and then release the lip for 10 seconds. On a notepad rate the degree of hypertonicity perceived.

Step 3. Repeat this procedure until the patient achieves a mean tone score that is at least 3 scale values improved over the baseline ratings, or "0" if the baseline score was a 2 or 3, over 10 consecutive trials.

Step 4. After each set of 10 trials, enter the mean result in a separate column on the y-axis grid of the chart, making certain to record the date of the session, number of trials (10), musculature treated (L), activity symbol (U/D$_1$), and calculated target criterion (?) in the respective cells of the column. Discontinuation of the exercise is advisable if the patient fails to demonstrate any observable trend of improvement after 30 consecutive trials. If this particular course is followed, the next lip exercise in sequence is nonetheless administered, albeit with guarded optimism. *Note:* As with tongue therapy, pulling the lip too forcefully and abruptly can be counterproductive and may yield negative effects.

Lip Hypertonicity Exercise No. 2

Step 1. Employ roughly the same baseline method as discussed in the preceding exercise, except that here the upper lip is in the spotlight. Thus, render a rating for the tone of this structure only, and tag the result on the chart with the symbol "BU/D_2." Proceed according to the rule advocated in Exercise no. 1.

Step 2. Once the patient is relaxed, grasp the upper lip and gently pull it fully upward toward the nose; hold it in that position for a count of 10 seconds and then release it for 10 seconds. On a notepad rate the degree of hypertonicity perceived. Follow the exact same method for establishing the criterion for advancement as that detailed in the preceding exercise.

Note: These two exercises are usually sufficient stimulation to improve lip hypertonia. Not unlike the responsiveness of the tongue musculature, the lips generally show signs of improvement within a few sessions. Whereas the prognosis for such results is considered good, in the event that the outcome of treatment is not satisfactory the patient should be taught to compensate as much as possible as subsequent exercises are introduced.

Jaw Hypertonicity

Note: Structurally, the mandible does not lend itself to tone reduction therapy as well as the tongue and lips. Use of acrylic bite blocks such as those shown in Figure 6–4 to help stabilize and maintain the jaw in desired positions can facilitate the exercises in this subsection. When working with patients who exhibit strong biting reflexes, construction of Citricon-based putty bite blocks like those shown in Figure 6–5 may prove more useful because they reduce the chances of tooth abrasion. These materials, however, must be tailored to the oc-

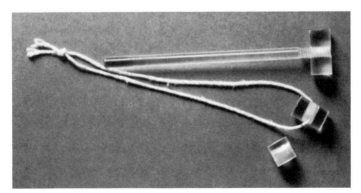

Figure 6–4. Acrylic bite block set (Dworkin, 1980 — Edgewood Press, Inc., Box 811, Nicholasville, KY 40356) composed of ½ inch by ½ inch, ¾ inch by ½ inch, and 1 inch by ½ inch rod-shaped blocks with compatible male threaded acrylic handle (12.5 cm long). Note that the female thread pierces through the rod to enable discretionary use of a string instead of the handle, as recommended for certain lip force physiology exercises, for example.

Figure 6–5.
Putty bite blocks tailored to an individual patient's occlusal status and attached to long cotton-tipped applicators.

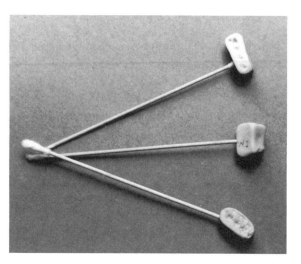

clusal pattern of each patient and are more expensive than the universally applicable acrylic blocks. They also tend to deteriorate over time, necessitating periodic replacement. Clinicians who prefer neither the acrylic nor the putty blocks may substitute corks of different lengths for the same purposes. When using the acrylic or cork blocks, cover them completely with finger cots for sanitary reasons, even though the blocks may be cleaned with soap and hot water before their insertion in the patient's mouth.

Construction of the putty blocks is relatively simple:

Step 1. Take a ball of putty about the size of a cherry and knead it in the hand for about 15 seconds.

Step 2. Place a small dent in the ball to accommodate two to three drops of liquid hardener (accelerator). Knead the hardener well into the putty for approximately 30 seconds, then mold the putty into the shape of a rod or rectangular log about 1 inch long by ½ inch wide.

Step 3. Position the ends between the upper and lower premolar teeth on either side of the mouth, then request the patient to bite down very gently so that a shallow impression of the teeth is created in the putty.

Step 4. Remove the block and allow it to stand for a minute or two so that it hardens completely before use.

Step 5. To prevent accidental swallowing and to enable easy insertion and removal during the exercise regimen, attach a handle to the block. Note in Figure 6–5 that the different blocks shown, all have wooden cotton-tipped applicators as handles. Once the putty is hardened, use a pointed end of a paperclip to bore a tiny hole about halfway through the center of the block on the side that faces the clinician when inserted. Take the wooden end of the applicator and slowly but forcefully twist it in the hole until it is securely fastened within the material.

Step 6. To identify the top and bottom sides for ease of use, etch with a ballpoint pen the letter "T" above the handle signifying the top side of the block.

Repeat this procedure to construct two more blocks: ¾ inch by ½ inch and ½ inch by ½ inch. Some patients prefer to be allowed to hold the handle during the exercises; for those capable of doing so, this should not be discouraged.

Jaw Hypertonicity Exercise No. 1

Step 1. To determine a baseline against which the treatment efficacy can be measured, position the ½-inch bite block between the patient's teeth as shown in Figure 6–6. Here a piece of string is threaded through the hole in the acrylic block in lieu of the acrylic handle that normally is screwed onto the block. Either set up will suffice as protection against accidental swallowing. For the sake of the Figure a finger cot was not placed over the block, but one should be used at all times. A piece of dental floss, roughly 12 inches long, serves well instead of the string. Instruct the patient not to bite down hard on the block, but rather to relax the jaw musculature as much as possible. Position the nail of the thumb on the lower incisor teeth and the nail of the middle finger against the upper incisor teeth next to one side of the block, thus creating a second block or wedge between the patient's teeth. With the other hand remove the bite block and replace it with another wedge of fingers from that hand. Now slowly spread the patient's jaws apart by increasing the distances between the fingers of these wedges; the patient is asked to try neither to resist nor to assist this effort with conscious contractions of the masticatory musculature. Once the jaws are spread apart so that the cutting edges of the teeth are at least 1 inch apart for 5 seconds, slowly decrease this distance by bringing the opposing fingertips into fully compressed contact with one another for an additional count of 5. Repeat this passive open/close jaw maneuver five times without a break between trials, mentally noting the degree of hypertonicity or inherent mandibular resistance present during each set of ex-

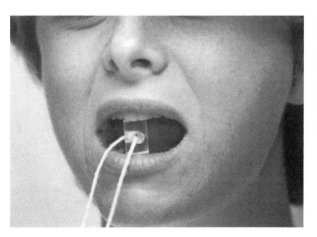

Figure 6–6.
Bite block in position for exercises of the lips or tongue, or both. The string can be substituted for the acrylic handle, which is especially recommended for tasks requiring a tight lip seal.

cursions. Record the perceived amount using the aforementioned +4 to −4 scale, and enter the mean result on the Tone Improvement Chart in the usual way. Make certain to tag this baseline entry with the appropriate musculature (J) and activity (BO/C$_1$) symbols. Proceed with the next step if this finding equals or exceeds "+1.5"; otherwise skip this regimen and move on to the exercises indicated next in the sequence of articulation subsystem treatments.

Step 2. Begin by positioning the ½ inch by ½ inch bite block between the patient's teeth and instructing him or her to try not to bite down consciously on the block. Use the stopwatch to cue the patient when 30 seconds have elapsed, at which time the trial is over. Allow 15 seconds rest and then measure the tone present using the finger wedge technique detailed in Step 1 above. Record the perceived tonal status on a notepad.

Step 3. Repeat this entire procedure until the patient achieves a mean tone score at least 3 scale values improved over the baseline rating, or "0" if the baseline score was a 2 or 3, over 10 consecutive measurements.

Step 4. After each set of 10 trials and finger wedge measures, enter the mean result in a separate column on the y-axis grid of the Tone Improvement Chart, making certain to record the date, number of trials (10), musculature treated (J), activity symbol (O/C$_1$), and calculated target criterion (?) in the respective cells of the column. Upon achievement of this criterion, advance to the next exercise. As usual, if the patient fails to demonstrate an observable trend of improvement after 30 consecutive trials, discontinue the exercise, but proceed nonetheless with cautious optimism as the next exercise in sequence is introduced.

Jaw Hypertonicity Exercise No. 2

Step 1. Follow the exact same baseline procedure as detailed in Exercise no. 1. Proceed with the next step if this finding suggests the continued need for tone reduction treatment; otherwise advance to the next indicated exercise subsection.

Step 2. Follow the identical overall treatment, scoring, and advancement methods recommended in the preceding exercise, except that here the ¾ inch by ½ inch bite block is used for passive jaw displacement. Note that data recorded on the Tone Improvement Chart will be represented by the activity symbol "O/C$_2$." Proceed with the next exercise as indicated.

Jaw Hypertonicity Exercise No. 3

Step 1. Follow exactly the same baseline procedure as detailed in Exercise no. 1, and proceed with Step 2 if so indicated.

Step 2. Again, follow the same protocol as employed in Exercise no. 1, except that here the 1 inch by ½ inch bite block is used. Remember that data collected here are to be represented on the Tone Improvement Chart by the activity symbol "O/C$_3$."

Note: These three exercises may prove helpful for some patients, particularly those with mild or moderate hypertonicity of the mandibular musculature. Patients with more severe involvement tend not to be as responsive to this regimen but may benefit from gentle bilateral massage of the belly of the masseter muscle, a chief elevator of the jaw. This muscle is the most accessible and manipulable of all the muscles of mastication, thus lending itself to the relaxing effects of massage therapy. If such a technique is attempted, it may be best to use small circular strokes with moderate finger pressure for roughly 30 seconds bilaterally before measuring the effects on muscle tone, as described in Exercise no. 1.

TREATMENT OF WEAKNESS

Weakness of a body part may be diffuse or localized, progressive or constant, and variable or stationary. Sometimes it is associated with pain. Determining whether the muscles composing the articulation subsystem possess "adequate" strength is a difficult process because normative data have not been abundantly published and methods to measure strength have not been standardized. In the speech physiology laboratory, tongue, lip, and jaw strength are routinely evaluated using force transducers that are typically interfaced with a microcomputer work station for differential appraisal. Clinicians outside the laboratory setting rely more on various resistance techniques, which afford perceptual measures of muscle strength. In either case the examiner is responsible for using common sense and experience when evaluating strength of a structure. That which constitutes "normal" or "abnormal" strength is subject to great debate and obviously varies from patient to patient: The yardstick used for one may be inappropriate for another. Nevertheless, if diagnosis, age, sex, presence of complicating illnesses, and level of cooperation are weighed and balanced, patients can be reasonably clustered into homogeneous groups for strength testing purposes. Interpretations of the data collected can then be confined to within-group comparisons, using performances of normal counterparts, relative to age and sex, to establish baselines. Along this line of reasoning it is well understood that normal males generally exhibit greater maximum force of the articulators than their female counterparts, and young children usually cannot achieve the levels registered by older children and adults.

Although tongue, lip, and jaw weakness have been observed in all the dysarthrias, these pathophysiologic features are most commonly presented by patients with spastic dysarthria, flaccid dysarthria, or mixed forms of dysarthria containing either or both of these subtypes. As discussed earlier, the spastic dysarthric patient usually exhibits bilateral weakness of the entire articulation subsystem, although the severity of such involvement may be highly variable from structure to structure, and more pronounced on one side than on the other. When treatments of tongue, lip, and jaw weakness are indicated for this type of patient, they are best introduced after completing the exercise regimen for coexisting hypertonicity.

The extent of articulation subsystem weakness in the flaccid dysarthric patient largely depends on the degree of involvement of the Vth, VIIth, and/or XIIth cranial nerves, which respectively supply the jaw, lip, and tongue musculature. Unlike the spastic dysarthric counterpart whose difficulties are almost always bilateral and widespread, this type of patient may frequently present with symptoms that are unilateral and isolated to only one or two of these articulators. The variability factor, however, relative to severity within and between involved structures is similarly not uncommon here. When treatments of tongue, lip, and/or jaw weakness are indicated for the flaccid dysarthric patient, they are best introduced before the initiation of any other articulation subsystem exercises prescribed. Coexisting hypotonicity is not treated directly, but is indirectly influenced during the strengthening programs.

When baseline testing reveals significant weakness of these articulators, regardless of the patient's diagnosis, strengthening exercises are usually indicated to restore as much muscle power as possible. Clinical research has shown a high positive correlation between the degree of weakness and the severity of articulatory imprecision in patients with different types of dysarthria. This clinician has discovered that attention paid to such weakness, by means of the exercise regimen that follows, almost always induces improved muscle strength as well as performances on all subsequent articulation subsystem exercises. On the other hand, experimentation with deliberate omission of the strengthening regimen has proved less rewarding overall for many patients. If such exercises are going to have a significant positive effect on muscle strength, this is usually evident after three or four intensive sessions. A trend in this direction is frequently observable during the first or second session, especially in patients with anything less than severe weakness at the outset of treatment. Those with severe to profound degrees of involvement tend to progress more slowly, but they too may be expected to show relative gains.

As a final reminder, when working to strengthen a given articulator, it is advisable to limit clinical stimulation of the structure to these exercises. Bombarding the tongue, for example, with tone reduction therapy at the beginning of a session, followed by strengthening exercises, followed sequentially with stints of force physiology and phonetic training to end the session may appear on the surface to be a well-spent clinical hour. This approach, though packed with stimulation, is usually counterproductive in that rarely do the tongue, lip, and jaw move in tandem through their indicated treatments. They are likely instead to respond differently in degree and time to these exercises. A given articulation treatment session may be composed of exercises for tongue hypertonicity, lip weakness, and abnormal jaw force physiology. The amount of time devoted to each disturbance may vary, depending on the severity of involvement and its perceived relationship with the articulatory imprecision exhibited by the patient. Another patient may be exposed to a completely different set of exercises, sequenced according to his or her idiosyncratic pathophysiologic profile and responses to such treatments.

Note: To administer the exercises in this subsection, resistance blocks and a crossbar apparatus need to be constructed, as described below.

Resistance Blocks for Tongue Strengthening

Figure 6–7 illustrates three different blocks constructed out of citricon putty and molded to ordinary tongue depressors. The block in the middle is designed for anterior and the other blocks for left and right lateral tongue strengthening.

Step 1. Begin each construction with an amount of putty roughly equal to the size of a walnut. Knead the putty in the hand for about 15 seconds and then create a small dent into which three or four drops of liquid hardener are placed.

Step 2. Knead the hardener well into the putty for approximately 30 seconds, then mold it onto a tongue depressor as shown, making certain that a relatively broad flat edge of putty is shaped at the end of the stick. The patient will use this edge as a source of resistance while pushing against it with the tip of the tongue. Note that the block in the middle is generally larger than the other two blocks. This is because the anterior strengthening exercises induce a flat tongue-tip maneuver, requiring a broader edge for tongue contact than that needed for the lateral exercises, which induce a more pointed tongue-tip posture.

Step 3. Once the putty is appropriately shaped and molded around the end of the stick, have the patient gently bite down into the putty just enough to establish shallow dental imprints for secure and easy placement during the exercises. For the anterior design the upper and lower central and lateral incisor teeth serve this purpose. For the lateral blocks the upper and lower (left and right) first and second premolar teeth create the impressions.

Step 4. To eliminate confusion as to which block is which, and which side is upper and which is lower, use a pen to note these distinctions on the stick. Figures 6–8 and 6–9 illustrate respectively the anterior and left lateral blocks in

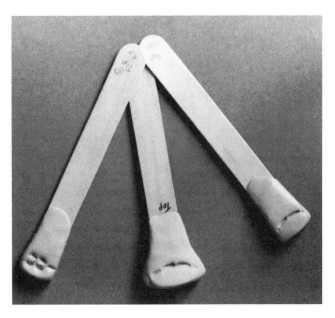

Figure 6–7.
Custom-made putty bite blocks for resistance tongue-strengthening exercises. The block in the middle is designed for the anterior vector, and the other two blocks for the right and left lateral vectors.

Figure 6–8.
Patient practicing with the putty resistance block tailored for isometric tongue strengthening in the anterior plane.

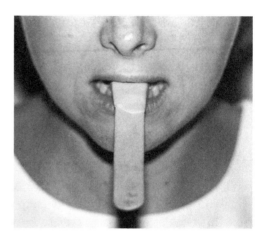

position as the patient pushes against the edges created, which now are in close proximity to the tongue-tip. These blocks are used during the treatment session for resistance training, and also can be taken home for practice.

Use of the flat edge of a tongue depressor and the index and middle fingers, as shown in Figures 6–10 and 6–11, can serve in place of the putty blocks. However, these exercise techniques are not as effective because they require that the clinician provide the counterforce during the exercises, thereby disenabling easy practice away from the clinic. These methods are valuable, nonetheless, as they are called on for subjective measures of anterior and lateral tongue strength throughout this treatment paradigm.

Crossbar for Tongue, Lip, and Jaw Strengthening

Figure 6–12 illustrates a crossbow-like apparatus constructed out of standard-size tongue depressors (sticks) in the following way:

Figure 6–9.
Patient practicing with the putty resistance block tailored for tongue strengthening toward the left lateral plane. Note that this is not truly an isometric task because the tongue musculature must change length and shape to participate effectively.

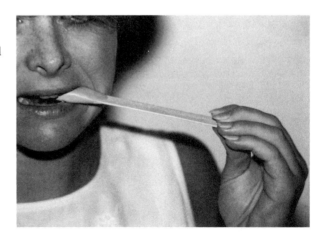

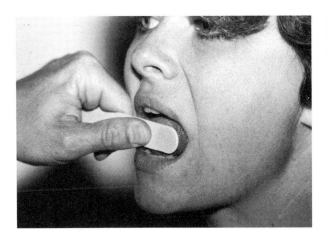

Figure 6–10.
Subjective isometric anterior tongue strength measurement using a wooden tongue depressor for resistance.

Step 1.   Two sticks are taped together at one end using a ½ inch by 3 inch piece of tape.

Step 2.   Transversely slide a single stick between the connected sticks until it meets resistance near the level of the tape. Draw a line on the top stick marking the position boundary of the crossbar, and then remove this wedge.

Step 3.   Two sticks are taped together at both ends as another crossbar. Slide this thicker wedge between the connected sticks, again until it meets the zone of resistance created by the tape. The outer boundary of this wedge should approximate the one drawn for the single wedge. Remove this wedge.

Step 4.   Three sticks are taped together at both ends to serve as a thicker wedge. Transversely slide it between the connected sticks to the point of resistance, and mark on the top stick the outer boundary of the crossbar. Remove this wedge.

Step 5.   Four sticks are taped together at both ends as yet a thicker wedge. Slide it into position until it meets resistance, and mark its outer boundary on

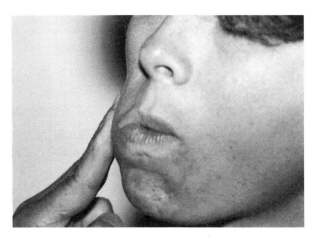

Figure 6–11.
Subjective (isotonic) right lateral tongue strength measurement using fingers for resistance.

Figure 6–12.
Crossbar apparatus constructed of wooden tongue depressors and tape for the purposes of tongue, lip, and jaw force physiology and strengthening training. Note the four-stick resistance wedge lined up appropriately with its marker.

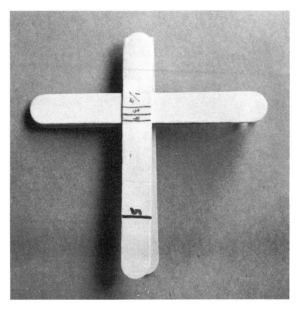

the top stick. Remove this wedge. Note that the numbers 1/2, 3, and 4 in Figure 6–12 represent these boundaries. The 4, for example, means that when the wedge consisting of four sticks is inserted as shown, its outer boundary should be positioned immediately below and equal to the number 4 line drawn. These wedges will be used later in force physiology therapy. For the strengthening program, an additional step is necessary to prepare the crossbar.

Step 6.   Five sticks are taped together at both ends for use as the maximum resistance wedge during one of the strengthening exercises. To use this wedge, slide it between the connected sticks so that its outer boundary is roughly 1½ inches from the open-ended tips of the sticks. Draw a line to mark this location for easy and consistent positioning during the exercise. *Note:* Whereas the wedges can be used in many different patients, the unit itself cannot because it comes into contact with the mouth.

Strengthening exercises are subdivided into three sections: Tongue, lip, and jaw musculature. Again, the putty blocks and crossbar apparatus should not be shared by patients. Each patient should have his or her own set of such materials.

Tongue-Strengthening Exercise No. 1

Step 1.   To establish baseline measures of anterior and lateral tongue strength, use the procedures illustrated in Figures 6–10 and 6–11, respectively. For the *anterior baseline measurement*, make certain that the upper and lower borders of the tongue depressor are positioned between the patient's upper and lower incisor teeth so that the flat edge is in close contact with the tip of the tongue at rest. Request that the patient push against this surface with the tongue-tip as hard as possible as the thumb exerts external resistance. Apply enough counterforce to prevent protrusion of the tongue-tip beyond the cutting edges of the teeth. As the patient pushes against the stick for about 5 seconds, rate the overall degree of force exerted. The Strengthening Chart (Figure 6–13) will be used ultimately to record the mean score. Note that the rating scale is identical to the one recommended for subjective measures of muscle tone. The zero level represents a *normal* amount of strength perceived. Scores above zero in the +1 to +4 range indicate respective levels of above-average strength. Scores below zero conversely denote graduated degrees of below-average strength. Repeat this anterior measure several times, with a 15-second rest period between trials, and enter on the y-axis grid the mean result. Be sure to record the date of baseline data acquisition, number of trials, musculature (T), and vector measured (BA$_1$) in the appropriate cells of the column.

Step 2. For *right lateral baseline measures,* make certain that the index and middle fingertips are pressed firmly against the patient's right cheek as he or she is requested to push the tongue-tip as hard as possible into the cheek with the objective of overcoming this external resistance. Apply sufficient counterforce to prevent the patient's cheek from bulging significantly outward. Note the degree of lateral force exerted over the course of 5 seconds. Repeat this procedure several times and follow the scoring and charting method recommended above for the anterior measurement, except that here use the activity (vector) symbol "BR$_1$" to represent these baseline findings. For *left lateral baseline measures,* follow exactly the same method as for the right side, except that these data are represented by the activity symbol "BL$_1$" on the Strengthening Chart. Proceed with the next step if the anterior mean baseline score is equal to or worse than "−1.5"; otherwise skip this exercise and move on to the next one.

Step 3. The resistance block for anterior vector strengthening, as shown in the middle of Figure 6–7, is used throughout this exercise. Position the tailor-made block in the patient's mouth and request that he or she press the tongue-tip lightly against the flat edge of the block. Then prompt the patient to sustain as hard a push as possible against this edge for a count of 5 seconds. Invariably and automatically this resistance technique induces a biting force that tends to prevent the block from being dislodged. It is worth noting here that patients may do their very best, or try their hardest to succeed, when they are encouraged by the clinician with each effort. Coaching the patient with sideline enthusiasm, such as "come on, *push, push, push,*" can be very effective.

Step 4. Repeat this procedure five times, allowing a rest period of 15 seconds between each effort. Five such efforts constitute one trial, at which time anterior strength is to be reanalyzed using the perceptual baseline technique described in Step 1 above and illustrated in Figure 6–10. Record this subjective impression on a notepad and continue with the exercise until the patient achieves a mean rating at least 3 scale values improved over the baseline rating, or "0" if the baseline score was −2 or −3, over 10 consecutive trials.

Step 5. After each set of 10 trials, enter the mean rating in a separate column on the y-axis grid of the Strengthening Chart (see Figure 6–13), making

STRENGTHENING CHART

Patient's name: _____

Birthdate: _____ Sex: _____

Speech diagnosis: _____
Medical diagnosis: _____
Clinician: _____
Facility: _____
Address: _____
_____

Comments:
_____
_____
_____

ACTIVITY KEY

1. Musculature: Tongue (T); Lip (L); Jaw (J)

2. Vectors: Anterior (A); Right (R); Left (L);
   Palatal (P); Open/Close (O/C)

Baseline (pre-treatment): B + feature symbol

TREATMENT RESPONSES

Dates:																				
+4																				
+3																				
+2																				
+1																				
0																				
-1																				
-2																				
-3																				
-4																				
No. of trials																				
Musculature																				
Vector																				
Target criterion																				

Very Strong ← Normal → Very Weak

Subjective Rating

SESSIONS

Figure 6–13. Blank Strengthening Chart to be used to increase the strength of articulators.

210

certain to record the date of data collection, number of trials (10), musculature in training (T), activity vector (A_1), and calculated target criterion (?) in the respective cells of the column. As always, if the patient fails to demonstrate a discernible trend of improvement after 30 consecutive trials, it may be best to discontinue and proceed with the next indicated exercise.

Note. Patients with significant weakness of the elevator mandibular musculature may struggle with this exercise because the position of the block may not remain stable. Interestingly, this side effect has not been observed by this clinician very often. Even severely involved spastic dysarthric patients have demonstrated consistent ability to work through the technique. If this should prove to be a problem for a given patient, however, the baseline technique can be substituted for the putty block as the exercise tool. This substitution method is also required for edentulous patients and those with poorly fitting dentures.

Tongue-Strengthening Exercise No. 2

Step 1.   Follow exactly the same baseline method as discussed in the preceding exercise, Step 1, except that for these data the anterior vector score is tagged with the activity symbol "BA_2," the right lateral score gets the "BR_2" symbol, and the left lateral rating is represented by the symbol "BL_2" on the Strengthening Chart. Here, if the left lateral finding is equal to or worse than "−1.5," proceed with the next step; otherwise move on to the next exercise.

Step 2.   The resistance block for left lateral vector strengthening, as shown in Figure 6–9, is used throughout this exercise. Position this tailor-made block in the patient's mouth and request that he or she press the tongue-tip lightly against the flat edge. Then encourage the patient to push as hard as possible against this edge for a sustained period of 5 seconds. Counting aloud may be appreciated feedback. Follow the same scoring, charting, and advancement procedures detailed in the preceding exercise for anterior strengthening, except that here all data acquired are tagged with the activity vector symbol "L_1." The baseline method illustrated in Figure 6–11 may be substituted as the treatment approach for patients whose dentition or mandibular musculature weakness prohibit use of the resistance block.

Tongue-Strengthening Exercise No. 3

Step 1.   Follow once again the baseline method of Exercise no. 1, but for these data the anterior, right, and left lateral vector scores are represented on the Strengthening Chart by the symbols "BA_3, BR_3, and BL_3," respectively. Here, if the right lateral finding is equal to or worse than "−1.5," proceed with the next step; otherwise move on to the next exercise.

Step 2.   The resistance block for right lateral vector strengthening is used for this exercise. Follow the exact same scoring, charting, and advancement procedures detailed for left lateral stimulation in the preceding exercise, except that these data are tagged with the activity vector symbol "R_1" on the chart.

Tongue-Strengthening Exercise No. 4

Step 1. To establish a strength baseline for the lingua-alveolar (palatal) vector, use the crossbar (Figure 6–12) and the five-stick wedge. Slide the wedge into its marked position near the end of the crossbar. To prevent the jaw from participating in this exercise, put the ¾ inch acrylic bite block, threaded with a piece of string or dental floss to protect it from being accidentally swallowed, between the upper and lower premolars on either side of the mouth and instruct the patient to maintain a light biting force on the block throughout the tongue exercise. Covering the block with a finger cot can reduce slippage.

Step 2. Place the end of the top stick (the one with the numerical markings) of the crossbar in the patient's mouth at the level of the upper alveolar ridge, as shown in Figure 6–14 for the four-stick wedge. Note that the upper incisor teeth will serve as resistance against top stick movement. This will position the undersurface of the bottom stick of the crossbar in close contact with the dorsum of the tongue-tip. Request that the patient use the tongue-tip to try to push the bottom stick up toward or into contact with the top stick if possible.

Step 3. Note the extent to which the patient's effort decreases the distance between the top and bottom crossbar sticks. A decrement scale in one-quarter units may prove useful for such scoring purposes. Simple conversions would allow these data to be entered on the existing Strengthening Chart (Figure 6–13) to track treatment effects. For this technique, when the patient is unable to decrease the distance between the crossbar sticks even one unit (or one-quarter of complete closure), a score of zero is rendered. Compressing the lower stick one-quarter of the way up is rated a "1," one-half closed is rated a "2," three-quarters closed is rated a "3," and complete contact with the upper stick receives a score of "4." Repeat this procedure three times and enter the mean baseline score on the chart, making certain to list the date, number of trials (3), musculature tested (T), and activity vector symbol (BP_1). If this finding is equal to or worse than "2," proceed with the next step; otherwise advance to the next indicated exercise in sequence.

Figure 6–14.
Tongue-strengthening exercise with crossbar apparatus. The vector is lingua-alveolar, and the target here is 4N, established using the four-stick resistance wedge. Note the string, which is attached to the ¾ inch by ½ inch acrylic bite block, located between the upper and lower first molars, used to stabilize and inhibit the jaw.

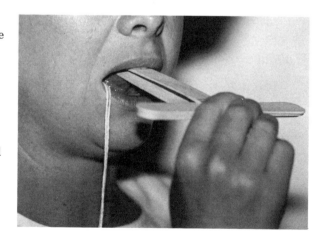

Note: Rough calibration maintains that a force equal to 9 Newtons (approximately 2 pounds) is required to overcome completely the resistance created by the five-stick wedge. This task can be construed as a maximum force exercise. This calibration figure, however, must be considered relative, not absolute. The tensile strength of the wood sticks may vary considerably from one another, and with repeated use saliva tends to hasten both weakening and warping, which can distort calibration and analysis of the patient's performances. When such breakdown appears evident it is wise to discard the unit, not the wedges, and make another one. A new unit may need to be constructed after every 50 trials of use. Finally, young children and severely involved patients of all ages may need to begin this exercise with less resistance: Perhaps the two- or three-stick wedge at the outset, with gradual increases as strength is improved. Female patients may require the same considerations. As a general rule of thumb relative to how much resistance with which to initiate this exercise program, if the patient can elevate the lower stick during baseline measure one unit or more, the wedge used for that trial may be adopted as the treatment tool. However, experimentation with the other wedges should be conducted to find the one most suited for initial exercise use: The greater the resistance from the start the better.

Step 4. Use the crossbar apparatus in the same fashion as outlined in the above step, except that here the patient is encouraged to push as hard as possible for a sustained period of 5 seconds, again with the ultimate objective of elevating the lower stick into contact with the upper one. As with the three preceding exercises, coaching is recommended to motivate the patient to perform to maximal potential. After the trial, record the patient's score on a notepad, following the rating method of Step 3, and allow the patient to rest for 15 seconds. Repeat this procedure until the patient achieves a mean rating that is at least 3 scale values improved over the baseline rating, or "0" if the baseline score was a 2 or 3, over 10 consecutive trials.

Step 5. After each set of 10 trials, enter the mean score in a separate column on the y-axis grid of the Strengthening Chart, making certain to list the date, number of trials (10), musculature (T), activity vector (P_1), and calculated target criterion (?) in the respective cells of the column. If the patient fails to demonstrate any trend of improvement after 30 consecutive trials, discontinue this exercise and advance to the next indicated exercise in sequence. *Note:* Use of a mirror for visual biofeedback may prove fruitful during this exercise.

Lip-Strengthening Exercise No. 1

Step 1. Establish baselines using a button (about the size of a nickel) and a 12 inch piece of string or dental floss. Loop the string through two buttonholes and tie a knot in the end. After instructing the patient to close the teeth, position the button against the teeth behind the midline of the lips, as shown in Figure 6–15, to measure *anterior lip strength*. In a tug-of-war fashion, pull on the string with moderate force as the patient is required to resist this effort to dislodge the button by vigorously contracting the circumoral musculature. Note that the lit-

Figure 6–15.
Anterior lip-strengthening task using a button on a string as the instrument of resistance.

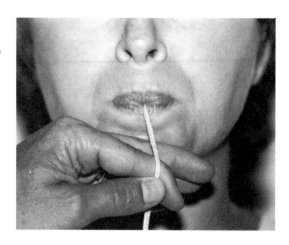

tle, ring, and middle fingers rest against the patient's chin as the string is tugged by the index finger and thumb. Try to maintain a steady tugging force that is sufficient to tax the patient but not great enough to break through the inherent lip seal too easily. Note the perceived degree of anterior lip strength using the +4 to −4 subjective rating scale of the Strengthening Chart. Repeat this procedure three times and enter the mean baseline result in a separate column on the y-axis grid, noting the date, number of trials (3), musculature tested (L), and activity vector (BA_1).

    Step 2. For *right and left lateral lip strength measures,* position the button behind the respective corners of the lips against the labial surfaces of the teeth as shown in Figure 6–16, and tug using the same method as above for anterior resistance. Repeat each side three times and enter the perceived baseline means in separate columns on the chart, making certain to tag the right and left lateral data with the activity vector symbols "BR_1 and BL_1," respectively. Proceed with

Figure 6–16.
Right lateral lip-strengthening task using a button on a string for resistance.

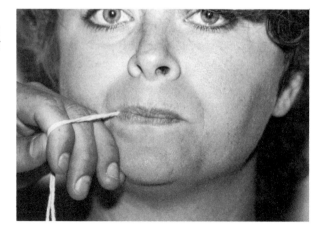

the next step if the anterior mean baseline score is equal to or worse than "-1.5"; otherwise skip the exercise and advance to the next one. *Note:* The size of the button may need to be decreased for very young patients.

Step 3. Follow the same button and string technique as above for anterior lip resistance appraisal, except that here the patient is encouraged to press the lips as hard as possible for a sustained period of 5 seconds, with the objective of winning the tug-of-war. Enthusiastic coaching can motivate the patient to try his or her best to perform maximally. After the trial, record the perceived score using the rating scale in the usual way, then allow the patient to rest for 15 seconds.

Step 4. Repeat this procedure until the patient achieves a mean rating that is at least 3 scale values improved over the anterior baseline rating, or "0" if the baseline score was -2 or -3, over 10 consecutive trials.

Step 5. After each set of 10 trials, enter the mean result in a separate column on the y-axis grid of the Strengthening Chart, listing the date of data acquisition, number of trials (10), musculature trained (L), activity vector (A_1), and calculated target criterion (?) in the respective cells of the column. Advancement to the next exercise is also indicated, although the prognosis remains guarded, if the patient fails to demonstrate any observable trend of improvement after 30 consecutive trials. Note that whether lip weakness is unilateral or bilateral, this anterior strengthening exercise is almost always indicated and helpful. Also, the tugging force should be commensurately adjusted to the patient's age, sex, and level of baseline impairment. Remember the objective is not to overthrow the patient, but rather to help improve lip strength by encouraging hard work.

Lip-Strengthening Exercise No. 2

Step 1. Reestablish a baseline for right lateral lip strength, following the same method outlined in the preceding exercise, noting that this finding is tagged with the activity vector symbol "BR_2" on the Strengthening Chart in a separate column. Proceed with the next step if this mean baseline score is equal to or worse than "-1.5"; otherwise move on to the next exercise.

Step 2. Follow the same button and string method shown in Figure 6–16 and discussed in the preceding exercise for lateral lip strength testing. Here, however, the patient is encouraged to press the lips together as hard as possible for a sustained period of 5 seconds, with the objective of resisting having the button pulled out from between the corner of the lips. Encouragement helps ensure that the patient tries to perform to the maximal extent possible.

Step 3. Follow the same method of scoring, charting, and advancement detailed in the preceding exercise for anterior lip strengthening, except that here the data collected are tagged on the chart with the activity vector symbol "R_1." This regimen is usually unnecessary in the absence of right facial paralysis or weakness.

Lip-Strengthening Exercise No. 3

Step 1. Reestablish a baseline for left lateral lip strength in virtually the same fashion as outlined in the preceding exercises. This finding, however, is represented by the activity vector symbol "BL_2" on the Strengthening Chart. Proceed with the next step if this mean result is equal to or worse than "-1.5"; otherwise advance to the next exercise.

Step 2. Follow the same button and string treatment method used in the preceding exercise, except that here the button is positioned in the left lip corner, and the data collected and charted are tagged with the activity vector symbol "L_1." The criterion for advancement is consistent with the preceding lip-strengthening exercises.

Lip-Strengthening Exercise No. 4

Step 1. Establish an additional baseline measure of anterior lip strength using the crossbar apparatus and the three-stick wedge. Slide the wedge into its marked position on the unit, then place the ½ inch acrylic bite block, threaded with string or dental floss to prevent it from being accidentally swallowed, between the patient's upper and lower premolars on either side. The block inhibits the jaw from participating in the lip activities. Instruct the patient to maintain a light, steady biting force on the block throughout the lip exercise. To reduce slippage of the block, it should be covered with a finger cot.

Step 2. Place the ends of the unit between the patient's lips as shown in Figure 6–17 for the two-stick wedge condition that may be initially easier for certain patients, and instruct him or her to try to press the sticks together with the lips. To rate this effort follow the method detailed in Tongue-Strengthening Exercise no. 4, Step 3, and proceed with the next step according to the same criterion. Note that rough calibration maintains that a force equal to 3 Newtons (approximately 325 g) is required to overcome completely the resistance created

Figure 6–17.
Lip-strengthening exercise with crossbar apparatus. The vector is (anterior) bilabial, and the target here is 3N, established using the three-stick resistance wedge. Note the string that, as in Figure 6–14, attaches to a bite block for jaw stability and inhibition.

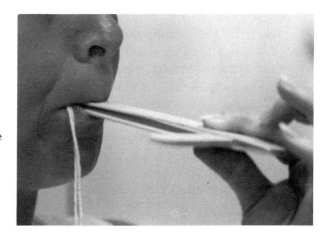

by the three-stick wedge. For some patients this level may be too difficult at the outset. A one- or two-stick wedge may be a better starting point in such patients, with gradual increases in resistance as lip strength is improved with exercise. As a general guide, if the patient can compress the sticks during baseline measures 1 unit (one-quarter of the way closed) or more, the wedge used for testing may be adopted for the exercise regimen. However, experimentation with the other wedges must be conducted to discover the one best fit for initial use in treatment: The greater the level of resistance from the start the better. Use the activity symbol "BA_2" to tag these baseline data on the Strengthening Chart.

Step 2. Use the crossbar apparatus in the same fashion as in the baseline method, except that here the patient is encouraged and coached to press the lips as hard as possible for a sustained period of 5 seconds, again with the ultimate objective of forcing the open ends of the unit into complete contact. Follow exactly the same scoring, charting, and advancement procedures recommended in Tongue-Strengthening Exercise no. 4, Steps 4 and 5, except that here use the activity symbol "A_2" to tag the data. This technique usually works very well as an adjunct to the anterior strengthening exercise and is thus indicated for most patients with lip weakness.

Supplemental Lip-Strengthening Exercise

The following techniques may be introduced as adjuncts to, but not substitutes for, the preceding four exercises.

Exercise 1. Assemble corks of different widths. Begin with the largest cork and have the patient hold it between the lips for 10 seconds. Once the patient demonstrates steady control of this cork, try the same task with the next largest cork, and so on until an adequate grip is demonstrated with the smallest cork. Finally, an ordinary toothpick can be introduced with the same objective. Tracking the patient's responses is necessary to measure treatment efficacy. For lateral strengthening, simply adjust the placement of the cork to the respective corner of the lips. If it is suspected that the jaw is engaged during these activities, use a ½ inch bite block to inhibit such participation.

Exercise 2. Place the ½ inch acrylic bite block between the patient's upper and lower premolars, and position the end of a tongue depressor between the lips, as shown in Figure 6–18. Request the patient to squeeze the lips together for 10 seconds, with the objective of causing the stick to become and remain perpendicular to the level of the lips for the duration of the trial. If the patient achieves this criterion, load the distal end of the stick with a single quarter. To maintain the level position of the stick and balance the quarter, the patient must make a lip force adjustment. If this task is accomplished, more than one quarter can be stacked on the end of the stick in any denomination desired, but gradual increases are usually most easily tolerated. Young patients in particular enjoy this exercise and may become so adept that they are able to manage five or more coins. As with all other exercises, employ methods of administration and charting that afford accurate and replicable measures of treatment efficacy. For lateral

Figure 6–18.
Lip-strengthening exercise using a wooden tongue depressor and bite block for jaw stability and inhibition. The objective is to contract the lip musculature sufficiently to position the stick parallel with the ground at the level of the lips.

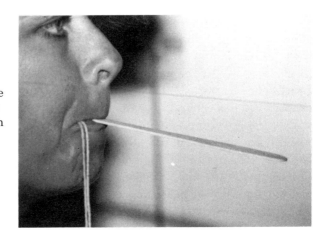

strengthening, the tongue depressor can be positioned in the respective corner of the lips, and the bite block should be moved to the central incisor teeth location. The block, of course, inhibits the contribution of the jaw to the exercise.

Exercise 3.   Position a piece of paper between the lips and request that the patient try to prevent it from being withdrawn by pressing the lips together as hard as possible. With a moderate amount of force, steadily tug on the paper as the patient attempts to resist the pull. The amount of resistance established can be rated and charted in the usual way, following the method employed in the first three primary exercises. For lateral strengthening, adjust the paper position to the respective lip corner. Because the jaw is unlikely to influence this activity, a bite block is probably unnecessary here.

Jaw-Strengthening Exercise No. 1

Step 1.   To establish a baseline for strength of jaw elevation, a most important vector for speech purposes, use the crossbar apparatus and the five-stick wedge. As usual, slide the wedge into its designated location, and position the ends of the unit between the patient's upper and lower central incisor teeth, as shown in Figure 6–19 for the four-stick wedge. As with the tongue and lip measures, for some patients the degree of resistance created by the five-stick wedge may be too great at the outset. In such instances, use of lesser wedge resistance is indicated at first, with gradual increases as strength is improved with exercise. Of course, baseline testing requires experimentation with all the wedges constructed to find the one best suited for treatment initially. Again, the most useful rule suggests that if the patient can compress the sticks one unit (one-quarter of the way closed) or more, the wedge used for that measure meets this criterion. Since more than one wedge may satisfy this objective, select the one for use initially that creates the most resistance.

Step 2.   Once the best fit wedge is selected and positioned, request that the

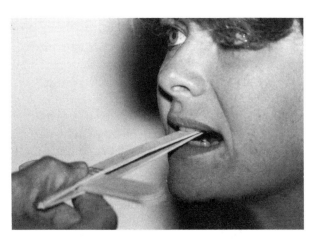

Figure 6–19.
Jaw-strengthening exercise
with crossbar apparatus. The
biting vector is targeted at 4N
here, established using the
four-stick resistance wedge.
Note that no bite block is used
for this task.

patient bite down as hard as possible with the objective of clamping shut the ends
of the sticks between the teeth. Note the extent to which the patient's effort decreases the distance between the sticks. Follow the same method for scoring and
charting this baseline result as that described for Tongue-Strengthening Exercise
no. 4, making certain, however, to list the musculature tested as "J" and the activity vector symbol as "BO/C_1" on the Strengthening Chart. If this finding is
equal to or worse than "2," proceed with the exercise; otherwise advance to the
next indicated articulation subsystem exercise in sequence.

 Step 3. Use the crossbar apparatus in the same fashion as that adopted for
the baseline measures above, except that here the patient is encouraged to bite
down as hard as possible for a sustained period of 5 seconds, with the ultimate
objective of compressing fully the ends of the sticks. As with all the strengthening exercises, the patient is coached and encouraged to perform with maximal effort. After the trial, record the score on a notepad, following the baseline rating
method, then allow the patient to rest for 15 seconds.

 Step 4. Repeat this procedure until the patient achieves a mean rating at
least 3 scale values improved over the baseline rating, or "0" if the baseline score
was 2 or 3, over 10 consecutive trials.

 Step 5. In the usual way, after each set of 10 trials, enter the mean score
in a separate column on the y-axis grid of the Strengthening Chart, listing accordingly the date of the session, number of trials (10), musculature trained (J),
activity vector (O/C_1), and calculated target criterion (?) in the respective cells of
the column. The criterion for discontinuation remains the same as always: If after 30 consecutive trials no discernible trend of improvement is evident, it is best
to move on to the next treatment indicated. Again, a mirror for visual biofeedback always proves helpful for these types of exercises. *Note:* If muscle strengthening does not result from these articulator exercises, the prognosis for improvement with the following force physiology training program necessarily shifts to
"guarded."

TREATMENT OF ABNORMAL FORCE PHYSIOLOGY

Force dyscontrol of the tongue, lip, and/or jaw musculature is commonly observed in all types of dysarthric patients and is causally related to their articulatory imprecision. The characteristics of such muscle-forcing abnormalities vary from patient to patient and structure to structure in accordance with the underlying diagnosis and resultant pathophysiology. The extent to which a given patient can learn to reorganize muscle forces and movements of these articulators, through specific oral gymnastic and phonetic exercises, will dictate the ultimate therapeutic objective to improve speech intelligibility. However, the best methods to habilitate or rehabilitate such controls have not been well researched or unequivocally determined. Techniques that prove facilitative for one patient may miserably fail with another, even in the face of the same overall diagnosis, let alone when the clinical histories are diverse. Factors such as the patient's age, sex, overall medical condition, language-cognitive-intellectual status, and emotional continence all may influence the nature of the motor dyscontrol as well as the most feasible treatments and their outcomes. The speech motor difficulties that characterize patients with different types of dysarthria were discussed in detail in Chapter 1 and thus are not reviewed here. As can be seen in Table 6–1, the need for force physiology training is virtually predictable for all dysarthric patients who present with disturbances of the articulation subsystem. Systematic administration of this training program is advised. Table 6–2 recommends such an approach. Note that when tone reduction or strengthening exercises are indicated, regardless of the degree of coexistent force dyscontrol of the same musculature, these treatments are always administered sequentially before the force

TABLE 6–2. Overall Sequence of Articulator Exercises Based on Degree of Neuromuscular Impairment

		EXERCISES				
Articulator Musculature Involved	Degree of Force Dyscontrol	Tone Reduction*	Strengthening*	Force Physiology	Phonetic Stimulation	Motor Speech Planning†
Tongue	Mild	First	Second	Third	Third	Fourth
	Moderate-Severe	First	Second	Third	Fourth	Fifth
Lips	Mild	First	Second	Third	Third	Fourth
	Moderate-Severe	First	Second	Third	Fourth	Fifth
Jaw	Mild	First	Second	Third	Fourth	Fourth
	Moderate-Severe	First	Second	Third	Fourth	Fifth

*If indicated; otherwise begin with force physiology training.
†Indicated with coexistent apraxia.
If tone reduction and/or strengthening exercises are not indicated, proceed directly to the force physiology training segment, which will benefit virtually all dysarthric patients who present with disturbances of the articulation subsystem. Naturally, the motor speech planning regimen is reserved for patients with apraxia. When apraxia coexists with dysarthria, introduction of this program is generally held in abeyance until completion of the physiologic exercise package. Pure apractic patients, on the other hand, would be treated from the start with the motor planning regimen.

physiology training program. If neither tone nor strengthening exercises are indicated for a given articulator, the treatment regimen focuses initially on the existing force dyscontrol. However, owing to potentially different degrees of neuromuscular involvement, idiosyncratic responses to previous treatments, or both, the tongue, lip, and jaw mechanisms may at any time be scheduled for a discrepant mixture of articulation subsystem exercises. The tongue, for example, may be undergoing the tone reduction program while simultaneously prescriptions are drawn for force physiology training of the jaw and select phonetic exercises for the lip musculature. How to divide the load of therapy relative to the time allotment to each articulator is not an easy question to address. Sometimes it is best to reserve the longest time for the most impaired musculature. When the degree of disturbance is uniformly distributed throughout the subsystem, treatment time per articulator may be more equitable. Extenuating circumstances, however, frequently prompt ongoing alterations of such plans. Clinicians may need to remain flexible on this subject.

As can also be seen from Table 6–2, if the patient presents with a mild degree of force dyscontrol, phonetic exercises aimed at the same musculature may be creatively coupled with the force physiology training regimen. This combination technique is most applicable to disturbances of the tongue and lip musculature inasmuch as there are many so-called "tongue" and "lip" sounds within the phonetic alphabet that may be employed for articulation practice. The jaw mechanism does not lend itself as well to such coupling because there are no true "jaw" sounds that can be selected for phonetic stimulation. When abnormal force physiology exceeds the mild degree, it is advisable to delay respective speech sound practice until attempts are made to prepare the articulation subsystem for such demands by administering in sequence all indicated physiologic exercises. Bypassing these prerequisite treatments in the hope of hastening the speech rehabilitation process has proved counterproductive for this clinician in the past. It may be myopic to neglect the role and importance of specific exercises designed to repair articulator force dyscontrols in dysarthric patients. Phonetic practice alone usually does not suffice to overcome these disturbances. Drilling these patients with traditional speech sound exercises to improve articulatory proficiency may not yield the best results in the final analysis. Frequently patients walk away from such sessions exhausted and "turned off" to therapy. Force physiologic treatments take time to administer and are somewhat taxing, both physically and financially, but in the long run they often reduce the length of the overall speech rehabilitation program, cut total costs, and (most important) contribute measurably to any articulation improvements achieved. The following sets of articulator exercises are therefore recommended in sequence for such purposes.

Tongue Force Physiology Exercise No. 1

Note. Depending on the patient's degree of jaw force control, either the previously described acrylic (Figure 6–4) or putty (Figure 6–5) bite blocks are used in this exercise. The putty blocks are indicated for patients with particularly unstable and strong biting forces and reflexes inasmuch as these materials are tailor-made for steady fit and are less abrasive to the dentition. However, because these blocks may yield to such strong forces, they do not necessarily restrict the jaw entirely from participating in or disrupting the tongue exercises, and they deteriorate over time. On the other hand, the acrylic blocks (1) are relatively handy, (2) are universally applicable across different exercises and patients, (3) are unyielding to biting forces and thereby inhibit potentially disruptive elevating jaw effects, and (4) are durable. Patients with mild to moderate jaw force dyscontrol generally do just fine with the acrylic blocks. If putty blocks are necessary, three should be constructed: ½ inch by ½ inch, ¾ inch by ½ inch, and 1 inch by ½ inch. Instructions on basic construction procedures were provided in the introduction to Jaw Hypertonicity Exercise no. 1 above. It is usually best to select the premolar region on either side of the patient's mouth as the site for the block impressions. Figure 6–20 illustrates the acrylic block in this location, which affords a good view of the tongue during the exercise regimen. Figure 6–21 shows how central positioning of a block can somewhat obscure this view. The patient's dental status and the clinician's preference usually contribute to the final decision regarding the primary site of block insertion. Remember, the acrylic blocks can be shifted to any comfortable location at any time. The putty blocks cannot because they are tailored to the occlusal surfaces in one given area of the mouth.

Step 1.   Place the ½ inch by ½ inch block in the patient's mouth in the usual way. Physically adept patients may be permitted to hold the block handle for added stability, comfort, and safety. Very young children and severely involved patients of all ages generally do better when the clinician manipulates the handle. To establish baseline ability, request that the patient raise the tip of the tongue to the alveolar ridge, hold it there for 2 seconds, lower it for an additional 2 seconds, and continue these alternating movements at the same speed for 30 seconds. Each round trip (Up/Down) will constitute a single trial. If the tongue-tip is moved without significant delay upon each verbal cue to raise it "up" and

Figure 6–20.
Here a ½ inch by ½ inch bite block is in position for lingua-alveolar valving mobility exercises. The block stabilizes the jaw and inhibits it from contributing to or interfering with the specific tongue movements isolated for practice.

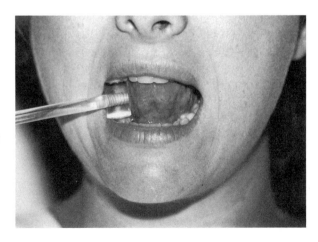

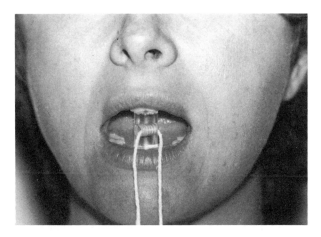

Figure 6-21.
Alternative positioning of the
bite block for lingua-alveolar
or bilabial valving mobility
exercises. The string is best for
practicing lip maneuvers
because it is less obtrusive
than the rigid acrylic handle.

lower it "down," if the movements are targeted with precision and completeness
to the upper alveolar ridge and back to the lower alveolar ridge accordingly, and
if the hold phases are steady, the trial is rated *correct.* Signs of motor dyscontrol
at any point in the cycle of the trial must be rated *incorrect.*

Step 2. Use a notepad to rate each trial throughout the 30-second task, allow 15 seconds for rest, and repeat this procedure two more times. Tally the mean
correct percentage of all trials and enter the baseline score on the Metronomic
Mobility Treatment Chart (Figure 6-22) in a separate column. Be sure to list the
date, minutes of therapy (1½), musculature tested (T), task (BU/D_1) and beats
per minute (30—every 2 seconds) in the respective cells of the column. Proceed
with the next step if this finding is equal to or less than 75 percent correct; otherwise skip this exercise and advance to the next one.

Step 3. Set the metronome to 30 bpm, position the ½ inch bite block in the
patient's mouth, and instruct him or her that the task is to raise and lower the
tongue-tip alternately to the respective alveolar ridges according to the beat: One
vector per beat continuously for 30 seconds. Explain the rating protocol. Permit
the patient to begin whenever desired, not unlike the game of jump rope in which
the player jumping, not the ones turning the rope, makes the decision when to
jump in. As soon as the patient begins, start the stopwatch or wristwatch so as to
monitor when 30 seconds have elapsed. The sound and sight of the metronome
should serve sufficiently to cue the patient to alternate the lingua-alveolar vector. The verbal cues may be provided in synch with the metronomic beats. Positioning the table mirror so that the patient can easily view and modify, if necessary, tongue movements is helpful. Keeping the metronome in close proximity to
the mirror to permit glimpses of the upcoming beats may also facilitate performances.

Step 4. Follow the same basic rating and scoring method described in Step
2, except that here we tally the mean correct percentage of all trials after 5 full
minutes of exercising, not including the 15-second rest periods between the 30-
second treatment segments. At the completion of each set of 5 minutes, which

METRONOMIC MOBILITY TREATMENT CHART

Patient's name: _____

Birthdate: _____ Sex: _____

Speech diagnosis: _____
Medical diagnosis: _____
Clinician: _____
Facility: _____
Address: _____
_____

Comments:
_____
_____
_____
_____
_____

ACTIVITY KEY

1. Musculature: Tongue (T); Lip (L); Jaw (J)

2. Task: Up/Down (U/D); Out/In (O/I);
   Left/Right (L/R); Close/Open (C/O);
   Pucker/Spread (P/S); Airflow (A)

3. Beats Per Minute: 30, 60, 90, 120 (150,
   200, variable [V])

4. Minutes of Therapy: Fill in amount

Baseline (pre-treatment): B + feature symbol

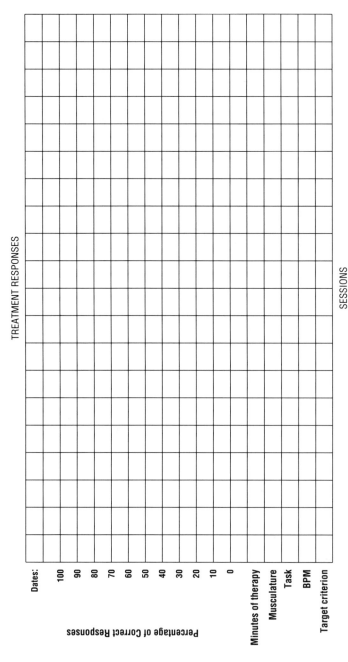

TREATMENT RESPONSES

Percentage of Correct Responses

Dates:

100
90
80
70
60
50
40
30
20
10
0

Minutes of therapy
Musculature
Task
BPM
Target criterion

SESSIONS

Figure 6–22. Blank Metronomic Mobility Treatment Chart to be used to improve the gross force control of articulators.

224

represents ten 30-second exercise segments, calculate this percentage, extract the result from the notepad, and enter this finding on the Metronomic Mobility Treatment Chart in a separate column.

Step 5. Repeat this procedure until the patient achieves a mean correct score that is at least 75 percent improved over the baseline score or 100 percent correct, whichever is less, over 10 consecutive minutes of therapy. Make certain that all data entries on the treatment chart are listed according to the appropriate date, minutes of therapy (5), musculature treated (T), task (U/D_1), bpm (30), and calculated target criterion (?) in the respective cells of the column. Discontinuation of the exercise is recommended if after 30 consecutive minutes of treatment there is no discernible trend of improvement. Advancement to the next exercise is still indicated, but with more caution than if the patient had met the above criterion.

Tongue Force Physiology Exercise No. 2

Step 1. To establish baseline, follow the exact same method as in the preceding exercise, except that here the "Up/Down" alternate tongue-tip vectors are governed not by a 30-bpm stimulus, but rather by 60 bpm. The rating, scoring, and charting procedures are also identical, except that these baseline data are represented by the task symbol "BU/D_2" and the bpm are listed as "60" on the Metronomic Mobility Treatment Chart. The next step is indicated when this result is equal to or less than 75 percent correct; otherwise proceed to Exercise no. 3. Note the need to adjust the scores relative to the number of bpm and the ultimate number of trials possible in any given evaluation and treatment segment.

Step 2. Follow the exact same treatment method employed and described in the preceding exercise, except that here a 60-bpm stimulus is used. The rating, scoring, charting, and advancement criteria remain the same, however. Make certain that all data entries on the treatment chart are represented by the task symbol "U/D_2" and the bpm are listed as "60" in their respective cells.

Tongue Force Physiology Exercise No. 3

Step 1. Again, establish a baseline following exactly the method recommended in Exercise no. 1, except that here the "Up/Down" alternate activities are set at 90 bpm. The rating, scoring, and charting procedures are also identical, with the exception that these baseline data are tagged with different task and bpm symbols: "BU/D_3" and "90," respectively. Be sure to adjust the scoring procedure to reflect the difference in bpm and the numbers of trials possible in each evaluation and treatment segment.

Step 2. Follow the exact same treatment method detailed in Exercise no. 1, except that here a 90-bpm stimulus is used. Maintain the identical rating, scoring, charting, and advancement criteria, however. Be sure to tag all data entries in the Metronomic Mobility Treatment Chart with the task symbol U/D_3 and to list the bpm as 90 in their respective cells of the column.

Tongue Force Physiology Exercise No. 4

Step 1. The ½ inch by ½ inch block is used yet again as in the preceding three exercises, except that here the "Up/Down" alternate tongue-tip vectors are ruled by a 120-bpm stimulus. The rating, scoring, and charting procedures detailed in the first of these exercises are followed here also, except that these baseline data are to be represented by the task symbol "BU/D$_4$" and the bpm listed as "120" on the treatment chart. Once again, be certain to adjust the scoring policy with respect to the bpm stimulus and the consequential increase in the possible number of trials each and every evaluation and treatment segment.

Step 2. Follow the exact same treatment method employed and described in Exercise no. 1, except that here a 120-bpm stimulus drives the segments of treatment. The rating, scoring, charting, and advancement criteria detailed before are maintained here. All data entries on the Metronomic Mobility Treatment Chart, however, are tagged with different task and bpm symbols from those used in the preceding exercises: "U/D$_4$" and "120," respectively.

Note. For patients who excel through Exercise no. 4, faster bpm stimuli may be attempted with the ½ inch block. Adjustments in the number of minutes of treatment and criteria adopted for advancement may be made at the discretion of the clinician, but should conform to the individual patient's potential and motivation to continue with the tasks. The next exercise in sequence is indicated for all patients, however, whether or not criteria were met on the preceding four exercises and regardless of any intentions to experiment with faster bpm stimuli.

Tongue Force Physiology Exercise No. 5

Step 1. The ½ inch by ½ inch block is used again, except that here the "Up/Down" gestures are governed not by a steady beat but by a variable rate. Once the block is in position, verbally cue the patient when to raise the tongue-tip as usual and when to lower it. The words "up" and "down" are easiest for such purposes. Use a stopwatch or second hand on a wristwatch to determine when to alternate the cue according to the different bpm stimuli practiced in the preceding four exercises. To establish baseline ability, the first 30-second evaluation segment might consist of the following continuous random sequence of verbal cues: "up" for 2 full seconds (30 bpm), "down" for 1 second (60 bpm), "up" for half of a second, "down" for two-thirds of a second, "up" for 1 second, "down" for 2 seconds, "up" for half of a second, "down" for two-thirds of a second, "up" for 1 second, "down" for 2 seconds, and so on until roughly 30 seconds elapse. Each trial is rated, scored, and charted in the exact same fashion as before, making certain that after three 30-second segments of baseline testing, preferably following different patterns of verbal cues, the data entered on the Metronomic Mobility Treatment Chart are tagged with the appropriate task (BU/D$_5$) and bpm (V) symbols. *Note:* Use of the notepad to rate correct/incorrect each and every trial is particularly important for this exercise owing to the random and variable speed of the task.

Step 2. Follow the same basic procedures described in the preceding step and in Exercise no. 1, except that here we tally the mean correct percentage of all trials after 5 full minutes of exercising, not including the 15-second rest period allowed between the 30-second treatment segments. It is preferable to randomize the length of time between the continuous "Up/Down" verbal cues per segment, not only to reduce the likelihood of order effects, but to make the exercise less monotonous. At the completion of each set of 5 minutes, the equivalent of ten 30-second segments, calculate in the usual way this percentage from the notepad recordings and enter the result on the treatment chart in a separate column.

Step 3. Repeat this procedure until the patient achieves a mean correct score at least 75 percent improved over the baseline score or 100 percent correct, whichever is less, over 10 consecutive minutes of therapy. Remember, as always, to list the appropriate date, minutes in treatment for that particular data entry (5), musculature treated (T), task (U/D$_5$), bpm (V), and calculated target criterion (?) in the respective cells of the column. Move on to the next exercise when indicated, as discussed earlier.

Tongue Force Physiology Exercise Nos. 6–10

This series is identical to the preceding five exercises in design and scope, with one exception: Here the ¾ inch by ½ inch bite block is used throughout the regimen. Remember to tag respectively these data with correct task symbols (U/D$_6$, U/D$_7$, U/D$_8$, U/D$_9$, and U/D$_{10}$) on the Metronomic Mobility Treatment Chart. All baseline data receive the prefix "B."

Tongue Force Physiology Exercise Nos. 11–15

This series is also identical to the first five exercises, except that here the 1 inch by ½ inch bite block is used throughout the regimen. Once again, these data should be represented respectively by the correct task symbols (U/D$_{11}$, U/D$_{12}$, U/D$_{13}$, U/D$_{14}$, and U/D$_{15}$) on the treatment chart. All baseline data receive the prefix "B."

Tongue Force Physiology Exercise No. 16

Step 1. To establish baseline ability, position the 1 inch by ½ inch bite block in the patient's mouth in the usual way. Request the patient to protrude the tongue centrally as far out of the mouth as possible, hold it there for 2 seconds, retract it as far back in the oral cavity as anatomically possible for an additional 2 seconds, and continue these alternating movements at the same speed for 30 seconds. Each round trip (Out/In) constitutes a single trial. As in the previous series of exercises, if the tongue is moved without significant delay upon each verbal cue to protrude it ("out") and retract it ("in"), if the movements are targeted with precision and completeness to the farthest anatomical boundaries for these vectors, and if the hold phases are steady, the trial is rated *correct*. Any signs of dyscontrol at any point in the cycle of the trial warrant an *incorrect* rating. Responses should be recorded for each trial throughout the 30-second task, allowing 15 seconds for rest. Repeat this procedure two more times. Tally the mean correct percentage of all trials and enter the baseline score on the Metronomic Mobility Treatment Chart in a separate column. List accordingly the date, minutes of therapy (1½), musculature tested (T), task (BO/I$_1$), bpm (30—every 2 seconds), and calculated target criterion (?) in the respective cells of the column. Proceed with the next step if this finding is equal to or less than 75 percent correct; otherwise skip this exercise and advance to the next one.

Step 2. Set the metronome to 30 bpm, position the 1 inch by ½ inch bite block in the patient's mouth, and instruct him or her that the task is to protrude and retract the tongue alternately to the farthest anatomical boundaries outside and within the oral cavity, respectively, according to the beat: 1 vector per beat continuously for 30 seconds. Explain the rating protocol. When the patient chooses to begin, start the stopwatch or wristwatch to monitor when 30 seconds have elapsed to end the segment. The sound and sight of the metronome should suffice as cues to the patient to protrude and retract the tongue alternately to the beat. If judged to be helpful, the verbal cues used in Step 1 ("Out/In") may be uttered in synch with the beats of the metronome. As always, a table mirror for visual biofeedback of these tongue movements is highly recommended. Follow the same basic rating and scoring method described in the preceding step, except that here we tally the mean correct percentage of all trials after 5 full minutes of exercising, not including the 15-second rest periods between the 30-second treatment segments.

Step 3. At the completion of each set of 5 minutes, which is equivalent to ten 30-second exercise segments, calculate this percentage, extract the result from the notepad, and enter this finding on the treatment chart in a separate column.

Step 4. Repeat this procedure until the patient achieves a mean correct score at least 75 percent improved over the baseline score or 100 percent correct, whichever is less, over 10 consecutive minutes of therapy. Make certain that all data entries on the chart are listed according to the appropriate date, minutes of therapy (5), musculature treated (T), task (O/I$_1$), bpm (30), and calculated target criterion (?) in the respective cells of the column. If the patient fails to demonstrate an observable trend of improvement after 30 consecutive minutes of treatment, discontinue the exercise and advance, as usual, to the next exercise.

Tongue Force Physiology Exercise No. 17

Step 1. Follow the exact same protocol as detailed in Step 1 of the preceding exercise, except that for this baseline measure the alternating tongue movements are cued at an equivalent speed of 60, not 30, bpm. That is, the tongue is protruded and held in this position for 1 second, then retracted and held there for an additional second, and so on for 30 continuous seconds, as usual. The identical rating, scoring, and charting methods of Exercise no. 16 are used here. Make certain, however, to tag these baseline data on the Metronomic Mobility Treatment Chart with the correct task (BO/I$_2$) and bpm (60) symbols. Proceed as indicated.

Step 2. Follow exactly the same protocol as detailed in Steps 2 to 4 of the preceding exercise, except that here the metronome is set to 60 bpm. The identical rating, scoring, charting, and advancement criteria are adopted from Exercise no. 16. When logging these treatment data on the chart, be sure to record the correct task (O/I$_2$) and bpm (60) symbols in the respective cells of the column. Proceed as indicated.

Tongue Force Physiology Exercise No. 18

Step 1. Again, follow the same baseline protocol as detailed in Exercise no. 16, except that here the alternating "Out/In" tongue movements are cued at an equivalent speed of 90 bpm. When scoring and charting these baseline data, according to the method used in Exercise no. 16, make certain to record the correct task (BO/I$_3$) and bpm (90) symbols on the Metronomic Mobility Treatment Chart. Proceed as indicated.

Step 2. Again, follow the exact same treatment protocol as detailed in Exercise no. 16, except that here the metronome is set to 90 bpm. The identical rating, scoring, charting, and advancement criteria are adopted from Exercise no. 16. Be sure that these treatment data receive the correct task (O/I$_3$) and bpm (90) symbols on the treatment chart. Proceed as indicated.

Tongue Force Physiology Exercise No. 19

Step 1. Follow the exact same baseline protocol as detailed in Exercise no. 16, except that here the tongue movements are cued at a speed equivalent of 120 bpm. That is, "out" for half of a second, "in" for half of a second, "out" for half of a second, and so on for 30 continuous seconds. Rate, score, and chart these baseline measures according to the methods employed in Exercise no. 16. Make certain, however, to record the correct task (BO/I$_4$) and bpm (120) symbols on the Metronomic Mobility Treatment Chart. Proceed as indicated. *Note:* As before, for patients who excel through Exercises 16–19, these alternating movements may be practiced at faster bpm stimuli before advancing to Exercise no. 20.

Tongue Force Physiology Exercise No. 20

Step 1. The 1 inch by ½ inch block is used again, except that for this baseline measure the "Out/In" gestures will be governed not by steady state cues but by a variable rate. Once the block is in position, verbally cue the patient when to protrude and when to retract the tongue in the usual way. Again, the words "out" and "in" are the best cues. Follow the protocol detailed in Exercise no. 5, Step 1, for the "Up/Down" task, except that here the task naturally is "Out/In." Make certain that when charting these baseline data the correct task (BO/I$_{20}$) and bpm (V) symbols are used. Proceed as indicated.

Step 2. Follow the same basic rating, scoring, charting, and advancement criteria recommended in the above step and Steps 2 and 3 of Exercise no. 5. Make certain that when charting these treatment data the correct task (O/I_{20}) and bpm (V) symbols are used.

Tongue Force Physiology Exercise No. 21

Step 1. To establish baseline ability, position the 1 inch by ½ inch bite block in the patient's mouth between the upper and lower second molars on either side. This placement is an easy adjustment from the usual premolar positioning if the acrylic block has been routinely used for these exercises. Construction of a new block will be necessary, however, if the patient has been using a putty block up to this point. To do so, simply follow the original instructions in the notation of Exercise no. 1, except that the impression is taken not in the premolar region but between the upper and lower second molars. Request that the patient protrude the tongue, as in the previous four exercises, immediately lateralize it to the right corner of the lips and hold it in that position for 2 seconds, swiftly glide it across the midline of the lips to the left corner and hold it there for an additional 2 seconds, and continue these alternating movements at the same speed for 30 continuous seconds. Each round trip (Left/Right) constitutes a single trial. As previously defined, the performance is to be rated *correct* if the tongue is moved without significant delay upon each verbal cue to move "left" and "right," if the movements are targeted with precision and completeness to the farthest anatomical boundaries for these vectors, and if the hold phases are steady. Any signs of dyscontrol at any point in the cycle of the trial warrant an *incorrect* rating. Using a notepad, rate each trial throughout the 30-second task, allow 15 seconds for rest, and repeat this procedure two more times.

Step 2. Tally the mean correct percentage of all trials and enter the baseline score on the Metronomic Mobility Treatment Chart in a separate column. Be sure to list the date, minutes of therapy (1½), musculature tested (T), task (BL/R_1), bpm (30—every 2 seconds), and calculated target criterion (?) in the respective cells of the column in which these data are represented. Proceed with the next step if this finding is equal to or less than 75 percent correct; otherwise skip this exercise and advance to the next one.

Step 3. Set the metronome to 30 bpm, position the 1 inch by ½ inch bite block in the patient's mouth, and instruct him or her, once again, that the task is to move the tongue from the left to the right lip corner alternately to the beat: One vector adjustment per beat continuously for 30 seconds. Explain the aforementioned rating criteria. As in the previous exercises, when the patient chooses to begin, start the stopwatch to monitor the 30-second time limit for each segment of treatment. Follow the same basic rating and scoring method outlined above, except that here we tally the mean correct percentage of all trials after 5 full minutes of exercising. At the completion of each set of 5 minutes, which is equivalent to ten 30-second exercise segments, calculate this percentage, extract the result from the notepad, and enter this finding on the treatment chart. Adopt the identical criterion for improvement and advancement that has been detailed in all the preceding exercises. Make certain to tag these treatment data with the correct task (L/R$_1$) and bpm (30) symbols on the Metronomic Mobility Treatment Chart, accordingly.

Tongue Force Physiology Exercise Nos. 22–24

This series is identical to the preceding exercise in design and scope except that for these three exercises the "Left/Right" movements are governed by 60, 90, and 120 bpm, respectively. Naturally these exercises are represented on the Metronomic Mobility Treatment Chart respectively by the task symbols "L/R$_2$, L/R$_3$, and L/R$_4$," likewise the associated bpm symbols are "60, 90, and 120." Baseline data receive the prefix "B," as always. As before, patients who advance through Exercise nos. 21–24 may benefit from practicing these same activities at faster bpm stimuli before advancing to Exercise no. 25.

Tongue Force Physiology Exercise No. 25

Follow the exact same variable rating protocol detailed in Exercise no. 5, except that here the task is "Left/Right." Make certain when charting these data that they are represented by the correct task (L/R$_5$) and bpm (V) symbols. Remember, baseline symbol entries always receive the prefix "B." Proceed with the next exercise as indicated by the patient's responses to this treatment.

Tongue Force Physiology Exercise No. 26

Step 1. To establish baseline ability, the crossbar apparatus shown in Figures 6–12 and 6–14 and discussed in Tongue Strengthening Exercise no. 4 is used, noting that we begin with the four-stick wedge. Rough calibration places resistance with this wedge at approximately 4 Newtons (400 g). For visual biofeedback during this exercise, use the table mirror at all times. First, place the ¾ inch by ½ inch bite block in the premolar region, as shown. With the acrylic block a string is preferable to the long handle for this exercise because it is less cumbersome. If the patient requires the putty block, the wooden applicator handle is not quite as obstructive as the acrylic one, making an adjustment unnecessary. After insertion of the block, position the end of the top stick of the crossbar in proximity to the upper alveolar ridge, so that the lower stick rests on or near the tip of the tongue.

Step 2. Instruct the patient that the task here is to use the tongue-tip to push the lower stick halfway up toward the upper stick and to try to maintain this position for 5 seconds while the cutting edges of the upper incisors ensure stability of the top stick as the lower stick is moved. With a rest period of 15 seconds between trials, have the patient perform this task five times. Each trial should be rated independently, using the score key at the bottom of the Force

FORCE PHYSIOLOGY TREATMENT CHART

Patient's name:

Birthdate: Sex:

Speech diagnosis:
Medical diagnosis:
Clinician:
Facility:
Address:

ACTIVITY KEY

1. Musculature: Tongue (T); Lip (L); Jaw (J)

2. Time: 5, 10, Variable (V) seconds

3. Vectors: Palatal (P); Close/Open (C/O)

Baseline (pre-treatment): B + feature symbol

Comments:

TREATMENT RESPONSES

Dates:																				
Variable																				
2N																				
1N																				
0.5N																				
0.25N																				
No. of trials																				
Musculature																				
Vector																				
Time																				
Target criterion																				

Maximum ← Force Levels → Minimum

SESSIONS

SCORE KEY

C = Correct and immediate achievement of target level

L = Latency of 2 or more seconds before achieving and holding target level

V = Variably achieves target level within same trial

F = Fails to hold target level after making contact

U = Unable to acheive target level

Figure 6–23. Blank Force Physiology Treatment Chart to be used to improve the fine force control of articulators.

232

Physiology Treatment Chart (Figure 6–23) to measure the patient's performance.

Step 3.   At the completion of each trial, enter in the y-axis grid of the chart, on the 2N line indicating the 2-Newton target, the score key letter (C, L, V, F, or U) that best describes the overall characteristics of the effort. To save space on the chart, all five baseline ratings can be clustered next to one another in the same column, making certain that the date, number of trials (5), musculature tested (T), vector (BP_1), and time (5 seconds) are accurately recorded in the respective cells of the column. Proceed with the next step if the patient fails to achieve a "C" rating on three or more of the trials; otherwise skip this exercise and advance to the next one. *Note:* The requirement here to decrease by 50 percent the distance between the wooden crossbar plates, under the four-stick wedge condition, is roughly equal to a 2-Newton force target.

Step 4.   Use the crossbar apparatus following the exact same method described above. Repeat this procedure until the patient achieves a "C" rating on at least eight of ten consecutive trials. Again, to save chart space, several letter scores can be clustered into the same column. Be sure to record also the date, number of trials for the column, musculature treated (T), vector (P_1), time of hold phase (5), and target criterion (80 percent) in the respective cells of the column. Move on to the next exercise when the patient either achieves this criterion or fails to demonstrate any observable trends of improvement over baseline after 30 consecutive trials.

Tongue Force Physiology Exercise No. 27

Step 1.   Follow exactly the same baseline data acquisition, rating, scoring, charting, and advancement methods detailed in the preceding exercise, except that here the *two*—not the four-stick wedge—is used for resistance. Be sure to record the vector symbol (BP_2) to represent these baseline data on the Force Physiology Treatment Chart. *Note:* The force target here is approximately 1 Newton, and all data entries are thus made on the 1N line of the chart.

Step 2.   Follow identically the treatment method of the preceding exercise, except that the two-stick wedge is used here. Be sure to tag these data with the vector symbol "P_2" on the treatment chart.

Tongue Force Physiology Exercise No. 28

Step 1.   Again, follow the exact same baseline methodology as in Exercise No. 26, except that here the one-stick wedge is used for resistance. The vector symbol "BP_3" is listed on the Force Physiology Treatment Chart to represent these baseline data. *Note:* The force target here is approximately 0.5 Newtons, and all data entries are thus made on the 0.5N line of the treatment chart.

Step 2.   Follow identically the rating, scoring, charting, and advancement criteria detailed in Exercise no. 26, remembering that for these treatments the one-stick wedge is used. Tag the data collected with the vector symbol "P_3" on the chart.

Tongue Force Physiology Exercise No. 29

Step 1. Follow the same basic method used in the preceding exercise, except that here the lower stick of the crossbar is pushed *one-quarter,* not one-half of the way up toward the upper stick and held in this position for the usual 5 seconds. When rating, scoring, and charting these baseline results, be certain to tag the data collected with the vector symbol "BP_4" on the Force Physiology Treatment Chart. *Note:* The requirement here to decrease by 25 percent the distance between the wooden crossbar plates, under the one-stick wedge condition, is roughly equal to a 0.25-Newton force target. All data entries here are thus made on the 0.25N line of the treatment chart.

Step 2. Follow the exact same method of Step 1 above. Repeat this procedure as usual for these crossbar exercises, following the rating, scoring, charting, and advancement criteria detailed in Exercise no. 26. These treatment data are tagged with the vector symbol "P_4" on the chart.

Tongue Force Physiology Exercise Nos. 30–34

Step 1. Follow respectively the exact same baseline methods of Exercise nos. 26–29, except that for these measures the hold phase is increased to 10 seconds. Note that the vector symbols "BP_{5-8}" should be used respectively to tag these baseline data on the Force Physiology Treatment Chart.

Step 2. Follow respectively the exact same rating, scoring, charting, and advancement criteria recommended in Exercise nos. 26–29. Be sure to tag these treatment data respectively with the vector symbols "P_{5-8}" on the treatment chart.

Tongue Force Physiology Exercise No. 35

Step 1. The crossbar apparatus, two-stick wedge, bite block, and table mirror set-up is used here. Once the block and crossbar are positioned in the usual ways, baseline measures are obtained relative to the patient's ability to demonstrate tongue force control under *variable* time and target conditions. Instruct the patient that the task is to push up on the lower stick with the tongue-tip as required in the preceding exercises, except that here the target will vary in the same trial, as will the length of the hold phases. Begin by requesting that the patient force the tongue-tip upward so that the crossbar sticks are *halfway* closed. Count silently for 2 seconds and immediately instruct the patient to force the sticks into *three-quarter* contact. Count silently for 3 seconds and immediately request that the patient position the sticks *one-quarter* of the way closed. Silently count for 5 seconds and instruct the patient to rest. A minimal rest period of 15 seconds is recommended. Thus, a total of three different force targets (1N, 1.5N, and 0.5N, respectively) and three different hold phases (2, 3 and 5 seconds, re-spectively) are sequentially ordered without a break between these targets. The instructions for this trial may play out like this:

> Once the sticks are in position, I am going to ask you to use your tongue-tip, like before, to push the lower stick up toward the upper stick. However, the degree of force that I want you to use will vary within the trial. When I instruct you to push to a certain degree, keep doing so until I give you the next cue to switch to a new degree. *Do not* change the degree of force you use unless and until I instruct you to do so. Ready? Okay, push the sticks halfway closed (count silently for 2 seconds); now push them three-quarters of the way closed (count silently for 3 seconds); now push them one-quarter of the way closed (count silently for 5 seconds); and now rest your tongue.

Step 2. The entire trial is rated, not the individual force segments, using the Score Key at the bottom of the Force Physiology Treatment Chart to charac-terize and measure the patient's performance. At the completion of each trial, en-ter on the y-axis grid of the chart, on the line marked "Variable," the letter from the key that best describes the total effort. Repeat this pretreatment measure-ment two more times, but adopt different force and hold phase targets from those used for the first trial above. The second trial may require the patient to com-press the sticks three-quarters of the way for 3 seconds, one-quarter of the way for 2 seconds, and then one-half of the way closed for 5 seconds, for a total of 10 seconds to end the trial. On the third baseline trial the patient may be prompted to push the stick one-quarter of the way up for 5 seconds, three-quarters closed for 2 seconds, and finally one-quarter again for the remaining 3 seconds. The let-ter scores for these two baseline trials can be clustered in the same column next to that for the first trial, to save chart space. Make certain that the date, number of trials (3), musculature tested (T), vector (BP$_9$), and time (V) information are accurately listed in the respective cells of the column.

Step 3. Proceed with the next step if the patient fails to obtain a "C" rat-ing on two or more of the trials; otherwise skip this exercise and advance to the next one. *Note:* During this exercise *do not* use as a target complete closure of the crossbar sticks, because it is very difficult to ascertain the actual and ongoing de-gree of tongue force exerted when the sticks are fully compressed. All that can be determined with certainty is that *at least* 2N of palatal vector tongue force is be-ing applied.

Step 4. Use the crossbar apparatus following the exact same method de-scribed above, except that here introduce novel force and hold phase targets throughout the treatment paradigm so as to reduce the possibility of contaminat-ing order effects. Limiting each trial to three targets is recommended, at least two of them being different from one another. Continue this procedure until the patient achieves a "C" rating on at least eight of ten consecutive trials. To save chart space, several letter scores can be clustered into the same column on the line marked "Variable," making certain that the date, number of trials, muscula-ture treated (T), vector (P$_9$), time of hold phase (V), and target criterion (80 percent) are recorded in their respective cells. Advance to the next exercise when the patient either achieves this criterion or fails to demonstrate any observable trend of improvement over baseline after 30 consecutive trials.

Lip Force Physiology Exercise No. 1

Note. As with the preceding Tongue Force Physiology training program, the patient's jaw force control will dictate whether the acrylic bite blocks can be used or whether tailor-made putty blocks will be necessary (see Tongue Force Physiology Exercise no. 1 for further information regarding these latter blocks).

Step 1. As shown in Figure 6–21, place the ½ inch by ½ inch bite block in the patient's mouth between the central incisor teeth. Note that the string is substituted for the acrylic handle to permit full lip closure around the block. The string protects against (unlikely) accidental swallowing of the block and can be held or pinned to the patient's shirt. To establish baseline ability, request the patient to conceal the presence of the block by bringing the upper and lower lip into full and complete contact, hold that position for 2 seconds, open the lips completely to reexpose the block for an additional 2 seconds, and continue these alternating lip movements at the same speed for 30 seconds without interruption. Each round trip (Close/Open) constitutes a single trial. If the lips move without significant delay upon each verbal cue to "close" and "open" around the block, if these movements are targeted with precision and completeness to the closed and back to the open position, and if the hold phases are steady, the trial is rated *correct*. Signs of motor dyscontrol at any point in the cycle of the trial must be rated *incorrect. Note:* Patients who struggle with the central block position may benefit from relocating the block to the premolar region. Cover the block with a finger cot.

Step 2. Use a notepad to rate each trial throughout the 30-second task, allow 15 seconds for rest, and repeat this procedure two more times. Tally the mean correct percentage of all trials and enter this baseline score on the Metronomic Mobility Treatment Chart (see Figure 6–22) in a separate column. Be certain to record the date, minutes of therapy (1½), musculature tested (L), task (BC/O$_1$), and bpm (30—every 2 seconds) in the respective cells of the column. Proceed with the next step if this finding is equal to or less than 75 percent correct; otherwise skip this exercise and advance to the next one.

Step 3. Set the metronome to 30 bpm, position the ½ inch bite block in the patient's mouth, and instruct him or her that the task is to close and open the lips alternately according to the beat: One vector per beat continuously for 30 seconds. Explain the rating protocol described in the above step so that the patient understands the rules of the exercise. The patient should be permitted to begin whenever desired, but once committed must continue without a break for the full 30 seconds. A stopwatch serves to warn the patient when the trial has ended. The metronome, if placed strategically near the table mirror, may further serve as feedback both visually and auditorily to alternate temporally these lip gestures. The verbal cues "close" and "open" may be provided in synch with the metronomic beats as yet additional stimuli sources. Follow the same basic rating and scoring method described in the preceding step, except that here we tally the mean correct percentage of all trials after 5 full minutes of exercising, not including the 15-second rest periods between the 30-second treatment segments.

Step 4. At the completion of each set of 5 minutes, which represents ten 30-second exercise segments, calculate this percentage, extract the result from the notepad, and enter this finding on the Metronomic Mobility Treatment Chart in a separate column. Repeat this procedure until the patient achieves a mean correct score at least 75 percent improved over the baseline score or 100 percent correct, whichever is less, over 10 consecutive minutes of therapy. Be sure to list the appropriate date, minutes of therapy (5), musculature treated (L), task (C/O$_1$), bpm (30), and calculated target criterion (?) in the respective cells of the column. As usual, discontinuation of the exercise is recommended if after 30 consecutive minutes of treatment there is no discernible trend of improvement. However, advancement to the next exercise is still indicated, but with guarded optimism. *Note:* This exercise is virtually identical in design to Tongue Force Physiology Exercise no. 1, with the exception that here the task involves "Close/Open" *lip* movements not "Up/Down" tongue-tip vectors.

Lip Force Physiology Exercise Nos. 2–5

Note. These exercises are virtually identical to the previously detailed Tongue Force Physiology Exercise nos. 2–5, except that here the task is "Close/Open" lip movements to 60, 90, 120, and variable bpm stimuli, respectively, with the ½ inch block in position. Follow the same data acquisition method and rating, scoring, charting, and advancement criteria for these exercises as were employed earlier for their tongue force counterparts. However, be certain that these treatment data are tagged respectively with the correct task (C/O$_2$, C/O$_3$, C/O$_4$, and C/O$_5$) and musculature treated (L) symbols on the Metronomic Mobility Treatment Chart. All baseline data, of course, are represented on the chart with the prefix "B" adjacent to the respective task symbols. Proceed as usual.

Lip Force Physiology Exercise Nos. 6–10

Note. This series is identical to the preceding lip exercises in design and scope with one exception: Here the ¾ inch by ½ inch bite block is used throughout the regimen. Remember to tag respectively these data with the correct task symbols (C/O$_6$, C/O$_7$, C/O$_8$, C/O$_9$, and C/O$_{10}$) on the treatment chart. All baseline data receive the prefix "B." Look back to Tongue Force Physiology Exercise nos. 6–10 for additional guidance: The only difference between those exercises and these is that here the "Close/Open" lip vector, not the "Up/Down" lingua-alveolar vector, is being treated. Proceed as usual.

Lip Force Physiology Exercise No. 11

Step 1. To establish baseline ability, position the ½ inch by ½ inch bite block in the patient's mouth in the usual way, substituting a string for the handle. Request that the patient pucker the lips as fully as possible, hold that position for 2 seconds, then smile broadly, holding that position for an additional 2 seconds, and continue these alternating lip movements at the same speed for 30 seconds without interruption. Each round trip constitutes a single trial. If the lips move free of significant delay upon each verbal cue to "pucker" and "spread," if these movements are targeted with precision and completeness to the full pucker and spread positions without interrupting jaw activity, and if the hold phases are steady, the trial is rated *correct.* Signs of motor dyscontrol at any point in the cycle of the trial must be rated *incorrect.* Follow the rating, scoring, charting, and advancement criteria detailed in Exercise no. 1 above, making certain to tag these baseline data with the correct task symbol (B P/S_1) on the Metronomic Mobility Treatment Chart.

Step 2. Adopt the exact same data acquisition method and rating, scoring, charting, and advancement criteria detailed in Steps 3 and 4 of Exercise no. 1, except that here the task is "Pucker/Spread" not "Close/Open." Be sure to tag these treatment data on the treatment chart with the correct task symbol (P/S_1).

Lip Force Physiology Exercise Nos. 12–15

Note. This series is identical to Exercise no. 11, except that for these four exercises the speed of the metronome is changed respectively to 60, 90, 120, and variable bpm. Tongue Force Physiology Exercise nos. 2–5 describe in detail these alterations and how they are employed in the treatment paradigm. For each of these lip exercises, follow the same rating, scoring, charting, and advancement criteria established in the preceding Lip Force Physiology Exercises. Be certain, however, to tag respectively these treatment data with the correct task symbols (P/S_2, P/S_3, P/S_4, and P/S_5) on the Metronomic Mobility Treatment Chart. All baseline data are naturally represented on the chart by the prefix "B" adjacent to the corresponding task symbols. Proceed as usual.

Lip Force Physiology Exercise No. 16

Step 1. To establish baseline ability, the crossbar apparatus is used as shown in Figure 6–17. Position the ¾ inch by ½ inch bite block in the premolar region, as usual. Begin with the four-stick wedge, which creates roughly 4 Newtons of resistance between the crossbar (wooden) plates. Place the ends of these plates between the patient's upper and lower lips and request him or her merely to rest but not press the lips on the plates.

Step 2. Instruct the patient that the task here is to use the lips to compress these plates *halfway* closed and to maintain this position for 5 seconds. The table mirror will provide adequate visual biofeedback regarding this target. With a rest period of 15 seconds between trials, have the patient perform this task five times. Each trial should be rated independently, using the Score Key at the bottom of the Force Physiology Treatment Chart (Figure 6–23) to measure the patient's overall performance. As before for the tongue force regimen, at the completion of each trial enter on the y-axis grid of the chart, on the 2N line indicating the 2-Newton target, the letter from the key (C, L, V, F, or U) that best describes the characteristics of the effort. If all five baseline scores are clustered next to one another in the same column, chart space will be preserved. Make certain that the date, number of trials (5), musculature tested (L), vector (BC/O_{11}), and time (5 seconds) are recorded in the respective cells of the column. Proceed with the next step if the patient fails to achieve a "C" rating on three or more of the trials; otherwise skip this exercise and advance to the next one. *Note:* The requirement to compress the crossbar plates to the halfway closed position, under the four-stick wedge condition, is roughly equal to a 2-Newton force target.

Step 3.   Use the same crossbar set-up again and follow identically the method of the preceding steps. Repeat this procedure until the patient achieves a "C" rating on at least eight of ten consecutive trials. Save chart space by chunking several letter scores into each column of data. Be sure to record as well the date; number of trials for the column, though this will be evident from the amount of letter entries; musculature treated (L); vector (C/O_{11}); time of hold phase (5); and target criterion (80 percent) in the respective cells of the column. Move on to the next exercise when the patient either achieves this criterion or fails to demonstrate any observable trend of improvement over baseline after 30 consecutive trials.

Lip Force Physiology Exercise No. 17

Step 1.   Follow exactly the same baseline data acquisition, rating, scoring, charting, and advancement methods described in the preceding exercise, except that here the *two-stick* wedge is used for resistance. Be sure to record the vector symbol BC/O_{12} to represent these baseline data on the Force Physiology Treatment Chart. *Note:* The force target here is approximately 1 Newton, and all data entries are thus made on the 1N line of the chart.

Step 2.   Follow identically the treatment method of the preceding exercise, except that the two- not the four-stick wedge is used here, which creates resistance roughly equal to 1 Newton when the crossbar plates are compressed to the halfway mark. Be sure to tag these data with the vector symbol "C/O_{12}" on the treatment chart.

Lip Force Physiology Exercise No. 18

Step 1.   Again, follow exactly the same baseline data acquisition, rating, scoring, charting, and advancement methods detailed in Exercise no. 16, except that here the *one-* not the four-stick wedge is used, which creates resistance roughly equal to 0.5 Newtons when the crossbar plates are compressed to the halfway mark. The vector symbol "BC/O$_{13}$" is listed on the Force Physiology Treatment Chart to represent these baseline data. *Note:* Because the force target here is approximately 0.5 Newtons, all data entries for this exercise are thus made on the 0.5N line of the chart.

Step 2. Follow the identical treatment method detailed in Exercise no. 16, remembering that for this exercise the one-stick wedge is used for resistance, and the vector symbol "C/O$_{13}$" is listed on the treatment chart.

Lip Force Physiology Exercise No. 19

Step 1. Follow the same basic method used in the preceding exercise, except that here the crossbar plates are compressed merely *one-quarter* (not one-half) of the way closed, and held for the usual 5 seconds in this position. When rating, scoring, and charting these baseline results, be certain to tag the data collected with vector symbol "BC/O$_{14}$" on the Force Physiology Treatment Chart. *Note:* The task here to decrease by 25 percent the distance between the crossbar plates, under the one-stick resistance condition, is roughly equivalent to a 0.25 Newton force target. All data entries for this exercise are thus made on the 0.25N line of the chart.

Step 2. Follow the exact same method of Step 1 above. Repeat this procedure, as usual, following the data acquisition method and rating, scoring, charting, and advancement criteria detailed in Exercise no. 16. These treatment data are tagged with the vector symbol "C/O$_{14}$" on the chart.

Lip Force Physiology Exercise No. 20

Note. This exercise is identical to Tongue Force Physiology Exercise no. 35 with the exception that here we measure and treat the "Close/Open" lip not the "Palatal" tongue vector at *variable* resistance levels within the same trial. Look to the detailed instructions of that exercise for data acquisition methods and rating, scoring, charting, and advancement criteria guidelines, making certain that the verbal command adjustments to the patient reflect this obvious difference in musculature and vector training. Additionally, all data entries on the Force Physiology Treatment Chart should be tagged with the correct musculature (L) and vector (C/O$_{15}$) symbols in their respective cells of the column. Proceed as usual.

Lip Force Physiology Exercise Nos. 21–25

Note. For this series follow respectively exactly the same baseline and treatment methods of Exercise nos. 16–20, except that here the hold phase is increased to 10 seconds for each trial. Note that the vector symbols "C/O$_{16-20}$" should be used respectively on the Force Physiology Treatment Chart to tag the data collected during these five exercises. As usual, when charting the baseline findings the prefix "B" is saddled on the corresponding vector symbols.

Jaw Force Physiology Exercise No. 1

Note. Because the exercises that fall in this subsection involve jaw force measures, bite blocks are not used as they were in the preceding Tongue and Lip Force Physiology Exercises. All exercises below are based on the "Close/Open" vector.

Step 1. To establish baseline ability, request that the patient bite down gently so that the upper and lower teeth are occluded completely, hold that position for 2 seconds, open the mouth to create a gap of about 1 inch between the cutting edges of the incisors and hold this position for an additional 2 seconds, and continue these alternating jaw movements at the same speed for 30 seconds without interruption. Each round trip (Close/Open) will as usual constitute a single trial. If the mandible moves without significant temporal delay upon each verbal cue to "close" and "open," if these movements are targeted with precision and completeness to the designated closed and open positions, and if the hold phases are steady, the trial is rated *correct*. Signs of motor dyscontrol at any point in the cycle of the trial must be rated *incorrect*. Use a notepad in the usual manner to rate each trial throughout the 30-second task, allow 15 seconds for rest, and repeat this procedure two more times.

Step 2. Tally the mean correct percentage of all trials and enter this baseline score on the Metronomic Mobility Treatment Chart (Figure 6–22) in a separate column. Be certain to record the date, minutes of therapy (1½), musculature tested (J), task (BC/O$_1$), and bpm (30—every 2 seconds) in the respective cells of the column. Proceed with the next step if this result is equal to or less than 75 percent correct; otherwise skip this exercise and advance to the next one.

Step 3. Set the metronome to 30 bpm and instruct the patient that the task is to close and open the jaw alternately, as in the above step, according to the beat of the metronome: 1 vector per beat continuously for 30 seconds. Explain the rating protocol described above, as always. Follow the same basic data acquisition method and rating, scoring, charting, and advancement criteria detailed in Lip Force Physiology Exercise no. 1, making the necessary instruction adjustments to reflect that here jaw, not lip, "Close/Open" vectors are being measured. On the Metronomic Mobility Treatment Chart be certain to list the correct musculature treated (J), task (C/O$_1$), and calculated target criterion (?) symbols in their respective cells of the data columns.

Jaw Force Physiology Exercise Nos. 2–5

Note. These four exercises are virtually identical to the previously detailed Tongue and Lip Force Physiology Exercise nos. 2–5, with the obvious exceptions that here the task is "Close/Open" *jaw* movements; we shift from 30 to 60, 90, 120, and variable bpm metronomic stimuli, respectively; no bite block is used in the segments. Follow the same data acquisition method and rating, scoring, charting, and advancement criteria for these exercises as were employed earlier for their tongue and lip force counterparts. Be certain, however, that these treatment data are tagged respectively with the correct task (C/O_2, C/O_3, C/O_4, and C/O_5) and musculature treated (J) symbols on the Metronomic Mobility Treatment Chart. All baseline data, of course, should receive the prefix "B" in the corresponding task cell. Proceed as usual.

Jaw Force Physiology Exercise No. 6

Step 1. As shown in Figure 6–19, Jaw Force Physiology will be tested and treated using the crossbar apparatus. To establish baseline ability, begin with the four-stick wedge, which creates roughly 4 Newtons of resistance between the crossbar plates. Place the ends of these plates between the patient's upper and lower central incisor teeth and request him or her merely to rest the teeth but not bite down on the plates.

Step 2. Instruct the patient that the task here is to use the jaw musculature to bite down on the plates so that they are compressed *halfway* closed and to maintain this position for 5 seconds. As usual, the table mirror provides useful feedback during the trial. Allowing a 15-second rest period between trials, have the patient repeat this task five times. Each trial should be rated independently following the same basic scoring, charting, and advancement procedures detailed in Lip Force Physiology Exercise no. 16, making the necessary adjustments to reflect the fact that the task here is "Close/Open" *jaw* not lip force movement control. Thus, on the Force Physiology Treatment Chart be certain to use the correct musculature (J) and vector (BC/O_6) symbols. Remember, this task roughly equates with a 2-Newton force target, thus requiring that all data entries be made on the 2N line.

Step 3. Use the same crossbar set-up again and follow identically the method of the preceding step. Repeat this procedure until the patient achieves the previously recommended standard of a "C" rating on at least eight of ten consecutive trials. Chart space can be saved by clustering several letter scores into each data column on the treatment chart. Be sure to tag these entries with the correct vector (C/O_6) symbol and target criterion (80 percent). Move on to the next exercise subsection when the patient either achieves this criterion or fails to demonstrate any observable trend of improvement over baseline after 30 consecutive trials.

Jaw Force Physiology Exercise Nos. 7–10

Note. This series is identical in scope and design to the baseline and treatment segments of Lip Force Physiology Exercise nos. 17–20, except that here the task is "Close/Open" *jaw,* not lip, vectors. Look to the details of those earlier reviewed exercises for data acquisition methods and rating, scoring, charting, and advancement criteria guidelines. Make certain that the correct musculature (J) and vector (C/O_{7-10}) symbols are used to tag these treatment data on the Force Physiology Treatment Chart. As usual, when listing baseline findings use the prefix "B" next to the corresponding vector symbols.

Jaw Force Physiology Exercise Nos. 11–15

Note. This series is identical in scope and design to the counterpart Lip Force Physiology Exercise nos. 21–25, again with the exception of the obvious task difference of "Close/Open" *jaw* not lip, vectors. Consult the details of those lip exercises for information on data acquisition procedures and rating, scoring, charting, and advancement criteria guidelines. The musculature (J) and vector (C/O_{11-15}) symbols need to be accurately listed on the Force Physiology Treatment Chart in their respective cells, as do the target criteria (?). All baseline entries in the vector cells are accompanied by the prefix "B."

This concludes the subsection on articulator physiology exercises. Table 6–3 provides a capsule summary of these treatments as recommended for the tongue, lip, and jaw musculature disturbances commonly observed in dysarthric patients, with articulation subsystem disturbances.

TREATMENT OF ARTICULATORY IMPRECISION

Up to this point in the chapter we have concentrated largely on methods by which to prime the articulators for the physiologic demands of phonetic drills. We now proceed with treatment regimens aimed directly at improving articulatory proficiency. The prognosis for improvement here is often highly related to the results of all previously administered speech subsystem treatments. In this subsection the focus is exclusively on how to train dysarthric and apractic patients who have imprecise articulation to produce more adequately the sounds that they significantly misarticulate. Whether the errors are of the distortion, substitution, or omission types, and whether or not the patient may have forgotten how sounds are made, all may benefit from isolated sound drills. Whereas we may aim for nearly normal productions, having to settle for much less is a virtual certainty with most patients. Because of space limitations the various and sundry methods by which sounds taught can be transferred or generalized to different contexts will not be addressed. Clinicians do well by having at their disposal an assortment of picture cue cards that can be used to elicit single words of varying lengths and complexity, phrases, sentences, and spontaneous speech.

Some clinical researchers have suggested that treatment of those sounds that are misarticulated need not include isolated practice, and that such drills with patients other than the severely disabled are superfluous. It is moot to debate this issue because it is generally true that the bulk of time spent in articulation therapy involves the use of word stimuli in various contexts. Further, words, sentences, phrases, and connected discourse articulation exercises are much more interesting and meaningful to patients of all ages than single sounds or even nonsense syllables.

It is usually best to establish a reliable baseline of articulation skills before initiating this segment of treatment. (For example, see Yorkston and Beukelman: *Assessment of Intelligibility of Dysarthric Speech* [1982]). Such testing will provide information on the consistency of the patient's errors and the phonetic

TABLE 6–3.   Capsule Summary of Physiology Exercise Sequence for Possible

Disturbance	1	2	3	4
Tongue hypertonicity	Forward pull	R/L Lateral Pulls	F, R/L Pulls	
Lip hypertonicity	Lower lip pull	Upper lip pull		
Jaw hypertonicity	Open/Close passive jaw maneuver w/1/2" bite block	Open/Close maneuver w/3/4" block	Open/Close maneuver w/1" block	
Tongue weakness	Anterior resistance w/custom designed putty block	Left lateral resistance w/custom putty block	Right lateral resistance w/custom putty block	Lingua-alveolar resistance w/crossbar apparatus & 5 stick wedge
Lip weakness	Anterior resistance w/button & string	Right lateral resistance w/button & string	Left lateral resistance w/button & string	Anterior resistance w/crossbar apparatus & 3 stick wedge
Jaw weakness	Closing resistance w/crossbar apparatus & 5 stick wedge			
Tongue force dyscontrol	Alternate lingua-alveolar vectors w/1/2" bite block at 30 bpm w/metronome	Ditto at 60 bpm	Ditto at 90 bpm	Ditto at 120 bpm
Lip force dyscontrol	Alternate Close/Open vectors w/1/2" bite block at 30 bpm w/metronome	Ditto at 60 bpm	Ditto at 90 bpm	Ditto at 120 bpm
Jaw force dyscontrol	Alternate Close/Open vectors at 30 bpm w/metronome but no bite block	Ditto at 60 bpm	Ditto at 90 bpm	Ditto at 120 bpm

Articulation Subsystem Disturbances

5	6–10	11–15	16–20	21–25	26–35
Ditto at variable bpm	Same as 1–5 except w/3/4″ block	Same as 1–5 except w/1″ block	Same as 1–5 except for Out/In vectors w/1″ block	Same as 1–5 except for left/right vectors w/1″ block	Lingua-alveolar vector w/crossbar apparatus at various resistance levels ranging from .25N to 2N at both 5-sec and 10-sec hold phase levels
Ditto at variable bpm	Same as 1–5 except w/3/4″ block	Same as 1–5 except for pucker/ spread vectors w/1/2″ block	Close/Open vectors w/crossbar apparatus at various resistance levels ranging from .25N to 2N at both 5-sec and 10-sec hold phases		
Ditto at variable bpm	Close/Open vectors w/crossbar apparatus at various resistance levels ranging from .25N to 2N at both 5-sec and 10-sec hold phases				

context in which the sounds that may be targeted for treatment are least vulnerable to breakdown. In some patients, errors will be fairly predictable and independent of boundary influences. Others may display inconsistent errors that are exacerbated by certain phonetic environments. Consequently, and not surprisingly, articulation therapy in the dysarthrias must be customed to fit the salient signs and symptoms of the individual patient. However, because basic techniques that may facilitate phoneme productions, in light of the underlying residual neuromuscular or motor planning deficits, are worth exploring, they are offered below for review.

The stimulation exercises in this subsection are designed for universal application. Any patient who struggles with articulatory imprecision and has completed prerequisite, indicated physiologic training may be a good candidate for these exercises. The primary purpose here is to teach *acceptable* sound productions. Articulatory proficiency is not the ultimate objective; rather, it is better and more realistic to strive for improved speech intelligibility, whether residually imprecise or not. Practicing target sounds should progress from simple productions, perhaps in isolation at first, through gradually more difficult levels involving words of increasing length and phonetic complexity. To establish a strong base of motivation, those sounds judged potentially easier to learn, as determined by the underlying pathophysiology and severity of dysfunction, might best be drilled in the earlier stages of the stimulation program: The inherently more difficult sounds may be phased-in judiciously as the patient experiences success at lower levels. Ultimately, word stimuli containing the target sounds are practiced in sentence, phrase, and conversation contexts.

Before delving into the specially designed exercises below, it is worth noting that patients who have journeyed with relative success through other subsystem treatments generally are well prepared to tackle the phonetic stimuli. Gains made earlier with any of the speech breathing, resonation, phonation, or articulator exercises usually lend critical support during phonetic training. The road is a lot tougher here for patients who have not achieved as much success with previous subsystem treatments. In either case, the patient should be approached with the same degree of clinical enthusiasm. The exercises, if indicated, are to be administered in the same fashion, irrespective of the underlying etiology or prognosis for improvement. However, because the treatment outcomes invariably differ from patient to patient, the criteria for advancement within the exercise regimen should reflect these anticipated results at the outset. This approach sets attainable goals for the patient, rather than ones that are unrealistic, and ensures a balance of motivation that is almost always helpful.

Prior to and periodically throughout the Phonetic Stimulation Exercise regimen, measure the patient's articulatory skills during connected discourse, using the Speech Characteristics Chart (see Figure 2–2) to record this baseline impression. Recall the importance of listing the date of data collection and the activity feature symbol (BA_1) in the appropriate cells of the column. Each new baseline entry receives a correspondingly new numeric subscript. The same chart should be used to record ongoing impressions of treatment efficacy. For these treatment data entries the prefix "B" is omitted from the activity feature cell.

Phonetic Simulation Techniques

Vowels

From an articulatory point of view, vowels are perhaps the simplest of the sound classes to produce and teach. They generally require much less complicated or gross adjustments of the tongue, lips, and jaw than sounds in the other classes. Because most patients experience at least some degree of success practicing vowel productions, irrespective of their responses to all previous speech subsystem treatments, it is often best to begin the phonetic stimulation program with the vowel sounds. Serving as the bridges between consonants in words, the vowels add power to the acoustic signal, making speech audible at great distances.

It is beyond the scope of this chapter to explore in detail the anatomy of the different vowels. Suffice it to say that all are voiced, and some are classified as "front" (i, ɪ, e, ɛ, æ), others are considered "back" (u, ʊ, ɔ, o, a), and there is also a "central" one as well (ə or ʌ). Terms such as high, mid, low, tense, and lax are also used to describe these sounds. For example, the /i/ is a "high-front-tense" vowel, whereas the /a/ is a "low-back-lax" one. Anatomical and physiologic descriptions permit slightly different views of these same sounds. To produce the /i/ the front part of the tongue should be positioned with tension high in the mouth. The /a/, on the other hand, is generated when the back of the tongue is held low and relaxed in the mouth. Diphthongs are created by coupling two vowels (aɪ, aʊ, jʊ, ɔɪ, and, to lesser degrees, ɛɪ, ou).

Let's examine how these sounds may be stimulated in isolation. Ultimately they will be practiced in various contexts with target consonants. When the patient is ready to advance to these levels, the best approach is usually a gradual one, beginning with VC or CV syllables and progressing sequentially to bisyllable, trisyllable, and multisyllable word stimuli as criteria are met along the way. Methods of sentence, phrase, and connected discourse usage are respectively introduced in the latter stages of the stimulation program, commensurate with the patient's responses to the other segments of articulation therapy. *Note:* The suggestions below deviate in design from all preceding exercises and only some of the vowels will be addressed. These techniques are provided merely to illustrate possible ways of eliciting production of the vowels in those dysarthric and apractic patients who are unable to do so without such assistance. Whether the results of these techniques yield normal responses, reasonably intelligible approximations of the targets, or barely acceptable compensatory productions, clinicians may then blend these newly acquired sounds into the consonant stimulation regimen. How best to interface these stimulation techniques with the overall treatment plan for a given patient will not be pursued.

Stimulation of the /a/

First, sit in front of the patient as shown in Figure 6–1, and demonstrate prolongations of this vowel, exaggerating lip and jaw excursions and the mouth-open posture so that the patient easily visualizes the anatomy of the sound. *Second*, request that he or she open the mouth and rest the tongue-tip behind the lower incisors, using the mirror for biofeedback. Then use a wooden tongue blade to depress the tongue gently, and request that the patient try to prolong the /a/ as long and as steadily as possible. If necessary, alter the position of the depressor until a relatively good vowel is produced. *Third*, have the patient prolong the vowel in the same fashion five times in a row with the aid of the tongue depressor, permitting a deep breath between trials. If all these productions are judged acceptable, repeat the task without the stick. *Fourth*, if all these productions are adequate, have the patient prolong the /a/ for 3 seconds, rest the following 3 seconds, and continue this alternating sequence for 30 seconds, without instructions relative to the speech-breathing dynamics to employ. *Fifth*, create any number of variations of this exercise theme and practice them all until the patient demonstrates at least 75 percent intelligible productions of the /a/ in isolation. If there are intelligible consonants in the patient's repertoire, now is a good time to interface those sounds with the /a/ in ways mentioned above (e.g., CV, VC, VCV, CVC, etc.). *Note:* If the patient cannot achieve the criterion for this sound, the prognosis diminishes for improvement of other vowel difficulties.

Stimulation of the /i/

First, request that the patient place the tongue-tip behind the lower incisors as for the /a/. *Second*, position the ends of two tongue blades between the teeth as shown in Figure 6–24 and instruct the patient to bite down gently on the sticks and smile so that the lip corners are spread apart. *Third*, if lip retraction is not pronounced, assist the patient by spreading further the lip corners with the thumb and index finger as illustrated. *Fourth*, have the patient try to prolong the /i/ as long and as steadily as possible. Follow the same basic guidelines for prac-

Figure 6–24.
To stimulate production of the vowel /i/, a two-stick wedge can be used to facilitate an adequate jaw position while simultaneously the fingers assist with lip positioning.

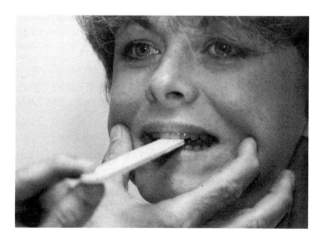

tice as suggested for the /a/ above. *Fifth,* introduce the /a/ and /i/ in a sequence exercise, in which the patient is required to alternate productions of these sounds according to different time frames and embedded within the various consonant environments possible at this point in the program.

Stimulation of the /u/

First, request that the patient place the tongue-tip behind the lower incisors in the usual way. *Second,* position the end of a long cotton-tipped applicator along the midline of the tip of the tongue, as shown in Figure 6–25, and instruct the patient to bite down gently and pucker the lips around the stick. *Third,* if lip puckering is insufficient, use the fingers as illustrated to squeeze the cheeks simultaneously to assist this posture. *Fourth,* have the patient try to prolong the /u/ as long and as steadily as possible. Follow the same method employed to stimulate and practice the preceding vowel. Note from Figure 6–26 that a stethoscope may be used to provide auditory biofeedback of vocal fold activity during vowel stimulation. Some patients, particularly those who continue to struggle with phonation subsystem dyscontrol, appreciate this method. The diaphragm of the scope can be placed on the clinician's larynx as well, for demonstration purposes. *Fifth,* once the criterion set for the /u/ has been met, a rolling exercise of the /i-u-a/ vowels often proves rewarding. Here's how it works: The patient takes as deep a breath as possible and begins the exercise by prolonging the /i/ for roughly 5 seconds, then glides without another breath or hesitation into production of the /u/ for an additional 5 seconds, and then finishes by gliding smoothly into a 5-second prolongation of the /a/. Alterations of the sequential order of the vowel train and/or the prolongation times are recommended as excellent exercise alternatives.

Stimulation of the /ɛ/ and /e/

First, request that the patient rest the tongue-tip behind the lower incisors. *Second,* use a tongue depressor to push the tongue-tip down to induce a hump in

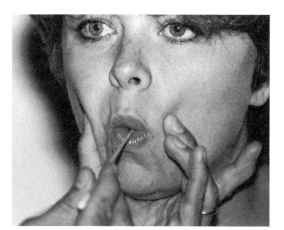

Figure 6–25.
Use of finger compression and a long cotton-tipped applicator to induce lip rounding for the production of the vowel /u/.

Figure 6–26.
Use of both a cotton-tipped
applicator stick and a stethoscope to
stimulate production of the vowel
/u/. The stethoscope can be
instrumental for voicing feedback
during the practice of any number of
sounds.

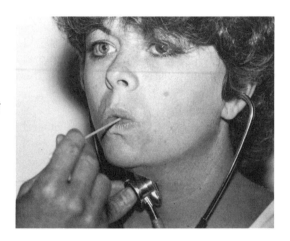

the blade and front regions. *Third*, instruct the patient to relax the lips and
tongue musculature as much as possible and try to prolong the /ɛ/ sound. In the
beginning, producing the sounds concurrently with the patient can be helpful
feedback. Adjust the pressure and position of the tongue depressor as necessary
to facilitate production. Through experimentation and practice the patient usually achieves adequacy. *Fourth*, employ the methods recommended above for
practice of this sound in different contexts. *Fifth*, to produce the /e/ the patient
starts with the /ɛ/ and glides to the /i/ sound without hesitation. *Sixth*, practice
this adjustment until the patient can generate at least a decent production, and
then add this sound to the list for creative rehearsal.

Stimulation of the /ɪ/ and /ʊ/

    First, demonstrate these sounds for the patient, pointing out that the re-
quirements for their production are similar to those for their tense cognates the
/i/ and /u/, respectively, except that here the lips and tongue musculature are
generally held in a more relaxed fashion. Vocal energy tends to be reduced as
well during these productions. *Second*, have the patient experiment by variably
lessening the articulator tension as the /i/ and /u/ are prolonged to see if by doing
so there is perceptible conversion to the /ɪ/ and /ʊ/ sounds. *Third*, follow the same
basic method of practice outlined for the preceding vowels. Be creative relative to
coupling these sounds in various sequences and combinations with the other vowels learned and consonants used thus far.

Stimulation of the /o/

    First, request that the patient open the mouth wide. *Second*, using the fin-
gers of one hand, gently compress both cheeks simultaneously while the fingers
of the other hand position the lips in a relaxed and rounded posture, as illustrated in Figure 6–27. *Third*, liken the requisite lip adjustments for this sound
to those that smokers employ to blow smoke rings. *Fourth*, instruct the patient to
try the sound, inhibiting premature lip puckering with those fingers on the lips,

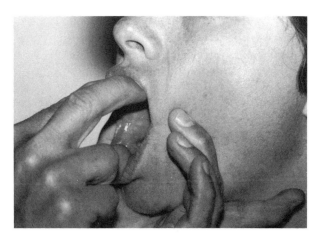

Figure 6–27.
Fingers in position to
stimulate production of the
vowel /o/. The distance
between the thumb and the
index and middle fingers
rounding the lips is gradually
decreased to induce the lip
protrusion required for precise
production. Simultaneously the
cheeks are squeezed to ensure
this requisite posture of the
lips.

and inducing, when desired, this effect with those fingers on the cheeks. *Fifth*,
follow the same basic practice methods earlier used for the other vowels.

Stimulation of the Diphthongs

This class of sounds is relatively easy to teach, if the component parts have
been learned. The /aɪ/ can be produced by gliding from the /a/ to the /i/. The /au/
results when gliding from the /a/ to the /u/. The /ɔɪ/ is generated with the /ɔ/ and
/i/ combination, and the /ju/ emanates by smoothly coupling the /i/ and /u/. Incor-
poration of these sounds into the list of practice material provides introduction to
many new word stimuli.

Note.   At the completion of vowel training, be sure to rate articulation in
various contexts, using the Speech Characteristics Chart to record these impressions. Compare these data with all previously collected and charted articulation
scores.

Consonants

Historically, the consonant sounds have been homogeneously clustered into
manner and place of production groups for ease of description and to facilitate
training. The "manner" categories essentially include nasals, plosives, fricatives,
affricatives, and glides. The "place" group is subdivided into bilabial, labio-dental, lingua-alveolar, lingua-velar, lingua-palatal, and lingua-dental sounds. As
these names imply, productions of the various consonant sounds require complex
adjustments of the vocal tract. Thus, as a group they are generally more difficult
to teach than the vowels. Naturally, some of the consonants are by design easier
than others to produce. Perhaps that is why consonant development gradually
emerges throughout the childhood years concurrently with the overall sensorimotor advancements. Because of time and space limitations, not all the consonants will be covered. The techniques of stimulation are designed to elicit isolated, adequate productions. Measures that might be taken to interface the

sounds taught with other sounds learned or unimpaired are not detailed. The sections below are subdivided by "place" of production, but are not necessarily presented in any order of importance or by ease of administration. Note that, as with the vowels earlier studied, prior to and periodically during consonant training it is advisable to rate the patient's articulation skills, using the Speech Characteristics Chart to record such impressions and track and measure any improvements made.

Stimulation of the Bilabials (/m/, /w/, /p/, /b/)

All things being equal relative to underlying physiologic support of the various speech subsystems, the bilabial sounds are good candidates for initial treatment because by comparison they are the simplest sounds to produce. Most dysarthric and apractic patients respond favorably to such stimulation. Of course, if there is persistent resonation subsystem leakage, notwithstanding earlier treatments, the /p/ and /b/ sounds may be stubborn but not necessarily impossible to improve, owing to their dependence on adequate intraoral air pressure and flow. Let's look at the /m/ and /p, b/ separately.

/m/. This bilabial nasal consonant is easy to teach if the patient can at least bring the upper and lower lips together. *First,* place the patient's fingertips on your lips and nose and prolong the /m/, enabling the vibratory sensation to be felt. *Second,* do the same thing with the patient's fingertips against the larynx for similar feedback. *Third,* have the patient look in the mirror and attempt to prolong the /m/ as long and as steadily as possible, feeling his or her own lips, nose and larynx for vibratory feedback and modification of production if necessary. Use of a stethoscope may prove additionally helpful for patients having trouble turning on or maintaining vocal fold activity during this effort. *Fourth,* if the patient is still struggling, create a tongue depressor bridge between the patient's and your lips, as shown in Figure 6–28. If the patient cannot press or maintain lip contact, despite previous lip force therapy, the stick may be steadied using manual assistance. Once this bridge is positioned and stabilized, prolong the /m/

Figure 6–28.
Wooden tongue depressor bridge between the lips of the clinician and the patient to stimulate production of the consonant /m/ by enabling transmission of vibration for tactile feedback.

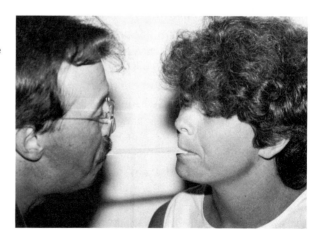

with sufficient intensity to transmit associated lip vibrations across the stick to the patient's lips for tactile feedback. *Fifth*, simultaneously place a small mirror beneath your nostrils to illustrate nasal airflow during this production as yet another form of feedback regarding the mechanics of this sound. *Sixth*, now request that the patient try again to prolong the /m/ and periodically urge him or her to use the fingertips to feel nasal, labial, and laryngeal vibrations. The clinician's concurrent productions are eventually faded as the patient demonstrates consistent success. *Seventh*, if necessary remove the bridge and tape the plastic nasal olive of the See-Scape Device,* described in detail in Chapters 3 and 4, to the patient's nostril as illustrated in Figure 6–29. Continue to practice /m/ productions, noting that upward float movement signifies nasal air emission, a requisite feature of the sound. *Eighth*, once consistent, adequate /m/ productions are achieved according to the criterion level chosen for the patient, couple this sound with any of the vowels and other consonants the patient is capable of producing for more complex speech stimulation.

/**p, b**/. These bilabial plosives are also easy to produce, provided the patient can generate sufficient intraoral air pressure. *First*, place a facial tissue in front of the lips to demonstrate the air puff associated with /p/ production. *Second*, place the patient's palm in front of the lips to permit tactile feedback of the same effect. *Third*, in lieu of the plastic nasal olive, connect a 2 inch piece of drinking straw to the rubber tubing of the See-Scape apparatus and position the open end of the straw between the lips. Demonstrate the plosive manner by repeating the /p/ several times, noting that with each production the float is propelled abruptly to the top of the tube. *Fourth*, have the patient attempt the sound following the three preceding steps for feedback of his or her own production. Note that poor lip seal may be assisted with the fingers. Any residual velopharyngeal incompetence, owing to less than ideal resonation subsystem treatment effects, may be reduced for purposes of /p/ practice by using a noseclip. *Fifth*, if

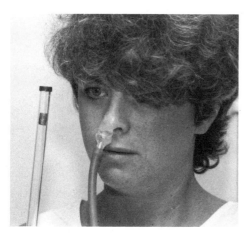

Figure 6–29.
Use of See-Scape Device to provide visual feedback of nasal air emission that may be associated with production of the consonant /m/. Taping the plastic nasal olive in position is less troublesome for both the clinician and the patient than having to hold the piece in place during the exercise. This technique is useful both when normal feedback of nasal consonant productions is so desired and when abnormal nasal air escape requires modification.

*See-Scape Device, Pro-Ed, 8700 Shoal Creek Blvd., Austin, Tx 78758.

the patient requires the clip, fasten a facial tissue to it in such a way that the tissue forms a drape that hangs down in front of the patient's lips. *Sixth*, request productions of the /p/ with the objective of causing the tissue to flutter outward with each implosion. Ultimately, as the patient comes to appreciate these performances, the noseclip, tissue, and See-Scape apparatus should be withdrawn for phonetic practice without such aids. *Seventh*, as usual, if and when this sound is achieved satisfactorily, it can be coupled with other sounds possible for intensive speech stimulation.

The voiced cognate /b/ is produced and can be taught in virtually the same fashion, except for the presence of vocal fold vibrations, which must be highlighted. Use of a stethoscope and tactile feedback techniques are often facilitative, although not usually necessary for isolated stimulation. Inherently driven by greater acoustic energy than its voiceless counterpart, the /b/ is sometimes an easier and more rewarding sound with which to begin this program.

Stimulation of the Labio-Dentals (/f/, /v/)

Perhaps this is the next easiest class of sounds to train. Because the /f/ and /v/ are fricative sounds, adequate production requires relatively good intraoral airflow and pressure, which of course depend on velopharyngeal competence. Residual degrees of mild to (even) moderate incompetence of this valving mechanism, despite previous therapy, does not necessarily negate the usefulness of phonetic training of these sounds. Severe residual incompetence, however, often restricts the prognosis for improvement. Some dysarthric patients distort these fricative sounds, or plosive-like substitutions may occur as the requisite, uninterrupted air current across the labio-dental valve cannot be maintained with delicate consistency. *First*, demonstrate that the /f/ is produced by placing the lower lip against the cutting edges of the upper incisor teeth. *Second*, place the patient's hand in front of your lips so that the continuous airstream associated with this sound can be felt. *Third*, while producing the sound again place the rubber tubing of the See-Scape apparatus in proximity to this airstream origin, as shown in Figure 6–30, so that the float can respond to the airflow by traversing the

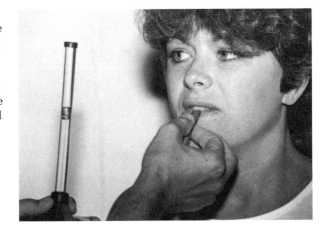

Figure 6–30. Positioning the open end of the rubber tubing of the See-Scape Device in proximity to the central incisor teeth during production of the consonant /f/. Note the Styrofoam float in the tube, which has moved upward in response to the airstream aerodynamics associated with this fricative sound.

tube. *Fourth*, have the patient attempt the sound by following the three preceding steps for feedback of his or her own production. Note that poor lip posturing can be assisted with the end of a tongue depressor or by using the fingers. If residual jaw force dyscontrol inhibits adequate mandibular posturing, construct a ¼ inch by 3 inch tubular bite block out of putty, position and hold it in the corner of the mouth between the upper and lower molar teeth, and have the patient gently bite down on the block to stabilize the jaw for /f/ production. Compensation for residual velopharyngeal incompetence may be accomplished with a noseclip, as discussed above for the /p/. *Fifth*, continue practice of the /f/ with and without the aids until the patient no longer would benefit from isolated stimulation. *Sixth*, as usual, ultimately couple the improved sound with other sounds learned or preserved for syllable and word stimulation.

The voiced cognate /v/ is produced and can be trained in virtually the same fashion, noting the difference established by the voice contribution. Invoke the techniques discussed above for voiced sound stimulation.

Stimulation of the Lingua-Dentals (/θ/, /ð/)

These sounds are also relatively easy to teach if the tongue-tip can be slightly protruded between or even against the anterior teeth. *First*, demonstrate production of the /θ/, and place the patient's hand in a position to feel the continuous air current created by the light lingua-dental valve. *Second*, place a small mirror in the path of this airstream to illustrate visually this airflow. *Third*, request that the patient protrude and gently bite down on the tongue-tip. *Fourth*, slide the end of a tongue depressor between the dorsum of the tongue and upper teeth, as shown in Figure 6–31, to stabilize this articulatory posture, and request the patient to try to pump air past the tongue against the cutting edges of the teeth to create this fricative sound. Use the mirror, the hand, and a piece of tissue for airflow feedback. If the patient cannot establish this valve without assistance, use a gauze pad for passive withdrawal of the tongue, with the patient instructed to install the requisite aerodynamics for the /θ/ as the compensatory place of production is artificially maintained. Eventually the patient must be

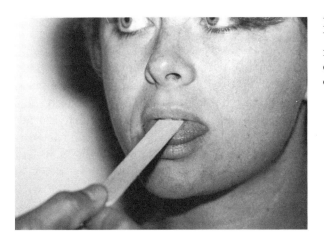

Figure 6–31.
Use of a tongue depressor to maintain interdental posture of the tongue during practice of the /θ/ sound.

weaned from such assistance for this sound to be of practical use. Fifth, as usual practice this production until it is ready for stimulation in complex phonetic environments.

The voiced cognate /ð/ is produced and may be taught in much the same ways, with the exception of also having to stimulate voice output, as explained for previous sound stimuli.

Stimulation of the Lingua-Alveolars (/t/, /d/, /n/, /l/, /s/, /z/)

These sounds are variable with respect to their manner of production: The /t, d/ are plosives, the /n/ is a nasal, the /l/ is a lateral, and the /s, z/ are fricatives. As a group the lingua-alveolars are more difficult to train than the preceding sound stimuli because comparatively they require more complex articulator shaping. The plosive and fricative pairs are particularly difficult to teach in the presence of residual physiologic deficits of the articulators, the velopharyngeal mechanism, or both.

/n/. This nasal consonant is generally fairly easy to teach if the patient can establish upper alveolar ridge contact with either the blade or tip of the tongue. *First*, demonstrate this sound by prolonging it. *Second*, place the patient's fingertips on your nose and larynx to feel the vibrations associated with the production. *Third*, place a small mirror under the nostrils to illustrate nasal airflow. The See-Scape apparatus, as shown in Figure 6–29, can also be used for such purposes as the sound is prolonged. *Fourth*, request that the patient open the mouth so that the alveolar ridge can be stimulated with firm upward pressure for 5 seconds using the index finger. *Fifth*, instruct the patient to press the tongue-tip with moderate force against this sensitized area, keep the teeth in relatively close contact, and try to prolong the /n/ sound. Use the same techniques as those of the preceding steps for feedback of the patient's own production. *Note:* If the patient is struggling with the tip-up posture, owing to residual tongue weakness and paresis, substitute a tip-down posture in which contact is made with the lower alveolar ridge, and the blade of the tongue is automatically positioned in the vicinity of the upper alveolar ridge. Having the patient vary, if necessary, tongue and jaw postures as the /n/ is prolonged may facilitate the best pronunciation possible. *Sixth*, once the patient achieves an acceptable production, practice the sound in isolation until it is ready for stimulation in complex phonetic contexts.

/t, d/. These plosive sounds are often misarticulated by dysarthric patients as fricative sounding errors because the tongue-tip fails to achieve a firm, steady valve with the upper alveolar ridge. The Tongue Force Physiology training program reviewed earlier may well have prepared the patient for the lingua-alveolar valving requirements of these two sounds as well as the /s, z/, which are addressed next. *First*, demonstrate the /t/ sound while the patient's hand is positioned to feel the air puff with each production. *Second*, point out the voiceless characteristic of the sound. *Third*, using the See-Scape apparatus and a straw as shown in Figure 6–32, once again illustrate the air implosion associated with this sound, as the float responds abruptly upward in the tube with each /t/ pro-

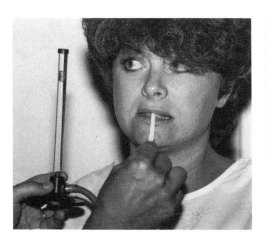

Figure 6–32.
Use of the See-Scape Device to demonstrate the plosive aerodynamics of the consonant /t/. Note that a piece of drinking straw is connected to the rubber tubing, in lieu of the plastic nasal olive, the end of which is positioned against the central incisor region to transmit intraoral air pressure and flow to the Styrofoam float for visual biofeedback.

duced. *Fourth*, sensitize the patient's alveolar ridge in the aforementioned way for /n/ stimulation. *Fifth*, instruct the patient to force the tongue-tip firmly against the sensitized alveolus, keep the teeth only narrowly apart, and try to articulate the /t/ sound using all the feedback techniques of the preceding steps to facilitate the performance. *Note:* If the tip-up technique is troublesome, try the tip-down maneuver, in which the blade of the tongue is postured for contact with the alveolar ridge. Many patients do well with this compensatory approach. In fact, this is not an uncommon articulatory posture for normal speakers. In addition, if residual velopharyngeal incompetence is a problem, the sound can at least be practiced with a noseclip. *Sixth*, keep practicing until the patient achieves consistent acceptable productions in isolation. Ultimately the goal is to interface the sound with vowels and other consonants for complex speech stimulation.

The voiced cognate /d/ can be taught in much the same fashion, highlighting the voicing difference through the usual feedback techniques.

/**s, z**/. For all speakers these fricatives are perhaps the most difficult sounds to master. They require fine adjustments of the tongue under high degrees of intraoral air pressure and flow. The slightest postural alteration or aerodynamic breakdown can be disastrous relative to quality and intelligibility of these sound productions. *First*, demonstrate prolongation of the /s/. *Second*, take a 2 inch piece of drinking straw, position one end against the central incisors, and repeat the sound to illustrate air friction, which is amplified through the chamber of the straw. *Third*, deliberately move the straw off center, around toward the lateral dentition, to demonstrate by loss of the amplified air current that the /s/ is produced by pushing air past a central groove of the tongue and through the incisor region. *Fourth*, connect the same straw to the rubber hose of the See-Scape apparatus, place the straw against the incisors once again, and prolong the /s/ to illustrate the airflow dynamics, as shown in Figure 6–33. The float travels sharply upward in response to this current and normally remains near or at the top of the tube throughout the production. *Fifth*, request that the patient bite down normally, smile so as to spread the lip corners, and hold these

Figure 6–33.
Production of the consonant /s/ transmitted through a straw, which is interfaced with the See-Scape Device for aerodynamic biofeedback of this fricative sound. Note the float fixed at the top of the tube in response to a normally produced /s/.

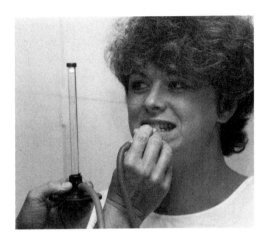

positions while experimenting with various tongue postures to discover the one that generates at least a decent sounding /s/. Remember to use the straw technique and the See-Scape apparatus for feedback of each effort. Such feedback is vital here, because minute adjustments of the tongue may evoke significant changes in the quality of the sounds produced that can prove very beneficial to observe both visually and auditorily. *Sixth*, continue practicing the /s/ until the patient achieves consistent acceptable productions in isolation. Complex syllable and word stimulation is next. Note that poor lip posturing can be assisted manually. If jaw dyscontrol persists despite previous physiologic training, have the patient bite down on a piece of paper to stabilize the jaw during production of the sound. A noseclip may be helpful for practice purposes if excess nasal air escape has not been successfully managed with the indicated resonation subsystem treatment regimen.

The voiced cognate /z/ can be taught in like fashion, excepting the need to emphasize the role of vocal fold valving for adequate production.

/l/. This lateral sound can be tricky to teach, especially when working with dysarthric patients who exhibit residual tongue force dyscontrol. For adequate production the tongue-tip must valve with the upper alveolar ridge as air flows steadily over the lateral borders of the dorsum. Acoustic energy is afforded through vocal fold vibrations. Tip-down posturing can be taught if only the blade of the tongue can be accessed for alveolar contact. *First*, demonstrate prolongation of the /l/. *Second*, sensitize the upper alveolar ridge as was done previously and request that the patient press the tongue-tip firmly against this area, keeping the teeth marginally apart. *Third*, thread a long cotton-tipped applicator across the tongue immediately behind this valve so that the stick extends over the lateral borders of the tongue, as illustrated in Figure 6–34. *Fourth*, request that the patient try to prolong the /l/ for as long and as steadily as possible, experimenting with slight tongue and jaw posturing modifications in the hope of promoting an acceptable production. *Fifth*, continue practicing this effect until the patient can demonstrate consistent adequate /l/ productions in isolation. Follow through with syllable and word stimulation in the usual ways.

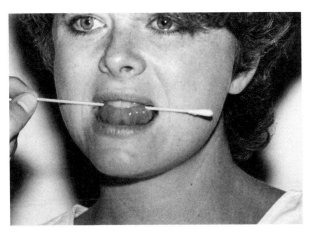

Figure 6–34.
A long cotton-tipped applicator
stick can be used in this
fashion during phonetic drills
of the lateral /l/. Extending
over and mildly depressing the
edges of the tongue, the stick
helps induce lateral airflow, an
important requirement for
adequate production of this
sound.

Stimulation of the Lingua-Velars (/k/, /g/)

Teaching this cognate pair of plosives can be trying. The required posterior
pumping action of the tongue against the velum is especially difficult for many
dysarthric patients with residual lingual force dyscontrol, velopharyngeal incompetence, or both. There is no surplus of compensatory articulation strategies for
these two sounds, although "glottal" stop and "pharyngeal" fricative productions
may be attempted. If the back of the tongue cannot achieve at least a mild degree
of valving with the velum, and if nasal air escape exceeds a moderate amount,
speech is potentially significantly affected. The precursor tongue force physiology
training regimen may prove indispensable to success with this stimulation program. *First*, demonstrate vigorously the /k/, and place the patient's hand in position to feel the air expulsion during such production. Use of a tissue and small
hand mirror may also provide feedback regarding the plosive aerodynamics of
this sound. *Second*, with a covered index finger stimulate the patient's velum
with gentle upward pressure for at least 5 seconds. A tongue depressor can be
substituted for the finger, but the degree of pressure applied cannot be as easily
regulated and perceived with this approach. Uncomfortable overstimulation can
occur as a result. *Third*, instruct the patient to retract the tongue so that the
back makes contact with the sensitized palatal area. If such valving is not volitionally demonstrated, use a plunger-type apparatus to try to push the tongue
back into this posture. The device shown in Figure 6–35 is a round plastic disk
glued to an acrylic bite block handle. A similar device can be constructed with
the putty material described earlier and a cotton-tipped applicator. To do so, take
a small amount of putty and add a few drops of liquid hardener. Knead the putty
and hardener for 15 to 30 seconds and shape it into a disk about the size of a
quarter in diameter and roughly ¼ inch thick. Once it is hardened, bore a tiny
hole in the center of the disk with the end of a paperclip, but *do not* pierce
through to the other side. Take the wooden end of the applicator and gently twist
it in this hole until it is sufficiently secure in the disk for plunging use. A drop or
two of superglue may lend additional support. Cover the disk and stick with a

Figure 6–35.
Plastic disk attached to acrylic bite block handle to form a plunger-like device for the purpose of facilitating lingua-velar valving as required for productions of the /k/ and /g/ consonants.

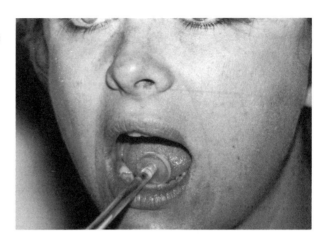

finger cot before using it in this fashion so as to prevent splintering effects or accidental swallowing of the material if breakage occurs. *Fourth,* once the tongue is either volitionally or artificially moved into contact with the velum, have the patient attempt production of the /k/ using all the aforementioned feedback techniques to stimulate acceptable output. If the plunger is being used, experiment with force and vector variations necessary to induce better production. *Fifth,* continue these practice methods until the patient no longer benefits from the isolated stimulation. If successful, advance to syllable and word applications in the usual ways.

The voiced cognate /g/ needs emphasis on the voice dimension using the vocal fold vibration feedback methods discussed earlier.

Stimulation of the Lingua-Palatals (/ʃ/, /ʒ/, /tʃ/, /dʒ/)
As can be plainly seen, the affricates /tʃ/ and /dʒ/ are partly composed of the fricatives /ʃ/ and /ʒ/. To stimulate the former pair into acceptable productions, the latter pair need first to be practiced and learned.

/ʃ, ʒ/. *First,* demonstrate the /ʃ/ by prolonging it with exaggerated lip-rounding activity. *Second,* place the patient's hand in a position to feel the airstream dynamics as the sound is prolonged. *Third,* use a small mirror to illustrate the turbulent airflow characteristics. The See-Scape apparatus can also be summoned for this purpose. Connect a 2 inch piece of drinking straw to the rubber tubing in the usual way and place the free end of the straw against the central incisors as the /ʃ/ is prolonged. The float moves sharply up the tube in response to the underlying aerodynamics and should remain there until the sound is terminated. *Fourth,* request that the patient bite down on the end of a cotton-tipped applicator, as shown in Figure 6–36. Simultaneously squeeze the cheeks firmly to facilitate a lip-rounding posture, which will enhance the /ʃ/ production. *Fifth,* instruct the patient to try to prolong the /ʃ/, adjusting as necessary the tongue posture throughout the effort until the best result is evident. This technique usually works very well, even with the most severely disabled patients. *Sixth,* continue practicing the sound this way, ultimately weaning the patient

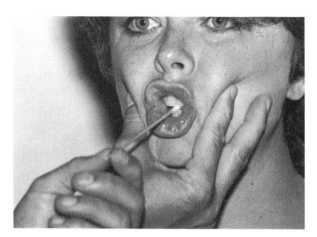

Figure 6–36.
The patient bites down gently on the cotton-tipped applicator to achieve and maintain adequate jaw position. Simultaneously the lips are induced into rounded posture by squeezing the cheeks with the fingers. Collectively, these techniques help stimulate production of the consonant /ʃ/.

from the stick and manual assistance if possible, until consistent adequate /ʃ/ production in isolation is demonstrated. Follow up with syllable and word stimulation in the usual ways.

Add the voice dimension to the treatment to stimulate production of the cognate /ʒ/. Use the methods employed and discussed earlier for voice feedback during this exercise.

/tʃ, dʒ/.   Couple the /t/ and the /ʃ/ to produce the /tʃ/. The /d/ and /ʒ/ articulated in close sequential order gives rise perceptually to /dʒ/. *First,* demonstrate the /t/ followed by the /ʒ/ sound with about 1 second between the individual productions. *Second,* repeat this approach a few times and then gradually bring the sounds closer and closer together until the end result is a distinct and explosive /tʃ/. *Third,* repeat this effort several times, placing the patient's hand so that the oral air puffs can be felt during these productions. Be certain to exaggerate lip rounding to convey the importance of this posture during practice of the sound. The See-Scape Device can also be used as it was separately with /t/ and /ʃ/ stimulation to illustrate here the explosive aerodynamic feature of the /tʃ/. Even a facial tissue held in front of the lips can provide such feedback. *Fourth,* request that the patient try to articulate first the /t/ and then the /ʃ/, separated by a brief pause. Prompt the gradual approximation of these sounds until a /tʃ/-like utterance is accomplished. Note that since many patients have a very hard time achieving this sound, the following inverted triangle technique may be facilitative.

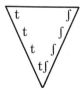

The patient is instructed to look at the triangle and start at the top line by articulating the /t/, waiting 7 seconds, and then producing the /ʃ/. Cues as to when to shift can be prompted by pointing to the target sounds throughout the trial. Gradually move down the triangle to the inverted apex, decreasing with each step the time gap between the /t/ and /ʃ/ productions. Practice these steps several times. This technique, in fact, is useful when coupling consonants and vowels for stimulation of syllable productions. *Fifth*, if these techniques are not successful, try having the patient repeat as rapidly as possible the /t/ followed on the sixth production by an attempt at /tʃ/; that is, /t-t-t-t-t-tʃ/. Practicing in this fashion has proved very helpful for a mildly spastic dysarthric patient who failed to generate an intelligible /tʃ/ until this technique was employed. *Sixth*, continue with the stimulation approach that works best until adequate consistent productions are evident in isolation. If possible, advance to more complex usage of the sound in the usual ways.

The voiced cognate /dʒ/ can be stimulated in much the same ways as its voiceless counterpart, except that the /d/ and /ʒ/ components are substituted as the stimuli.

Notes on Treatment of Articulatory Imprecision

Before proceeding with the final subsection of this chapter, the phonetic stimulation epilogue below warrants consideration.

First, use of table mirror and tape recorder throughout these exercises will prove invaluable for feedback to the patient. *Second*, learning to accept approximations or compensatory productions of the target sounds is perhaps the hardest clinical chore, not only for the patient but also for the clinician. If the end result of stimulation is a sound that is less severely distorted and more intelligible than it was before intervention, this effect should be accepted. *Third*, if the patient needs to employ an assortment of compensatory strategies to produce target sounds, these techniques should not be discouraged. Rather, clinicians do well by encouraging them. Patients, for example, may need always to use their hands to assist lip and jaw posturing during certain sound productions. *Fourth*, when a target sound is not improving despite valiant clinical efforts, look to easier vectors with which to experiment as compensatory approaches to production of the target. For example, the lingua-dental place of articulation may serve as an acceptable substitute for the lingua-alveolar vector when practicing the plosives /t/ and /d/. *Fifth*, remaining mindful of residual disturbances of other speech subsystems often helps temper expectations and instructions for articulatory proficiency. For example, when severe respiration difficulties persist, despite a full course of intervention, the patient may at best achieve a few syllables per breath. Urging frequent breaths to drive the articulation subsystem may yield better results than pushing the patient to maximize the possible effects of any single breath. *Sixth*, understanding the complete clinical neurologic profile of the patient, particularly with respect to language, cognitive, perceptual, and psychoemotional disturbances that may coexist in any combination in a patient who presents with motor speech disorders, may help balance the design of the overall speech intervention plan as well as the criteria adopted for advancement within and between the exercises. *Seventh*, when target sounds have been improved through isolated exercise, creatively stimulate their employment in connected discourse situations. Contrived sentences, commensurate in complexity with the patient's overall articulatory profile, short and long phrases, reading passages, and extemporaneous speaking situations are all excellent conditions to help transfer the ability to produce isolated sounds in more meaningful contexts. *Eighth,* realizing when to cease and desist phonetic stimulation is critical. It is never effective to exhaust a patient with tortuous exercises that elicit little if any trend of improvement. The decision to move on to other activities must be at the discretion of the clinician in concert with perceptions of how the patient is responding to the treatments being applied. The rule of thumb recommended throughout this text for other speech subsystem treatments may prove beneficial here as well: If after 30 consecutive trials (or minutes in some instances) of an exercise the patient does not demonstrate any observable trend of improved performance, it may be best to proceed to the next indicated step. This does not mean that treatment is discontinued if the criterion adopted for advancement has not been met. Rather, as long as the patient shows persistent signs of progress (within this time frame), prolongation of the exercise regimen may indeed be indicated. *Finally,* some patients do not improve regardless of the integrity of the treatment plan or their strong motivation to make gains. Nonverbal communication systems may be fruitful alternatives or augmentation for those whose severe unintelligibility restricts potential for *verbal* speech improvements.

TREATMENT OF MOTOR SPEECH PLANNING DEFICITS

This subsection is largely reserved for work with apractic patients. Although the exercises here may be adapted for use with other populations, they are designed to facilitate speech motor programming skills in individuals with relatively well preserved speech effectuation profiles. Before this regimen is begun, as with any suspected disorder, differential diagnostic testing is essential to define the full extent of the problem (e.g., see Dabul's *Apraxia Battery For Adults* [1979] and the *Dworkin-Culatta Oral Mechanism Examination* [1980]). Detailed descriptions of apraxia of speech were presented in Chapter 1, thus eliminating the need for such review here. Apractic patients generally do not struggle with associated respiration and resonation subsystem disturbances, and only occasionally exhibit clinically significant problems with coordinated voice motor control. Their primary difficulties are with articulation and prosody, as mentioned earlier in the chapter. Here we will focus on the former area. In the next chapter the latter disturbance will be addressed.

Over the years several clinicians have studied methods of treatment of apraxia of speech. The resounding common theme in the reports of these investigators is the importance of establishing a hierarchy of intervention strategies in which at the bottom limited, automatic speech is massaged; in the middle gradually more complex articulatory sequencing control is stimulated; and at the top volitional-purposive extemporaneous speech is practiced and reinforced. Pairing motoric gestures with the prosody of speech has been found helpful. Finger, hand,

and foot tapping all have been explored as (theoretical) methods of reorganizing neuromotor planning control. Melodious speaking in unison with hand-tapping activity to a special or familiar rhythmic pattern has similarly been attempted with apractic patients with some therapeutic success. It has been hypothesized that these gesture-assisted speech activities are helpful because they may evoke motor speech programming cooperation of the unimpaired cerebral hemisphere as well as spared centers within the damaged hemisphere, which may possess special melodic and rhythmic capabilities that are receptive to such stimulation. Whether or not these rhythmic-motoric exercises actually have penetrating central nervous system effects is still uncertain. What is clear, however, is the fact that their application effectively slows the rate of speech, increases prosodic sufficiency, and (perhaps most important) induces attention to the syllable components of words produced. The exercise plan in this subsection is based on the success this clinician has had using a nongestural, external temporal pacing stimulus provided by a standard metronome. As a device that helps the patient achieve temporal consistency in the initiation and organization of speech motor activities and calls attention to the need for precise, slower than normal rate, the metronome offers many advantages as a tool in the treatment of apraxia. Because the stimulation is externally driven, the patient is free to concentrate on speech motor control, yet still benefit from the effects of rhythmic pacing. In addition, an optimal rate can often be ascertained in the treatment regimen, which can be reinforced and replicated with conviction not only in therapy, but whenever and wherever speech may be practiced.

Reiterating the recommended sequence of articulation subsystem treatments for apractic patients we find (1) nonspeech oral motor planning activities, if oral (nonspeech) praxis is disturbed; (2) simple phonetic motor planning stimulation; and (3) complex phonetic motor planning stimulation. Note that segments of the preceding articulatory precision exercises may be necessary precursors to this regimen if the patient has forgotten the manner and place of articulation for certain sounds. Also realize that if there is coexistent significant dysarthria, the patient will require the aforementioned physiologic treatments that correspond to the nature of the associated deficits and the speech subsystems involved. These exercises are best ordered before the speech motor planning regimen.

The Metronomic Mobility Treatment Chart (Figure 6–22) will be used throughout the exercises recommended below to track patient responses. The criterion for advancement from one exercise to the next will not be etched in stone. In the past, 95 percent improvement over baseline levels over two to four consecutive treatment sessions was found useful in clinical research projects with apractic patients. More recently, looking at correct responses over a specific number of trials, not sessions, has proved efficient and productive. Clinicians ultimately need to adopt the standards with which they are most comfortable and that the individual patient merits. In this subsection a slightly different approach is taken and recommended. The discontinuation rule of thumb enumerated earlier will be invoked here as well: If after 30 consecutive trials of a given exercise the patient fails to demonstrate any observable trend of improvement to justify continuation, advance to the next indicated step. Prior to and periodically throughout this exercise regimen, use the Speech Characteristics Chart (see Figure 2–2) to rate the patient's articulatory proficiency, prosody, and contextual speech features. These data can be used for ongoing measures of treatment effects. Finally, before administering the treatment regimen indicated, be certain to obtain baseline measures of all anticipated tasks. These data afford additional information for the evaluation of treatment efficacy.

Note: Use of the *Index of Metronomic Levels* in Chapter 2 may prove helpful when administering the following motor planning exercises.

Nonspeech Oral Motor Planning Exercises

These exercises are designed for the patient with both *speech* and *oral* apraxia. Generally, speech and nonspeech praxis treatments can be coupled at the discretion of the clinician. When severe disturbances present, however, it is sometimes more prudent to order nonspeech treatments first. Success at this level may ultimately hasten progress when phonetic stimulation is initiated. Note that because breakdowns are likely to occur during these exercises, possibly requiring discussions along the way, the clock should be stopped to permit reviews of the difficulties. Data entries on the treatment chart, however, must reflect full time equivalents spent actually practicing the task.

Tongue Exercise No. 1

Step 1. To establish baseline ability, cue the patient to open the mouth and raise the tongue-tip to the alveolar ridge, hold that position for 2 seconds, lower it for 2 seconds, protrude it for 2 seconds, retract it for 2 seconds, and continue these alternating movements in this order until 32 seconds have elapsed for a total of four complete trials. On a notepad, rate these trials independently relative to the percentage of correct responses. The trial is judged *correct* if it is free of signs or symptoms of oral apraxia—groping, struggling, false starts, restarts, hesitancies, and/or failures to achieve and hold target vectors.

Step 2. Repeat the task three times with a rest of 15 seconds between each, tally the total percentage correct, and enter the result on the Metronomic Mobility Treatment Chart. Be certain to record the date, minutes of testing (2), musculature (T), task (BU/D, O/I$_1$—representative of first baseline Up/Down, Out/In maneuvers), and bpm (30—every 2 seconds) in the respective cells of the data column. A score of less than 75 percent indicates the need for Step 3; otherwise go on to the next exercise.

Step 3. Explain the purpose of the exercise and the rating criteria. Set the metronome to 30 bpm and request that the patient perform the same "U/D–O/I" tongue-tip maneuvers to the beat—1 vector per beat. Verbally cue the patient with each beat in the beginning: i.e., to the beat verbalize "up," "down," "out," "in," "up," "down," "out," "in," and so on in this order until 32 seconds have elapsed, which would allow a maximum of four complete trials (U/D, O/I equals one trial). Ultimately, as the patient learns the task, relative to the sequence of vectors, verbal cueing should be faded so that the only stimulus is the rhythmic beat of the metronome. Follow the same basic rating and scoring procedure recommended in Steps 1 and 2, except that chart entries are made after 5 full minutes of treatment.

Step 4. Tally the percentage of correct trials and record the result on the Metronomic Mobility Treatment Chart, making certain to list the appropriate date, musculature treated (T), task (U/D, O/I$_1$), and bpm (30) in the respective cells of the data column. Continue with this exercise until the patient achieves a percentage correct score that is at least 75 percent improved over the baseline score or 100 percent correct, whichever is less, over 10 consecutive minutes of treatment. Be sure to enter this calculated target criterion on the chart in the respective cell at the bottom of the anticipated data column. Advance to the next exercise at that time.

Tongue Exercise No. 2

Step 1. Repeat the same basic procedure as in the baseline measure of the preceding exercise, except that here increase the speed of tongue movements to the equivalent of 60 bpm or 1 vector per second. Rate, score, and chart the results accordingly, making certain to list the task as "BU/D, O/I$_2$" and the bpm as "60."

Step 2. Follow the treatment method of the preceding exercise, except that the metronome is set at 60 bpm, increasing tongue movements to 1 vector per second. Employ the same rating, scoring, charting, and advancement criteria, listing the task as "U/D, O/I$_2$" and the bpm as "60" on the Metronomic Mobility Treatment Chart in the appropriate cells of the data column.

Lip Exercise No. 1

Step 1. Establish baseline by having the patient open the mouth so that a ½ inch by ½ inch bite block can be positioned between the upper and lower incisors or molars, whichever is preferable and less obtrusive for the patient. Then cue the patient to close the lips firmly, hold that position for 2 seconds, open them completely for 2 seconds, smile broadly for 2 seconds, pucker for 2 seconds, and continue these alternating movements in this order until 32 seconds have elapsed for a total of four complete trials. As before, on a notepad rate these trials independently relative to the percentage of correct responses. Use the same rating and advancement criteria detailed in the preceding Tongue Exercise no. 1, Steps 1 and 2.

Step 2. Repeat the task three times, allowing a rest period of 15 seconds between each time, tally the total percentage correct, and enter the score on the Metronomic Mobility Treatment Chart. Remember to list the appropriate musculature tested (L), task (BC/O, S/P$_1$), and bpm (30) for these baseline data. Proceed accordingly.

Step 3. Set the metronome to 30 bpm and request the patient to perform the same "C/O–S/P" lip maneuvers to the beat—1 vector per beat. In the beginning, with each beat verbally cue the patient in the following way: "close," "open," "smile (spread)," "pucker," "close," "open," "smile," "pucker," and so on in this order until 32 seconds have elapsed. Fade the verbal cues as the task is learned, allowing the metronome to serve as the only external source of pacing. Follow the same rating, scoring, charting, and advancement methods of the preceding nonspeech exercises, making certain that on the chart the correct musculature treated (L), task (C/O, S/P$_1$), bpm (30), and calculated target criterion are entered in their respective cells.

Lip Exercise No. 2

Step 1. Repeat the same basic procedure as in the baseline measure of the preceding exercise, except that here increase the speed of lip movements to the equivalent of 60 bpm or 1 vector per second. Proceed as usual, listing on the Metronomic Mobility Treatment Chart the appropriate symbol for this task (BC/O, S/P$_2$).

Step 2. Follow the treatment method of the preceding exercise, except that the metronome is set at 60 bpm, increasing lip movements to 1 vector per second. Employ the same rating, scoring, charting, and advancement criteria, using the appropriate task (C/O, S/P$_2$) and bpm (60) symbols on the treatment chart.

Jaw-Airflow Exercise No. 1

Step 1. Establish baseline by requesting that the patient open the mouth, hold that position for 2 seconds, bite down and hold that position for 2 seconds, blow a steady stream of air for 2 seconds, and continue these alternating activities in this order until 30 seconds have elapsed for a total of five complete trials. Use the notepad to rate these trials independently relative to the percentage of correct performances. The same rating, scoring, charting, and advancement methods detailed in the preceding Tongue Exercise no. 1, Steps 1 and 2 should be employed here as well. Be certain to list the appropriate musculature tested (J), task (BO/C, A$_1$), and bpm (30) symbols on the Metronomic Mobility Treatment Chart. Proceed as usual.

Step 2. Set the metronome at 30 bpm and request the patient to perform the same alternating maneuvers, verbally cuing each one: "open," "close," "blow," "open," "close," "blow," and so on in this order until 30 seconds have elapsed. Fade the verbal cues as the task is learned, leaving the metronomic beat as the sole source of pacing. Follow the basic rating, scoring, charting, and advancement methods of the preceding exercises, using, however, the correct musculature (J), task (O/C, A$_1$), and bpm (30) symbols on the treatment chart to represent these baseline data.

Jaw-Airflow Exercise No. 2

Step 1. Repeat the same basic procedure as in the preceding baseline measurement, except that here increase the speed of activity to the equivalent of 60 bpm. Proceed as usual, listing the appropriate symbol for this task (BO/C, A$_2$) on the Metronomic Mobility Treatment Chart.

Step 2. Follow the same treatment method of the preceding exercise, but set the metronome at 60 bpm, increasing these alternate activities to one per beat. Employ the rating, scoring, charting, and advancement criteria as before, listing the appropriate task (O/C, A$_2$) and bpm (60) symbols on the treatment chart. Proceed with the next subsection of exercises when indicated.

Speech Motor Planning Exercises

The exercises that follow are designed sequentially to improve speech motor programming ability in the apractic patient. They should be practiced in front of a mirror for visual feedback of articulator adjustments. Throughout the regimen, use of a tape recorder for periodic auditory feedback of performances can be very helpful. The progressive hierarchy of the tasks, relative to phonetic complexity, is self-evident and should be adopted for all patients. Baseline measures, of course, dictate where in the sequence to begin with any given patient. Most apractic patients who present without coexistent dysarthria are essentially introduced to motor speech therapy at this level, inasmuch as the many other speech subsystem treatments discussed throughout this text are usually not indicated.

Before the initiation of the first exercise below, to start the program it is always best to explain the overall purpose of the treatment plan. Discussion about the usefulness of the metronome should be held. Highlight the fact that tapping a finger, hand, or foot in unison with the beat of the metronome sometimes proves helpful and should be attempted if so desired. Periodically review the Motor Speech Planning Treatment Chart (see Figure 6–37) so that the patient can keep track of ongoing responses to the exercises. Many patients enjoy and appreciate the effects of metronomic pacing to the extent that they purchase a unit for home use; patients leaning in this direction should be encouraged to buy one.

Finally, because many apractic patients also suffer from aphasia, the instructions, guidance, and criteria for advancement levels must be structured with consideration of the severity of this coexistent disorder. When necessary and possible, the patient's significant others may prove instrumental in facilitating the treatment plan, not only at the clinic but also in the home environment. Paying close attention to the discontinuation rule of thumb recommended throughout the text is of critical importance with this population. Remember that data entries on the treatment chart must reflect, as usual, time spent actually exercising. Time-outs stop the treatment clock and are not factored into the scores recorded.

MOTOR SPEECH PLANNING TREATMENT CHART

Patient's name: _____

Birthdate: _____ Sex: _____

Speech diagnosis: _____

Medical diagnosis: _____

Clinician: _____

Facility: _____

Address: _____
_____
_____

Comments:
_____
_____
_____
_____
_____

ACTIVITY KEY

1. Speech task: Consonant-Vowel syllable sequence (CV);
   Consonant-Vowel-Consonant syllable combination (CVC);
   Single Syllable complex word combination (X);
   Bi-syllable word repetition (B);
   Tri-syllable word repetition (T);
   Multi-syllable word repetition (M);
   Sentence productions (S)

2. Beats Per Minute: 30, 60, 90, 120 (150, 200, variable [V])

3. Minutes of therapy: Fill in time

   Baseline (pre-treatment): B + feature symbol

TREATMENT RESPONSES

Percentage of Correct Responses

Dates:

100
90
80
70
60
50
40
30
20
10
0

Minutes of therapy

Activity symbol

BPM

Target criterion

SESSIONS

Figure 6–37. Blank Motor Speech Planning Treatment Chart to be used to improve the control of articulator posturing and sequences of movements in apractic patients.

269

CV Syllable Sequence Exercise No. 1

Step 1. Establish baseline ability by having the patient alternate production of the CV syllable sequence /pʌ-tʌ/ several times, with a 2-second pause between the syllables: /pʌ/ for 2 seconds, /tʌ/ for 2 seconds, /pʌ/ for 2 seconds, and so on. On a notepad, rate the pairs of productions, not the individual syllables, as either *correct* or *incorrect*. A correct rating should be rendered when a pair of productions is free of the abnormal articulatory and prosodic features that characterize apraxia of speech: (1) groping; (2) transpositions, either reiterative or anticipatory; (3) omissions or substitutions; and (4) false starts, restarts, prolongations, pauses, or hesitancies.

Step 2. Repeat this procedure three times, altering the CV syllable pairs each time, and tally from the notepad scores the total number of pairs produced without error. Calculate the correct percentage and enter this baseline result on the Motor Speech Planning Treatment Chart, making certain to record the date, minutes of trials (?), task (BCV_1), and bpm (30—every 2 seconds) symbols in their respective cells of the data column. A score of less than 75 percent correct indicates the need for Step 3 below; otherwise proceed with the next exercise.

Step 3. Explain the rating criteria before starting treatment. Set the metronome at 30 bpm and instruct the patient to repeat the CV syllable pair /pʌ-tʌ/ to the beat—one syllable per beat continuously for 30 seconds. The clock starts when the patient begins and terminates when 30 seconds have elapsed. Discourage the patient from stopping before 30 seconds. Placing a stopwatch in view or a verbal cue about time remaining often helps guide the patient. On a notepad, rate each pair of CV syllables independently, altering the pairs periodically to reduce boredom and possible order effects, following the scoring criteria of Step 2 above.

Step 4. At the completion of 5 full minutes of treatment, the equivalent of ten 30-second segments, not including rest periods, tally the total percentage of correct productions from the notepad and enter this result in a separate column on the y-axis grid of the treatment chart. Be sure to list the date, minutes of treatment (5), task (CV_1), and bpm (30) in the respective cells of the data column.

Step 5. Continue with the exercise until the patient achieves a percentage correct score that is at least 75 percent improved over the baseline level or 100 percent correct, whichever is less, over 10 consecutive minutes of treatment. Advance to the next exercise at that time. Be sure to list the target criterion on the chart. Adopt the discontinuation rule if and when no improvement trend is observed. *Note:* Real words are often best for practice material. The following CV syllable word pairs are recommended for this exercise regimen: may-ray, day-gay, hay-way, lay-jay, by-my, lie-die, sigh-shy, boo-new, do-who, zoo-chew, now-how, row-show, be-me, pea-tea, key-lee, saw-paw, fee-see, and so on.

CV Syllable Sequence Exercise Nos. 2–4

These exercises are identical in design to the one above, except that for these three the two-syllable sequences are alternately produced at metronomic speed equivalents of 60, 90, and 120 bpm, respectively. When charting these treatment data, be sure to use the correct task (CV_{2-4}) and bpm (60, 90, or 120) symbols. The prefix "B" is always used in the activity cell to symbolize that the data represent baseline ability. Faster rates may be practiced when indicated, before advancing to the next set of exercises.

CV Syllable Sequence Exercise No. 5

Step 1. Establish baseline ability by requesting that the patient alternate production of the CV syllable sequence /pʌ-tʌ-kʌ/ several times, with a 2-second pause between the syllables. On a notepad, rate the three-syllable train productions, not the individual parts, as either *correct* or *incorrect,* using the aforementioned scoring criteria. Repeat this procedure three times, altering the CV syllables that compose the train each time, and tally the total number of trains produced without error.

Step 2. Calculate the correct percentage and enter the baseline result on the Motor Speech Planning Treatment Chart in the usual way. Be sure to record the correct task (BCV_5) and bpm (30) symbols. A score of less than 75 percent correct indicates the need for Step 3; otherwise proceed with the next exercise.

Step 3. Set the metronome at 30 bpm and instruct the patient to repeat the CV syllable sequence /pʌ-tʌ-kʌ/ to the beat—one syllable per beat continuously for 30 seconds in the usual way. Following previously used rating, scoring, charting, and advancement criteria, rate each full train of syllables independently, altering the composition of the train periodically.

Step 4. At the completion of 5 full minutes of treatment, tally the total percentage of correct productions from the notepad and enter this result in a separate column on the y-axis grid of the treatment chart. Be sure to list the task (CV_5), bpm (30), and calculated target criterion in the appropriate cells of the column. *Note:* Use any of the CV syllable words recommended at the end of Exercise no. 1 to construct trains for practice here; e.g., /boo-lay-pea/.

CV Syllable Sequence Exercise Nos. 6–8

These exercises are identical in design to the one above, except that for these three the three-syllable sequences are alternately produced at metronomic speech equivalents of 60, 90, and 120 bpm, respectively. When charting these data, be sure to use the correct activity (CV_{6-8}) and bpm (60, 90, or 120) symbols. As always, the prefix "B" is used to tag baseline data. Faster rates may be tried if indicated for a given patient before advancing to the next set of exercises.

CVC Syllable Combination Exercise No. 1

Step 1. Establish baseline ability by requesting that the patient alternate production of the CVC syllable sequence /pʌb-tʌg/ several times, with a 2-second pause between the syllables. On a notepad, rate the combined effort, not the individual words, as either correct or incorrect according to the scoring criteria detailed in the CV Syllable Sequence Exercise no. 1, Steps 1 and 2. Repeat this procedure three times, selecting different CVC word combinations each time, and tally the percentage of correct word pair productions.

Step 2. Enter this baseline result on the Motor Speech Planning Treatment Chart, making certain, as usual, to record the date, minutes of testing (?), task (BCVC$_1$), and bpm (30) symbols in the respective cells of the data column. A score of less than 75 percent correct indicates the need for Step 3 below; otherwise proceed with the next exercise.

Step 3. Set the metronome at 30 bpm and instruct the patient to repeat the CVC syllable sequence /pʌb-tʌg/ to the beat—one syllable per beat continuously for 30 seconds in the usual way. Following the aforementioned rating, scoring, charting, and advancement criteria, rate each word pair combination independently, altering the word pairs periodically.

Step 4. At the completion of 5 full minutes of treatment, tally the total percentage of correct productions from the notepad and enter the result on the treatment chart. Be sure to list the task (CVC$_1$), bpm (30), and calculated target criterion on the chart, accordingly. *Note:* The following CVC words can be paired in random fashion for this exercise: nub, hub, cub, rub, sub, tub, mud, dud, bud, feed, seed, lead, head, need, mug, tug, bug, rug, jug, hug, pun, none, sun, shun, bun, gun, kite, light, fight, height, might, roach, coach, putt, but, mutt, gut, cut, shut, dog, log, jog, hog, fog, pin, gin, fin, zip, rip, ship, chip, pit, mit, hit, sit, wit, tot, pot, lot, jot, dot, ban, van, tan, fan, ran, man, lap, nap, gap, sap, chap, bib, bob, boob, babe, did, dude, died, dad, and so on.

CVC Syllable Combination Exercise Nos. 2–4

These exercises are identical in design to those above, except that for these three the CVC word pairs are alternately produced at metronomic speed equivalents of 60, 90, and 120 bpm, respectively. When charting these data, use the correct task (CVC$_{2-4}$) and bpm (60, 90, or 120) symbols. When the prefix "B" is listed in the activity cell, the data recorded represent baseline ability. Faster rates, as usual, can be practiced before advancement to the next set of exercises.

CVC Syllable Combination Exercise No. 5

Step 1. Establish baseline ability by requesting the patient to alternate production of the CVC syllable sequence /nub-jug-might/ several times, with a 2-second pause between the syllables. On a notepad rate the three-word train as a unit, not its individual parts, as either *correct* or *incorrect* following the aforementioned scoring criteria. Repeat this procedure three times, selecting different CVC word stimuli each time, and tally the total number of correct trains produced.

Step 2. Enter the percentage correct baseline score on the Motor Speech Planning Treatment Chart in the usual way. Tag these data with the correct task

(BCVC$_5$) and bpm (30) symbols. Proceed according to the advancement criterion outlined in the first CVC exercise above.

Step 3. Set the metronome at 30 bpm and instruct the patient to repeat the CVC word train /nub-jug-might/ to the beat—one word per beat continuously for 30 seconds in the usual way. Follow the same basic rating, scoring, charting, and advancement methods detailed earlier. Be certain that all data charted here are tagged with correct task (CVC$_5$), bpm (30), and calculated target criterion information.

CVC Syllable Combination Exercise Nos. 6–8

These exercises are identical in design to the preceding one, except that for these three the CVC word trains are alternately produced at metronomic speed equivalents of 60, 90, and 120 bpm, respectively. The correct task (CVC$_{6-8}$) and bpm (60, 90, or 120) symbols represent these data, and the prefix "B" signifies baseline abilities. Faster rates can be practiced, if indicated, before proceeding with the next set of exercises.

Single-Syllable Complex Word Combination Exercise No. 1

Step 1. Establish baseline ability by requesting the patient to alternate production of the complex word pair /ask-mist/ several times, with a 2-second pause between the syllables. As usual, on a notepad rate the two-word combination as an independent unit, following the previously defined *correct/incorrect* dichotomous scoring criteria. Repeat this procedure three times, selecting different complex word pairs each time (e.g., bunk-shaft, blend-flirt) and tally the total number of pairs correctly produced.

Step 2. Enter the percentage correct baseline score on the treatment chart in the usual way. Tag these data with the correct activity (BX$_1$) and bpm (30—every 2 seconds) symbols. A score of less than 75 percent correct indicates the need for Step 3; otherwise proceed with the next exercise.

Step 3. Set the metronome at 30 bpm and instruct the patient to repeat the complex word pair /ask-mist/ to the beat—one word per beat continuously for 30 seconds. Follow the same basic rating, scoring, charting, and advancement methods detailed earlier. Tag all data on the treatment chart with the correct task (X$_1$), bpm (30), and calculated target criterion information. *Note:* The following complex words can be paired in random fashion for this exercise: tank, rank, sank, bunk, mink, fink, drink, guilt, belt, malt, bolt, felt, gift, drift, theft, shift, rift, art, dart, cart, fort, hurt, bent, rent, pent, sent, went, disc, risk, mask, desk, fray, from, freeze, fruit, freak, friend, grant, grass, green, great, pride, prom, prove, price, proof, block, bleek, black, bloom, blind, floss, flirt, floor, flake, flip, glad, gleam, glove, glide, glass, trace, train, trail, trade, track, thrash, throb, throat, thrust, thread, scram, scroll, scrape, script, scratch, screen, skid, skill, skim, skunk, skate, scall, spray, spring, sprout, sprint, and so on.

Single-Syllable Complex Word Combination Exercise Nos. 2–4

These exercises are identical in design to the preceding one, except that for these three the complex word pairs are alternately produced at metronomic speed equivalents of 60, 90, and 120 bpm, respectively. The correct task (X_{2-4}) and bpm (60, 90, or 120) symbols must be listed in the respective cells of all data columns. The calculated target criterion should also be recorded on the Motor Speech Planning Treatment Chart. Of course, the prefix "B" in the activity cell symbolizes that the data are baseline scores. Faster rates can be practiced as always before proceeding with the next set of exercises.

Bisyllable Word Repetition Exercise No. 1

Step 1. Establish baseline ability by requesting the patient to repeat the word /pencil/ several times, with a 2-second pause between productions. On a notepad, rate each production as correct or incorrect using the scoring criteria previously established for this subsection of exercises. Repeat this procedure three times, selecting a different bisyllable word each time (e.g., giraffe, laundry, yellow, shrinkage), and tally the total number of correct productions.

Step 2. Calculate the percentage correct score and enter the result on the Motor Speech Planning Treatment Chart in the usual way. Be certain to tag these baseline data with the correct task (BB_1) and bpm (30—every 2 seconds) symbols. A score of less than 75 percent correct indicates the need for Step 3; otherwise advance to the next exercise.

Step 3. Set the metronome at 30 bpm and instruct the patient to repeat the bisyllable word /pencil/ to the beat—one syllable per beat continuously for 30 seconds. Follow the same basic rating, scoring, charting, and advancement methods previously detailed. Tag all data on the treatment chart with the correct task (B_1), bpm (30), and calculated target criterion information. *Note:* The following bisyllable words should be used as alternates throughout this exercise regimen: giraffe, laundry, yellow, shrinkage, pretty, bible, reason, baseball, happy, oven, money, frequent, heaven, softly, speaking, stomach, finger, sadness, jealous, peanut, lemon, falty, wristwatch, washer, picture, fancy, foolish, thicket, zipper, lengthy, puppet, closet, monkey, chosen, catcher, cupcake, garbage, never, costly, rabid, random, and so on.

Bisyllable Word Repetition Exercise Nos. 2–4

These exercises are identical in design to the preceding one, except that for these three the bisyllable words are repeated at metronomic speed equivalents of 60, 90, and 120 bpm, respectively. The correct task (B_{2-4}) and bpm (60, 90, or 120) symbols need to be listed in their respective cells of all data columns, as do the target criteria. Use of the prefix "B" in the activity cell symbolizes baseline data. Faster rates can, as always, be practiced before proceeding with the next set of exercises.

Trisyllable Word Repetition Exercise No. 1

Step 1. To establish baseline ability, request that the patient repeat the word /tornado/ several times, allowing a 2-second pause between repetitions. On a notepad, rate each production independently, using the *correct/incorrect* scoring dichotomy and criteria outlined earlier. Repeat this task three times, selecting a different stimulus word each time (e.g., icicle, different, cinnamon, laughable), and tally the total number of correct productions from the notepad scores.

Step 2. Calculate the percentage correct and enter this baseline result on the Motor Speech Planning Treatment Chart in a separate column in the usual way. Be certain to list the correct task (BT_1) and bpm (30) symbols in the respective cells of the data column. Proceed with Step 3 if the score here is less than 75 percent correct; otherwise advance to the next exercise.

Step 3. Set the metronome at 30 bpm and request that the patient repeat the trisyllable /tornado/ to the beat—one syllable per beat continuously for 30 seconds. On a notepad, rate each repetition independently as either correct or incorrect, again following the rating criteria detailed earlier.

Step 4. At the completion of 5 full minutes of practice, altering periodically the trisyllable word target, tally the total number of correct productions, calculate the percentage correct, and enter this result on the treatment chart. Be sure to list the correct task (T_1) and bpm (30) symbols in the appropriate cells of the data column.

Step 5. Continue with this procedure until the patient achieves a percentage correct score at least 75 percent improved over baseline level or 100 percent correct, whichever is less, over 10 consecutive minutes of treatment. Be sure to list this calculated target criterion on the Motor Speech Planning Treatment Chart in the appropriate cell at the bottom of the anticipated data column. At that time advance to the next exercise. Of course, the discontinuation rule should be invoked if necessary. *Note:* The following words can be used as alternate trisyllable stimuli throughout this regimen: basketball, lollipop, telephone, magazine, halloween, rational, parakeet, dependent, salary, banana, chocolate, substitute, manager, Washington, president, believer, sharpening, jewelry, terminal, medical, hospital, different, icicle, laughable, carpenter, condition, celery, restaurant, cinnamon, and so on.

Trisyllable Repetition Exercise Nos. 2–4

These exercises are identical in design to the one above, except that for these three the word repetitions are produced at metronomic speed equivalents of 60, 90, and 120 bpm, respectively. When charting these treatment data be certain to list the task (T_{2-4}) and bpm (60, 90, or 120) symbols as well as the calculated target criteria. The prefix "B," as always, is used in the activity cell to signify baseline data, accordingly. Faster speeds may be practiced before advancing.

Multisyllable Word Repetition Exercise No. 1

Step 1. To establish baseline ability, have the patient repeat the word /automatic/ several times, with a 2-second pause between repetitions. On a notepad, rate each production independently using the *correct/incorrect* scoring system as before. Repeat the task three times, selecting a different multisyllable word each time, and tally the total number of correct productions from the notepad scores.

Step 2. Calculate the percentage correct score and enter the result on the treatment chart as usual. In the respective cells of the data column be certain to list the correct task (BM_1) and bpm (30) symbols. Proceed with Step 3 if this baseline score is less than 75 percent correct; otherwise advance to the next exercise.

Step 3. Set the metronome at 30 bpm and request that the patient repeat the multisyllable word /automatic/ to the beat—one syllable per beat continuously for 30 seconds. On a notepad, rate each repetition independently as either correct or incorrect, as so often before in this treatment subsection.

Step 4. At the completion of 5 full minutes of practice, tally the total number of correct productions, calculate the percentage correct, and enter this result on the Motor Speech Planning Treatment Chart in the usual way. Be sure to list the correct task (M_1) and bpm (30) symbols.

Step 5. Continue with this procedure until the patient achieves a percentage correct score at least 75 percent improved over baseline level or 100 percent correct, whichever is less, over 10 consecutive minutes of treatment. Be sure to record on the chart the calculated target criterion. At that time advance to the next exercise. *Note:* The following words should be used as multisyllable alternates throughout the regimen to reduce the potential for boredom and possible order effects: automobile, examination, possibility, justification, graduation, encyclopedia, visitation, anthropology, catastrophe, statistical, alphabetical, refrigerator, comfortable, television, apraxia, stimulation, generalize, watermelon, articulation, magnificent, seriously, positively, available, psychology, entertainment, vocabulary, overwhelming, immediately, accumulate, physiology, irresistible, insignificant, bibliography, and so on.

Multisyllable Word Repetition Exercise Nos. 2–4

These exercises are identical in design to the one above, except that for these three the word repetitions are produced at metronomic speed equivalents of 60, 90, and 120 bpm, respectively. Remember, when charting these treatment data be certain to list the correct task (M_{2-4}) and bpm (60, 90, or 120) symbols as well as calculated target criteria. The prefix "B," as always, renders the entry baseline data. Faster speeds may be practiced before advancing.

Sentence Exercise No. 1

Step 1. To establish baseline ability, have the patient read, or if necessary repeat aloud, the sentence /I enjoy banana pudding/ with a 2-second pause between all syllables. Allow several trials of the sentence, but rate each one independently using the *correct/incorrect* scoring criteria defined earlier. Repeat the task three times, selecting a different short sentence each time (see options below), and tally the total number of correctly produced sentences.

Step 2.   Calculate the percentage correct score and enter the result on the Motor Speech Planning Treatment Chart as usual. In the respective cells of the data column be certain to list the correct task (BS$_1$) and bpm (30) symbols. Proceed with Step 3 if this baseline finding is less than 75 percent correct; otherwise advance to the next exercise.

Step 3.   Set the metronome at 30 bpm and request that the patient read aloud or repeat the sentence /I enjoy banana pudding/ to the beat—one syllable per beat until the sentence is completed. Rate the entire sentence, guided by the correct/incorrect scoring criteria for this regimen. Repeat this procedure, periodically altering the sentence used.

Step 4.   At the completion of 5 full minutes of practice, tally the total number of correctly produced sentences, calculate the percentage correct, and enter this result on the treatment chart in the usual way. Make certain to list the correct task (S$_1$) and bpm (30) symbols.

Step 5.   Continue with this procedure until the patient achieves a percentage correct score that is at least 75 percent improved over baseline level or 100 percent correct, whichever is less, over 10 consecutive minutes treatment. Be sure to record this calculated target criterion on the chart, as usual. Advance to the next exercise at that time. *Note:* The following sentence examples can be used as alternate stimuli throughout this exercise:

1. The girl has a wonderful vocabulary.
2. Answer the telephone, please.
3. Wash your hands before dinner.
4. I need to use the bathroom.
5. We had better shut the window.
6. It is positively beautiful outdoors.
7. Children like to watch television.
8. Graduation day is a week away.
9. The position is available.
10. Sue won the presidential election.
11. Are you ready to go shopping?
12. The box contained three sweaters.
13. This restaurant requires reservations.
14. The refrigerator is empty.
15. In the summer it is fun to go swimming.

Sentence Exercise Nos. 2–4

These exercises are identical in design to the preceding one, except that for these three the sentences are produced at metronomic speed equivalents of 60,

90, and 120 bpm, respectively. When charting these treatment data, be certain to list the correct task (S_{2-4}) and bpm (60, 90, or 120) symbols as well as the calculated target criteria. The prefix "B" in the activity cell signifies baseline data. Faster speeds may be practiced if so indicated for a given patient.

Supplemental Exercise

Patients who travel successfully through at least some of the sentence exercises will benefit from a technique that weans them from metronome dependency. *First,* set the metronome at the maximal speed (30, 60, 90, or 120 bpm) achieved in the preceding sentence exercises. *Second,* select a sentence for practice and recite the syllables in tandem with the beat. *Third,* after two complete sentence productions, immediately stop the metronome and have the patient try the same sentence without the beat stimuli. Do not encourage any particular rate of syllable production. *Fourth,* if articulatory breakdowns occur, set the metronome in motion instantly and instruct the patient to follow the beat, as usual. *Fifth,* continue repeating the sentence until productions have at least resumed baseline level, and fade the metronome again. *Sixth,* request the patient to try the sentence at the most comfortable rate. Encourage finger, hand, or foot tapping as a possible means of internal pacing if the patient still struggles with the task. *Seventh,* repeat these steps as necessary until the patient is able to generate various sentences with at least 75 percent accuracy over 10 consecutive minutes of practice without the metronome. Discontinue the program, as always, when no discernible trend of improvement is evident after 30 consecutive minutes of practice.

Comments on Treatment of Speech Motor Planning

Patients journeying through this regimen are, by design, forced into rhythmic, almost robot-like articulation and prosody. The target pace is generally slower than normal, which enables most patients to monitor articulator activities, plan for upcoming sound combinations, and discriminate against error productions by immediate self-correction. As patients gain confidence in their ability to handle complex articulatory demands with fewer breakdowns, there is a tendency for such improvements to evolve into more natural-sounding and spontaneous conversational speech patterns. Treatment of associated prosodic insufficiency often provides the needed boost for this successful transition.

The primary objective of this phase of intervention for the apractic patient is to retrain voluntary control of both isolated and sequential articulator movements for the purpose of improving articulatory accuracy. A metronome is used throughout the program for external rhythmic stimulation of these speech motor events, although internal rhythm established by the patient's own movements such as finger, hand, and foot tapping is not discouraged during the exercises. The benefit of using continuous, uninterrupted rhythmic clicks like those provided by the metronome in the treatment of speech programming difficulties of apractic patients has not been studied widely. Some clinical researchers have suggested that tracking such an external source of stimulation can be stressful and even cause adverse articulation effects. It has been suggested that requiring the patient to time the sequences of articulator movements with the ongoing clicks of a metronome may be too demanding of, and disruptive to, the cortical speech programming mechanism. The research and clinical experiences of this clinician do not lend support to these hypotheses. Whereas the advantages of internal rhythmic stimulation are indeed taught and emphasized in the program of intervention recommended here, the addition of external pacing stimuli to the regimen has been found helpful with many different apractic patients. Serendipitously discovered in most of these individuals is their automatic preference for the metronome over body rhythm techniques when practicing speech motor control. Curiously, though, many of these same people do employ finger- or hand-tapping methods during extemporaneous speech away from the reach of a metronome. One may speculate that the metronome exercises not only stimulate accurate articulator postures and sequences of movements for speech purposes, but also may help develop the internal rhythmic-temporal mechanisms that drive the cortical speech programmer.

Treatment does not stop upon completion of the exercises in this subsection. Rather, we capitalize on the articulation subsystem gains as treatment focus is immediately shifted to the residual suprasegmental (pitch, loudness, duration, and silence) and prosody (rhythm, stress, and intonation) disturbances that may continue to plague speech intelligibility. Methods by which to modify abnormalities of these important speech parameters are addressed in detail in the next chapter. However, it is almost always most fruitful to delay introduction of such treatments until apractic patients have been sufficiently drilled to try to improve articulator motor planning capabilities. Waiting until then often ensures the best chances for success with the prosody subsystem treatment program.

This concludes the motor speech planning exercise subsection. Table 6–4 offers a sequential synopsis of the recommended treatment techniques for patients with apraxia.

Case illustrations are provided next to close the chapter. These patients help demonstrate the possible flow of articulation subsystem treatments in the real clinical world.

Illustrative Case No. 1

This 52-year-old white female presented to the speech pathology service with a history of tinnitus, loss of acuity and perceptions of roaring sounds in her left ear, unbalanced gait, and speech difficulties, which had slowly progressed over a period of 2 years. Audiologic testing showed moderate left sensorineural hearing loss, tone decay, and speech discrimination difficulty. Laryngologic examination illustrated left vocal fold atrophy and associated paralysis in the abducted position. CT scans and plain skull x-rays revealed an enlarged left internal acoustic meatus, suggestive of a neuromal mass. Clinical neurologic testing detected the following mild to moderate abnormal signs and symptoms: (1) sen-

TABLE 6–4. Capsule Summary of Motor Planning Exercise Sequence for Oral

Disturbance of Focus	1	2	3	4	5
Nonspeech oral motor planning difficulty (oral apraxia)	Alternating up/down–out/in tongue activities at 30 & 60 bpm with metronome	Alternating close/open–spread/pucker lip activities at 30 & 60 bpm with metronome	Alternating open/close jaw followed by prolonged airflow activities at 30 & 60 bpm with metronome		
Voice motor planning difficulty (apraxia of phonation)	Isolated vowels at 30, 60, 90 & 120 bpm with metronome	Two vowel sequences at 30, 60, 90, & 120 bpm with metronome	Three vowel sequences at 30, 60, 90 & 120 bpm with metronome	Alternating vowel-/h/ productions at 30, 60, 90, & 120 bpm with metronome	
Speech motor planning difficulty (apraxia of speech)	Two CV syllable sequences at 30, 60, 90, & 120 bpm with metronome	Three CV syllable sequences at 30, 60, 90, & 120 bpm with metronome	Two CVC word sequences at 30, 60, 90 & 120 bpm with metronome	Three CVC word sequences at 30, 60, 90 & 120 bpm with metronome	Two monosyllable word sequences at 30, 60, 90, & 120 bpm with metronome

sorimotor impairment of the entire left face, involving the forehead, eyelid, and circumoral musculature on that side; (2) left ptosis and reduction of the nasolabial groove on the same side; (3) weakness and paralysis of the left half of the mandible musculature; (4) weakness, paralysis, and atrophy of the left half of the velum; (5) weakness, paralysis, and atrophy of the left half of the tongue; (6) ataxic gait; (7) coarse nystagmus; and (8) irregular alternate motion rates of the left limbs. The chief clinical speech evaluation findings included (1) mild to moderate articulatory imprecision, (2) mild to moderate hypernasal resonance, and (3) hoarse vocal quality with associated pitch and loudness variation restrictions. These clinical impressions led to the speech diagnosis of *flaccid dysarthria* with associated limb and trunk ataxia, owing to a unilateral left acoustic neuroma involving the V, VII, VIII, IX, X, and XIIth cranial nerves and the inferior cerebellar peduncle and cerebellum on the same side. Below we focus on the articulation subsystem treatments administered in sequence. These exercises were introduced after successful resonation and phonation subsystem therapy, which included the fitting of a palatal-lift appliance and Teflon-glycerin vocal fold augmentation surgery.

First, the tongue-strengthening exercise program was sequentially administered in full. Note that tonal therapy is not indicated because treatment of hypotonia is indirectly accomplished through effective strengthening and force physiology exercises. As can be seen from Figure 6–38, *A,* we began with the anterior tongue-strengthening regimen on 4/11 following baseline testing and achieved

Apraxia, Apraxia of Phonation, and Speech Apraxia

6	7	8	9	10
Bisyllable word repetitions at 30, 60, 90 & 120 bpm with metronome	Trisyllable word repetitions at 30, 60, 90, & 120 bpm with metronome	Multisyllable word repetitions at 30, 60, 90, & 120 bpm with metronome	Sentence repetitions at 30, 60, 90, & 120 bpm with metronome	Sentence repetitions with and without metronome

criterion, as denoted by the asterisk, after just 30 trials of treatment. Left vector training was next. That too was successful after 30 treatment trials; right vector training, seemingly more dependent on left musculature contribution, was introduced next but was terminated with only modest gains. Strengthening the palatal vector was then begun on 4/20 using the crossbar apparatus. The criterion for improvement was not met after 50 trials. We discontinued the tongue-strengthening regimen at that time.

Second, the lip-strengthening exercise program was initiated on 4/25, beginning with the anterior seal vector as shown in Figure 6–38, *B.* This training was discontinued on 4/27 with only mild gains, as was left lateral strengthening on 5/03; right lateral strengthening was not indicated according to baseline ability. Additional anterior lip-strengthening also fell short of the target criterion, and was discontinued on 5/05.

Third, the jaw-strengthening regimen began on 5/10 and was discontinued the next session short of the criterion for improvement, as shown in Figure 6–38, *C.*

Fourth, the tongue force physiology training program was instituted on 4/25, immediately after achievement of the criterion for improvement during the palatal vector strengthening regimen. As can be determined from Figure 6–39, *A,* on 4/27 the patient achieved the criterion set for the first exercise protocol using the ½ inch by ½ inch bite block during lingua-alveolar valving maneuvers at 30 bpm. On 5/03 the criterion was met for the 60-bpm condition. Baseline ability

Text continued on page 287.

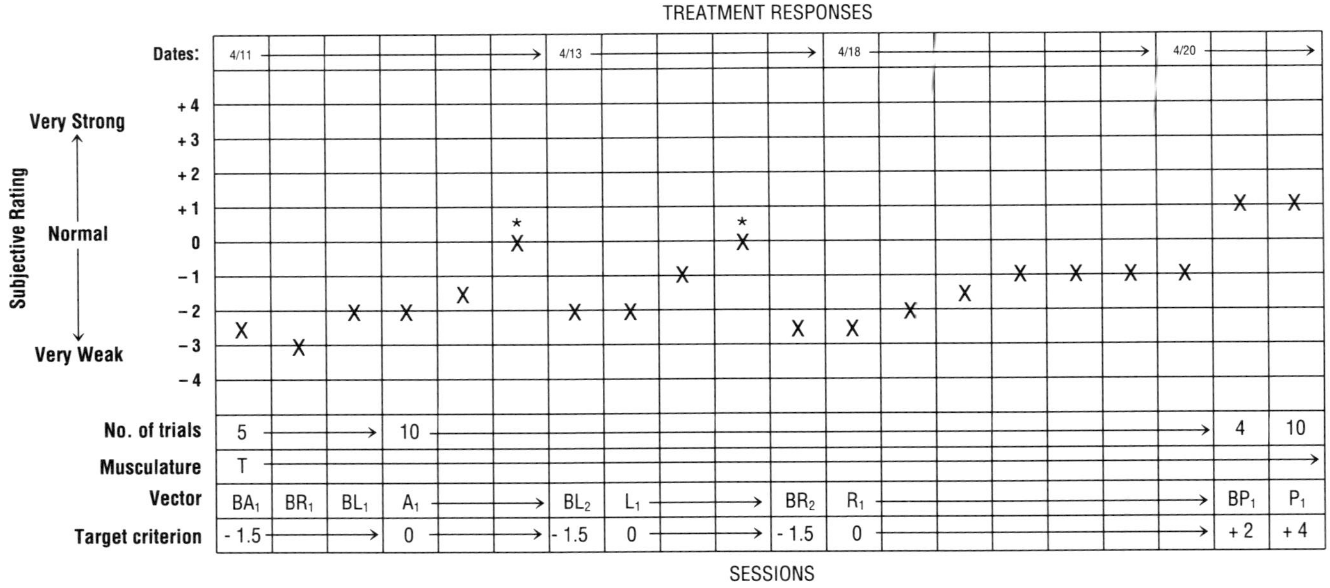

Figure 6–38. A through C, Tongue, lip, and jaw strengthening chart illustrating a flaccid dysarthric patient's responses to such therapy. An asterisk indicates that the criterion for improvement was met for the exercise task listed in the cell at the bottom of the column. This objective was achieved on two of the tongue-strengthening vectors: anterior and left lateral. Neither the lip- nor the jaw-strengthening programs resulted in comparable relative gains.

STRENGTHENING CHART

Patient's name: T.T.   (continued)

Birthdate: Sex:

Speech diagnosis:

Medical diagnosis:

Clinician:

Facility:

Address:

Comments:

_____

_____

_____

ACTIVITY KEY

1. Musculature: Tongue (T); Lip (L); Jaw (J)

2. Vectors: Anterior (A); Right (R); Left (L);
   Palatal (P); Open/Close (O/C)

Baseline (pre-treatment): B + feature symbol

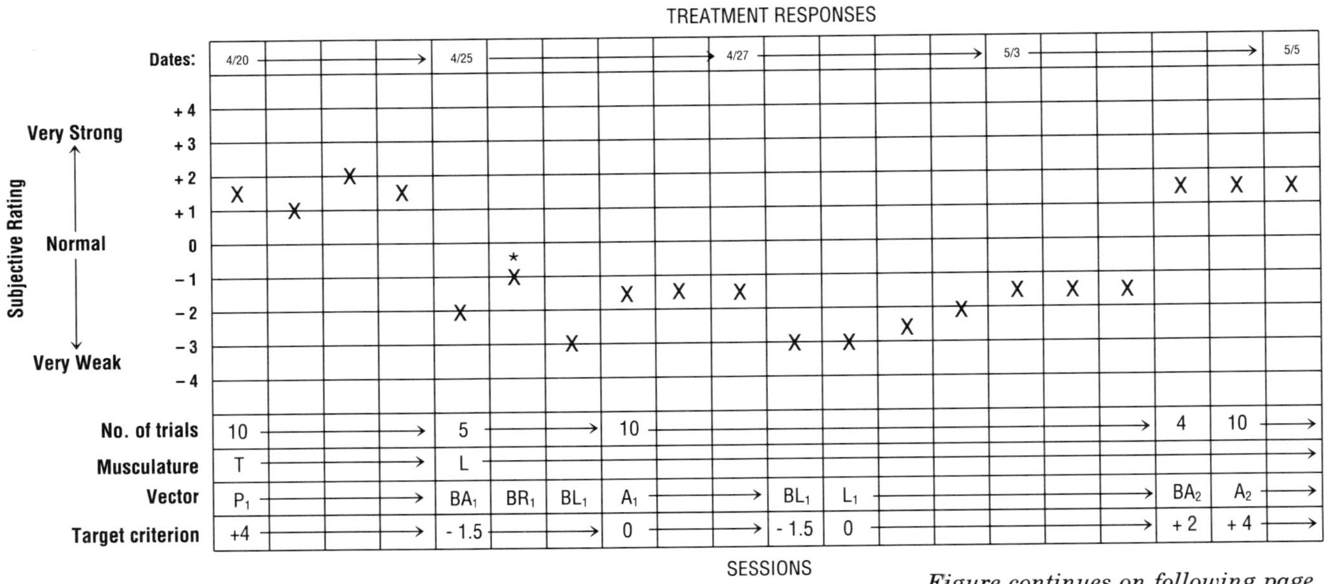

TREATMENT RESPONSES

Dates:	4/20	4/25	4/27	5/3	5/5
+4					
+3					
+2	X	X			X
+1	X	X			X
0 (Normal)		*X			X
−1		X		X X	
−2		X	X	X X	
−3			X	X	
−4			X		

No. of trials	10	5	10		4 / 10
Musculature	T	L			
Vector	P₁	BA₁ BR₁ BL₁	A₁ BL₁	L₁	BA₂ A₂
Target criterion	+4	−1.5	0	−1.5 0	+2 +4

SUBJECTIVE RATING
Very Strong ← Normal → Very Weak

SESSIONS

B

Figure continues on following page

Figure 6–38, B.

STRENGTHENING CHART

Patient's name: T.T. (continued)
Birthdate: Sex:

Speech diagnosis:
Medical diagnosis:
Clinician:
Facility:
Address:

Comments:

ACTIVITY KEY

1. Musculature: Tongue (T); Lip (L); Jaw (J)

2. Vectors: Anterior (A); Right (R); Left (L); Palatal (P); Open/Close (O/C)

Baseline (pre-treatment): B + feature symbol

TREATMENT RESPONSES

Dates:	5/5 →	5/10 →	→	5/12 →	
+4					
+3	X			X	X
+2	X X	X	X		
+1		X			
0					
−1					
−2					
−3					
−4					
No. of trials	10 →	4	10	→	
Musculature	L →	J		→	
Vector	A₂ →	BC₁	C₁	→	
Target criterion	+4 →	+2	+4	→	

Very Strong ↔ Normal → Very Weak

Subjective Rating

SESSIONS

C

Figure 6–38, *C.*

284

METRONOMIC MOBILITY TREATMENT CHART

Patient's name: T.T.   Sex: Fe
Birthdate: 10/28/33

Speech diagnosis: Flaccid dysarthria
Medical diagnosis: Left acoustic neuroma
Clinician: Dworkin
Facility: Private practice
Address: Anywhere, USA

ACTIVITY KEY

1. Musculature: Tongue (T); Lip (L); Jaw (J)

2. Task: Up/Down (U/D); Out/In (O/I);
   Left/Right (L/R); Close/Open (C/O);
   Pucker/Spread (P/S); Airflow (A)

3. Beats Per Minute: 30, 60, 90, 120 (150,
   200, variable [V])

4. Minutes of Therapy: Fill in amount

Baseline (pre-treatment): B + feature symbol

Comments:

TREATMENT RESPONSES

Percentage of Correct Responses

Dates:	4/25						4/27		5/3					

SESSIONS

Minutes of therapy	1 1/2	→	5			1 1/2	5		1 1/2	→	5		
Musculature	T											
Task	BU/D₁	BU/D₂	BU/D₃	BU/D₄	BU/D₅	BU/D₁	U/D₁	BU/D₂	U/D₂	BU/D₃	BU/D₄	U/D₄
BPM	30	60	90	120	V	30		60		90	120	
Target criterion	75%	75%	75%	75%	100%	75%	100%	75%	100%	75%	75%	100%

A

Figure 6–39. A and B, Chart illustrating effects of lingua-alveolar (U/D) valving exercises under different rate conditions for the flaccid dysarthric case sample. Note that all baseline measures on 4/25 corroborated the need for treatment. The criteria for improvement or advancement were met under the 30 (4/27), 60 (5/3), 90 (5/3), and variable (5/12) bpm movement rates. However, at 120 bpm the patient did not demonstrate an observable improvement trend, thus requiring discontinuation of that exercise on 5/5.

Figure continues on following page

285

METRONOMIC MOBILITY TREATMENT CHART

Patient's name: T.T.   (continued)

Birthdate: Sex:

Speech diagnosis:

Medical diagnosis:

Clinician:

Facility:

Address:

ACTIVITY KEY

1. Musculature: Tongue (T); Lip (L); Jaw (J)

2. Tasks: Up/Down (U/D); Out/In (O/I);
   Left/ Right (L/R); Close/Open (C/O);
   Pucker/Spread (P/S); Airflow (A)

3. Beats Per Minute: 30, 60, 90, 120 (150,
   200, variable [V])

4. Minutes of Therapy: Fill in amount

   Baseline (pre-treatment): B + feature symbol

Comments:

TREATMENT RESPONSES

Percentage of Correct Responses

Dates:	5/5			5/10			5/12			
100								*	*✕	
90								✕	✕	
80				✕					✕	
70					✕					
60			✕			✕				
50	✕		✕				✕			
40		✕								
30										
20										
10										
0										
Minutes of therapy	5	→	1 1/2	5						
Musculature	T									
Task	U/D₄	→	BU/D₄	U/D₅						
BPM	120	→	V							
Target criterion	100%	→	75%	96%						

SESSIONS

Figure 6–39, *B.*

for the 90-bpm condition exceeded threshold, thus negating direct intervention. On 5/05 (Figure 6–39, *B*) the 120-bpm status was withdrawn, owing to poor treatment effects. Several minutes of practice under the variable beat stimuli condition led to improvement to criterion on 5/12. Because of time and space limitations the patient's responses to Tongue Force Physiology Exercise nos. 6–25 will not be illustrated. Suffice it to say that she went on to achieve the criteria set with all the bite blocks for all the metronomic conditions, except the 120-bpm targets. This speed was very difficult to accomplish irrespective of the lingual vector practiced. Figure 6–40 reveals the effects of fine force physiology training using the crossbar apparatus. This program began on 5/17 and continued through 5/24. Note that on 5/19 the criterion was met for the 2N target. On this same date the patient went on to demonstrate criterion for the 1N target as well. The 0.5N and 0.25N targets were not exercised owing to excellent baseline performances. On 5/24 the patient was tested on all four of these targets under the 10-second holding phase condition. Results negated the need for intervention, as indicated by the asterisks. Variable fine force control was also demonstrated with success during that baseline testing session.

Fifth, the lip and jaw force physiology training programs were initiated on 5/10 and 5/17, respectively; the results are not detailed here. The patient sailed through the 25 lip exercises over the course of just three sessions, achieving criteria on all but the 120-bpm targets. The 15 jaw exercises were similarly mastered in three sessions, including the 120-bpm targets.

Sixth, after success with the tongue force physiology regimen on 5/24, phonetic stimulation was initiated for consonants, with special focus on the lingua-alveolars, lingua-velars, and lingua-palatals in various combinations and contexts. Lip sounds were phased in upon termination of the final lip force control exercise on 5/19. Phonetic practice continued for roughly 2 months, twice weekly. Excellent gains were realized in this time. The patient went from an articulation subsystem, perceptual baseline rating of 3.5 on the 7-point interval scale, indicating mild to moderate articulatory imprecision, to a post-treatment improved score of 2.0 on the same scale. She was enrolled in the prosody subsystem treatment program next to work on some of the suprasegmentals as well as the features of prosody.

Illustrative Case No. 2

This 23-year-old black male arrived at the speech pathology service 18 months after a left CVA, which resulted in the following salient clinical diagnoses: (1) right hemiparesis, (2) moderate apraxia of speech and concomitant mild aphasia, and (3) moderate unilateral right upper motor neuron dysarthria. Connected discourse was marked by variable articulatory breakdowns, including abnormal additions, omissions, substitutions, and distortions; frequent episodes of anticipatory sound, syllable, and word transpositions; false starts and repetitions; and classic articulatory groping behaviors. These error patterns tended to worsen with increased length and complexity of the speaking tasks. In addition, there

FORCE PHYSIOLOGY TREATMENT CHART

Patient's name: T.T.

Birthdate: 10/28/33   Sex: Fe

Speech diagnosis: Flaccid dysarthria

Medical diagnosis: Left acoustic neuroma

Clinician: Dworkin

Facility: Private practice

Address: Anywhere, USA

ACTIVITY KEY

1. Musculature: Tongue (T); Lip (L); Jaw (J)

2. Time (s): 5, 10, Variable (V) seconds

3. Vectors: Palatal (P); Close/Open (C/O)

Baseline (pre-treatment): B + feature symbol

Comments:

TREATMENT RESPONSES

	Dates:	5/17	→	5/19	→	5/24	→
	Variable						
	2N	v,f,f, / v,v	f,f,f, / v,f	v,v, / v,f,fu	c,v, / v,f,c	c,c,c, / v,v	c,c,c, / c,c	c,*c,v	c,*c,c, / v,c	c,*c,c, / v,c
Maximum	1N					v,v,c, / c,v	*c,c, / c,v,v	c,*c,c, / c,c		
Force Levels	0.5N						*c,c,c, / c,c	*c,c,c, / c,c	*c,c,c, / c,c	*c,c,c, / c,v
	0.25N								c,v	c,v
Minimum	No. of trials	5						3
	Musculature	T						↑
	Vector	BP₁	P₁	BP₂	P₂	BP₃	BP₄	BP₅	EP₆	BP₇	BP₈	BP₉
	Time	5 sec.						10 sec.		V
	Target criterion	8 of 10						↑

SESSIONS

SCORE KEY

C = Correct and immediate achievement of target level

L = Latency of 2 or more seconds before achieving and holding target level

V = Varibly achieves target level within same trial

F = Fails to hold target level after making contact

U = Unable to acheive target level

Figure 6–40. Fine tongue force physiology training responses. The lingua-alveolar (P) vector was targeted for practice under different resistance conditions. During the 5-second hold phase paradigm the criteria for improvement were met for all resistance levels, as denoted by the asterisks. Baseline performances during the 10-second as well as variable time hold phase paradigms exceeded threshold, negating the need for intervention.

was a mildly perceptible degree of hypernasality and nasal air emissions. Although language evaluations yielded equivocal results, some difficulties were detected during mental arithmetic tasks, spelling of lengthy words, and measures of word fluency and short-term memory for digits.

In addition to right hemiparesis of moderate degree, the clinical neurologic examination revealed: (1) right central facial and lingual weakness and paresis of moderate degrees, and (2) equivocal yet mildly perceptible velopharyngeal incompetence. All other results were insignificant. CT scans at the time of the CVA showed a substantial left hemispheric infarct predominantly involving Broca's area. Extension of the lesion into the left precentral gyrus and associated white matter perhaps helps explain contralateral corticospinal (limb) and corticobulbar (face, tongue, and possibly velopharyngeal) tract signs and symptoms, although such can and do result from higher cortical lesions alone. Below we review the articulation subsystem treatments administered in sequence. In fact, the patient began the speech therapy program at this level. The language, resonation, and prosody subsystem difficulties were not initially addressed in the treatment program, but held in abeyance to make way for intensive articulation focus.

First, owing to underlying hypertonicity of the tongue musculature, tone reduction therapy was prescribed. Figure 6–41 illustrates the patient's responses to intervention. Note the baseline measurement of +2.5 on 9/14. At the completion of the regimen on 9/18, the criterion for improvement of anterior (front) muscle tone was met, as denoted by the asterisk. Lateral (R/L) tone treatment was initiated next, and the criterion for improvement was achieved during the next session, 9/22. No further treatment was indicated, as the patient demonstrated on 9/30 acceptable baselines to end the regimen. Tonal therapy for the lip (L) musculature was not indicated, as evidenced by the last two baseline scores on Figure 6–41. However, because weakness was moderately evident, lip-strengthening exercises were initially introduced along with tone therapy for the tongue. Within four sessions, roughly 80 trials, the patient achieved the improvement criteria set for anterior, right, and left lateral lip strength. The lip force physiology training program was begun next, in concert with the tongue-strengthening regimen.

Second, tongue strengthening, not illustrated here, was initiated on 9/30, supported by the tone baseline score, which suggested overall maintenance of improved levels. The patient moved methodically but slowly through this regimen. Anterior vector strengthening required more than 100 trials to achieve the criterion established. The patient was unable to demonstrate significant gains when exercising the left lateral vector, which may depend mostly on the strength of the contraction of the right half of the tongue musculature. After 30 trials with no discernible improvement, we advanced to right lateral vector strengthening. The patient fell just shy of achieving the criterion set: Baseline ability was −2.0 and post-treatment was −1.0. These results prompted introduction of the force physiology training program.

Third, lip and tongue force physiology training was very helpful. The metronomic mobility exercises were especially rewarding in that they not only improved underlying force dyscontrol of these neuromuscularly impaired articula-

TONE IMPROVEMENT CHART

Patient's name: G.B.

Birthdate: 11/17/62   Sex: M

Speech diagnosis: Apraxia of speech/ spastic dysarthria

Medical diagnosis: Left CVA and right hemiparesis

Clinician: Dworkin

Facility: Private practice

Address: Anywhere, USA

ACTIVITY KEY

1. Musculature: Tongue (T); Lip (L); Velum (V); Jaw (J)

2. Activity: Forward tongue pull (F); Lateral tongue pull (R/L); Up/Down lip pull (U/D); Open/Close jaw excursions (O/C); Velar Massage (A/P)

Baseline (pre-treatment): B + feature symbol

Comments:

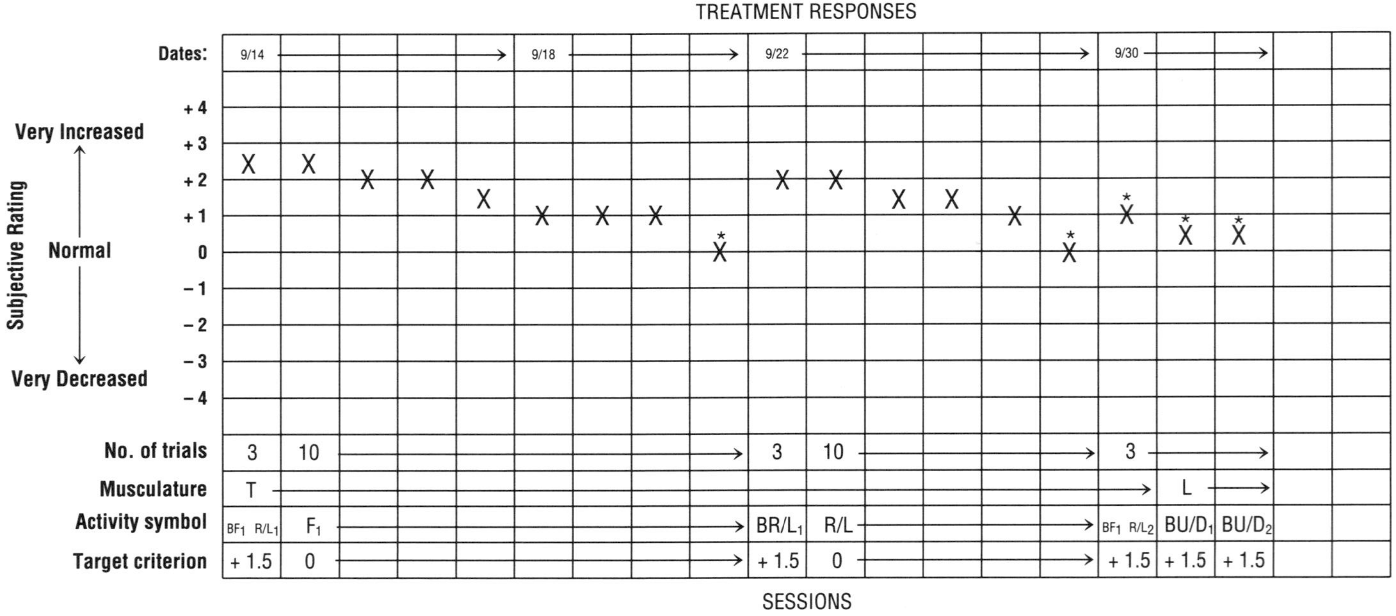

TREATMENT RESPONSES

SESSIONS

Figure 6–41. Chart illustrating the effects of tone reduction therapy for the tongue musculature in a patient with a mixture of apraxia of speech and unilateral spastic dysarthria. Note that for both forward (F) and lateral (R/L) passive resistance treatments the criteria for improvement were met, as denoted by the asterisks. Baseline measures of lip tonicity were judged within normal limits, negating intervention requirements.

tors but also facilitated overlying motor planning deficits. The lip musculature responded more quickly to the regimen, completing to criteria all the 25 exercises within 12 treatment sessions, a total of roughly four hours of intensive drills. Major obstacles occurred at the 120-bpm stimuli, and initially with the crossbar apparatus tasks. Less substantial were the results achieved with the tongue musculature. None of the 120-bpm tasks were completed to criterion, which surprised us in view of the patient's success with all the 90-bpm targets. As with the lips, crossbar training of the tongue was difficult, although signs of gradual yet erratic gains reinforced continuation of the exercises until the criteria were undoubtedly met. More than 7 full hours of intensive stimulation elapsed before tongue force physiology treatments were completed with good overall results.

Fourth, speech motor planning activities were delayed until the completion of all articulator physiologic exercises. Neither voice nor nonspeech oral motor planning treatments were indicated. Figure 6–42, *A* and *B* illustrates the patient's pretreatment skills across the motor speech planning task hierarchy. On the basis of these data we began the regimen at the two CV syllable sequence level (CV_3) at 90 bpm on 11/08 (see Figure 6–42, *B*). Note that at the beginning of the session on 11/11 the patient achieved the criterion for improvement (70 percent over 10 consecutive minutes of therapy), and thus the 120-bpm stimulus was introduced (see Figure 6–42, *C*), owing to poor baseline measures (BCV_4). This task was discontinued on 11/15 when the patient met the criterion for advancement. On the same date the three CV syllable sequence treatment paradigm (CV_5) was initiated at 30 bpm, followed by the 60- and 90-bpm targets, all of which were completed near the close of the session on 11/18. Note that the 90-bpm target baseline score (BCV_7) negated the need for therapeutic stimulation. On 11/22 the 120-bpm target plagued the patient. We discontinued practice, and looked past the Thanksgiving holiday to the CVC word pairs, which were introduced on 12/01 at 30 bpm (see Figure 6–42, *D*). The criterion for improvement was achieved on 12/03, and subsequent baseline measures at 60 and 90 bpm exceeded the threshhold of 75 percent correct. Although the patient made small gains during the 120-bpm word pair (CVC_4) practice, he was unable to meet the criterion. On 12/08 we discontinued the approach and introduced the three CVC word sequence exercise at 30 bpm (CVC_5). Not only did the patient achieve the criterion in the very next session, but his baseline scores on the 60, 90, and 120 bpm tasks negated the need for further practice. On 12/15 complex word pairs were stimulated at 30 bpm (X_1). As can be seen from the illustration, the patient struggled with this task until the 1/05 session (see Figure 6–42, *F*) when it was discontinued way short of the criterion for improvement. As required by design we advanced to the 60-bpm regimen (X_2). With additional practice, apparently, the patient learned to master this pace. Response generalization was evident on 1/12 when the 90- and 120-bpm baseline measures exceeded the threshold for treatment, as did all the bisyllable and most of the trisyllable baseline scores that followed. Notwithstanding the adverse research design implications of such effects, the carry-over into untreated conditions was welcome relief to the patient. We stimulated the trisyllable (T_4) words at 120 bpm as shown in Figure

Text continued on page 300.

MOTOR SPEECH PLANNING TREATMENT CHART

Patient's name: G.B.   Sex: M

Birthdate: 11/17/62

Speech diagnosis: Apraxia of speech / spastic dysarthria

Medical diagnosis: Left CVA and right hemiparesis

Clinician: Dworkin

Facility: Private practice

Address: Anywhere, USA

ACTIVITY KEY

1. Speech task: Consonant-Vowel syllable sequence (CV);
   Consonant-Vowel-Consonant syllable sequence (CVC);
   Single Syllable complex word combinations (X);
   Bi-syllable word repetition (B);
   Tri-syllable word repetition (T);
   Multi-syllable word repetition (M);
   Sentence productions (S)

2. Beats Per Minute: 30, 60, 90, 120 (150, 200, variable [V])

3. Minutes of Therapy: Fill in time

Baseline (pre-treatment): B + feature symbol

Comments:

TREATMENT RESPONSES

A

Percentage of Correct Responses (vertical axis: 0–100)

Dates:	11/8																	
Minutes of therapy	3																	
Activity symbol	BCV₁	BCV₂	BCV₃	BCV₄	BCV₅	BCV₆	BCV₇	BCV₈	BCVC₁	BCVC₂	BCVC₃	BCVC₄	BCVC₅	BCVC₆	BCVC₇	BCVC₈	BX₁	BX₂	BX₃	BX₄
BPM	30	60	90	120	30	60	90	120	30	60	90	120	30	60	90	120	30	60	90	120
Target criterion	75%																	

SESSIONS

Figure 6–42. **A** to **H,** Apractic patient's responses to a speech motor planning treatment regimen. Note that on 11/8 all baseline measures confirmed the need for the complete intervention package, which was initiated on the same date with the two CV syllable sequence stimuli tasks (CV₃) at the metronomic pace of 90 bpm. Each entry on the chart that contains an asterisk has met the criterion for improvement on the corresponding task (activity) listed in the cell at the bottom of the column.

Acrylic Bite Blocks, Edgewood Press, Box 811, Nicholasville, KY 40356.

See-Scape Device, Pro-Ed, 8700 Shoal Creek Blvd., Austin, TX 78758.

MOTOR SPEECH PLANNING TREATMENT CHART

Patient's name: G.B. (continued)

Birthdate: _____   Sex: M

Speech diagnosis: _____

Medical diagnosis: _____

Clinician: _____

Facility: _____

Address: _____

Comments: _____

ACTIVITY KEY

1. Speech task: Consonant-Vowel syllable sequence (CV);
   Consonant-Vowel-Consonant syllable sequence (CVC);
   Single Syllable complex word combinations (X);
   Bi-syllable word repetition (B);
   Tri-syllable word repetition (T);
   Multi-syllable word repetition (M);
   Sentence productions (S)

2. Beats Per Minute: 30, 60, 90, 120 (150, 200, variable [V])

3. Minutes of Therapy: Fill in time

Baseline (pre-treatment): B + feature symbol

TREATMENT RESPONSES

Dates:	11/8															11/11		
Activity symbol	BB₁	BB₂	BB₃	BB₄	BT₁	BT₂	BT₃	BT₄	BS₁	BS₂	BS₃	BS₄	BCV₁	BCV₂	BCV₃	CV₃		
BPM	30	60	90	120	30	60	90	120	30	60	90	120	30	60	90			
Target criterion	75%															70%		
Minutes of therapy	3															5		

Percentage of Correct Responses

SESSIONS

B

Figure continues on following page

Figure 6–42, *B.*

MOTOR SPEECH PLANNING TREATMENT CHART

Patient's name: G.B. (continued)

Birthdate: _____ Sex: M

Speech diagnosis: _____

Medical diagnosis: _____

Clinician: _____

Facility: _____

Address: _____

ACTIVITY KEY

1. Speech task: Consonant-Vowel syllable sequence (CV);
   Consonant-Vowel-Consonant syllable sequence (CVC);
   Single Syllable complex word combinations (X);
   Bi-syllable word repetition (B);
   Tri-syllable word repetition (T);
   Multi-syllable word repetition (M);
   Sentence productions (S)

2. Beats Per Minute: 30, 60, 90, 120 (150, 200, variable [V])

3. Minutes of Therapy: Fill in time

Baseline (pre-treatment): B + feature symbol

Comments:

_____

TREATMENT RESPONSES

Percentage of Correct Responses

Dates:	11/11		11/15			11/18			11/22
Minutes of therapy	3	5	3	5	3	5	3	5	3
Activity symbol	BCV₄	CV₄	BCV₅	CV₅		BCV₆	CV₆	BCV₇	BCV₈
BPM	120	120	30	30		60	60	90	120
Target criterion	75%	35%	75%	53%		75%	88%	75%	75%

SESSIONS

Figure 6–42, C.

c

294

MOTOR SPEECH PLANNING TREATMENT CHART

Patient's name: G.B. (continued)

Birthdate: Sex: M

Speech diagnosis:

Medical diagnosis:

Clinician:

Facility:

Address:

ACTIVITY KEY

1. Speech task: Consonant-Vowel syllable sequence (CV);
   Consonant-Vowel-Consonant syllable sequence (CVC);
   Single Syllable complex word combinations (X);
   Bi-syllable word repetition (B);
   Tri-syllable word repetition (T);
   Multi-syllable word repetition (M);
   Sentence productions (S)

2. Beats Per Minute: 30, 60, 90, 120 (150, 200, variable [V])

3. Minutes of Therapy: Fill in time

Baseline (pre-treatment): B + feature symbol

Comments:

TREATMENT RESPONSES

Percentage of Correct Responses

Dates:	11/22				12/1				12/3					
Minutes of therapy	5				3		5		3					
Activity symbol	CV₈				BCVC₁	CV₁				BCV₂	BCVC₃	BCVC₄		
BMP	120				30					60	90	120		
Target criterion	100%				75%	100%					75%			

SESSIONS

D

Figure continues on following page

Figure 6–42, *D*.

295

MOTOR SPEECH PLANNING TREATMENT CHART

Patient's name: G.B. (continued)

Birthdate: Sex: M

Speech diagnosis:

Medical diagnosis:

Clinician:

Facility:

Address:

ACTIVITY KEY

1. Speech task: Consonant-Vowel syllable sequence (CV);
   Consonant-Vowel-Consonant syllable sequence (CVC);
   Single Syllable complex word combinations (X);
   Bi-syllable word repetition (B);
   Tri-syllable word repetition (T);
   Multi-syllable word repetition (M);
   Sentence productions (S)

2. Beats Per Minute: 30, 60, 90, 120 (150, 200, variable [VI])

3. Minutes of Therapy: Fill in time

Baseline (pre-treatment): B + feature symbol

Comments:

TREATMENT RESPONSES

Percentage of Correct Responses

Dates:	12/3	12/8		12/10							12/15			
100								*X	*X	*X				X
90							*X	X	X	X			X	X
80							*X							
70			X		X							X		
60		X	X	X	X						X			
50	X	X									X			
40														
30														
20														
10														
0														
Minutes of therapy	5		3	5							3		5	
Activity symbol	CVC₄		BCVC₅	CVC₅							BCVC₆	BCVC₇	BCVC₈	BX₁	X₁
BPM	120		30								60	90	120	30
Target criterion	100%		75%	100%							75%		100%

SESSIONS

Figure 6–42, *E.*

MOTOR SPEECH PLANNING TREATMENT CHART

Patient's name: G.B. (continued)

Birthdate: Sex: M

Speech diagnosis:

Medical diagnosis:

Clinician:

Facility:

Address:

ACTIVITY KEY

1. Speech task: Consonant-Vowel syllable sequence (CV);
   Consonant-Vowel-Consonant syllable sequence (CVC);
   Single Syllable complex word combinations (X);
   Bi-syllable word repetition (B);
   Tri-syllable word repetition (T);
   Multi-syllable word repetition (M);
   Sentence productions (S)

2. Beats Per Minute: 30, 60, 90, 120 (150, 200, variable [V])

3. Minutes of Therapy: Fill in time

Baseline (pre-treatment): B + feature symbol

Comments:

TREATMENT RESPONSES

Percentage of Correct Responses

Dates:	12/15			1/5			1/8			1/12			
100												*×	*×
90											*×		
80							×		*×				
70			X			×		*×					
60	X	X		X	×							
50													
40													
30													
20													
10													
0													
Minutes of therapy	5	→		3	5		→			3	→		
Activity symbol	X₁	→		BX₂	X₂		→			BX₃	BX₄	BB₁	BB₂	BB₃
BPM	30	→		60			→			90	120	30	60	90
Target criterion	100%	→		75%	100%		→			75%				

SESSIONS

Figure 6–42, *F*.

Figure continues on following page

F

MOTOR SPEECH PLANNING TREATMENT CHART

Patient's name: G.B. (continued)

Birthdate: Sex: M

Speech diagnosis:

Medical diagnosis:

Clinician:

Facility:

Address:

ACTIVITY KEY

1. Speech task: Consonant-Vowel syllable sequence (CV);
   Consonant-Vowel-Consonant syllable sequence (CVC);
   Single Syllable complex word combinations (X);
   Bi-syllable word repetition (B);
   Tri-syllable word repetition (T);
   Multi-syllable word repetition (M);
   Sentence productions (S)

2. Beats Per Minute: 30, 60, 90, 120 (150, 200, variable [V])

3. Minutes of Therapy: Fill in time

Baseline (pre-treatment): B + feature symbol

Comments:

TREATMENT RESPONSES

Percentage of Correct Responses

SESSIONS

Dates:	1/12	1/14					1/19					1/21	
100		*X	*X										
90	*X	*X	X								*X		
80	*X				X	X	X	X		*X			X
70				X	X	X			X			X	
60				X	X					*X	X		
50				X					X				
40													
30										*X	X		
20													
10													
0													
Minutes of therapy	3	→	5						3	→	5		
Activity symbol	BB₄	BT₁	BT₂	BT₃	BT₄	T₄			BM₁	BM₂	BM₃	BM₄	BS₁
BPM	120	30	60	90	120				30	60	90	120	30
Target criterion	75%			→	100%				75%			→	100%

G

Figure 6–42, *G.*

MOTOR SPEECH PLANNING TREATMENT CHART

Patient's name: G.B. (continued)

Birthdate: Sex: M

Speech diagnosis:

Medical diagnosis:

Clinician:

Facility:

Address:

ACTIVITY KEY

1. Speech task: Consonant-Vowel syllable sequence (CV);
   Consonant-Vowel-Consonant syllable sequence (CVC);
   Single Syllable complex word combinations (X);
   Bi-syllable word repetition (B);
   Tri-syllable word repetition (T);
   Multi-syllable word repetition (M);
   Sentence productions (S)

2. Beats Per Minute: 30, 60, 90, 120 (150, 200, variable [V])

3. Minutes of Therapy: Fill in time

Baseline (pre-treatment): B + feature symbol

Comments:

TREATMENT RESPONSES

Dates:	1/21									1/26						

Percentage of Correct Responses

Minutes of therapy	5	3	5	
Activity symbol	S₁	BS₂	BS₃	BS₄	S₄
BPM	30	60	90	120	
Target criterion	100%	75%		96%	

SESSIONS

Figure 6–42, *H.*

299

6–42, *G*, but on 1/19 failed to make significant enough gains to justify continuation. Because the multisyllable word stimuli were performed with few errors across all metronomic conditions, but the sentence stimuli were troublesome, we began sentence treatments (S_1), which continued until 1/26 (see Figure 6–42, *H*) when the criterion was met at 120 bpm (S_4). The supplemental exercise was administered next with good success, to conclude the articulation subsystem treatment program. Focus was then placed on improving residual prosodic insufficiency, which contaminated contextual speech efforts despite gains made thus far. It should be noted that at the start of the patient treatment program articulation, prosody and contextual speech were perceptually rated 4, 5, and 4.5, respectively, on the Speech Characteristics Chart. Post-articulation therapy measures yielded these three parallel ratings: 2.5, 3.5, and 3.

SUGGESTED READINGS

Berlin, C. (1976). On: Melodic Intonation Therapy for aphasia by Sparks and Holland. *Journal of Speech and Hearing Disorders, 41*, 298–300.

Crickmay, M. C. (1966). *Speech therapy and the bobath approach to cerebral palsy.* Springfield, IL: Charles C Thomas.

Dabul, B. (1979). *Apraxia Battery for Adults.* Tigard, OR: CC Publications.

Dabul, B., & Bollier, B. (1976). Therapeutic approaches to apraxia. *Journal of Speech and Hearing Disorders, 41*, 268–276.

Daniel, B., & Guitar, B. (1978). EMG feedback and recovery of facial and speech gestures following neural anastomosis. *Journal of Speech and Hearing Disorders, 43*, 9–20.

Darley, F. L. (1984). Apraxia of speech: A neurogenic articulation disorder. In H. Winitz (Ed.), *Treating Articulation Disorders: For Clinicians by Clinicians*. Baltimore, MD: University Park Press.

Deal, J., & Florence, C. (1978). Modification of the eight-step continuum for treatment of apraxia of speech in adults. *Journal of Speech and Hearing Disorders, 43*, 89–95.

Dworkin, J., & Culatta, R. (1980). *Dworkin-Culatta Oral Mechanism Examination.* Nicholasville, KY: Edgewood Press.

Dworkin, J. P. (1984). Specific characteristics and treatments of the dysarthrias. In H. Winitz (Ed.), *Treating Articulation Disorders: For Clinicians by Clinicians*. Baltimore, MD: University Park Press.

Dworkin, J., Abkarian, G., & Johns, D. (1988). Apraxia of speech: The effectiveness of a treatment regimen. *Journal of Speech and Hearing Disorders, 63*, 280–294.

Dworkin, J., Petrucci-coley, T., & Abkarian, G. (1989). A therapeutic research approach to treatment of apraxia of phonation. *Poster at annual convention of American Speech & Hearing Association.*

Fairbanks, G. (1960). *Voice and Articulation Drill Book.* New York: Harper & Row.

Fisher, H. B. (1975). *Improving Voice and Articulation.* Boston: Houghton Mifflin.

Helm, N. A. (1979). Management of palilalia with a pacing board. *Journal of Speech and Hearing Disorders, 44,* 350–353.

Ince, L., & Rosenberg (1963). Modification of articulation in dysarthria. *Archives of Physical Medicine and Rehabilitation, 54,* 233–236.

Keith, R., & Aronson, A. (1975). Singing as therapy for apraxia of speech and aphasia: Report of a case. *Brain and Language, 2,* 483–488.

Miller, N. (1986). *Dyspraxia and its management.* Rockville, MD: Aspen Pub.

Nakano, K., Zubick, W., & Tyler, H. (1973). Speech defects of Parkinsonian patients: Effects of levodopa therapy in speech intelligibility. *Neurology, 23,* 365–370.

Netsell, R. (1985). Construction and use of a bite block for evaluating and treating speech disorders. *Journal of Speech and Hearing Disorders.*

Netsell, R., & Cleeland, C. (1973). Modification of lip hypertonia in dysarthria using EMG feedback. *Journal of Speech and Hearing Disorders, 38,* 131–140.

Robin, D., & Luschei, E. (1991). Measurement of tongue strength and endurance in normal and articulation disordered subjects. In C. Moore, K. Yorkston, & D. Beukelman (Eds.), *Dysarthria and apraxia of speech: Perspectives on management.* Baltimore: Paul H. Brooks, Pub.

Rosenbek, J., & Lapointe, L. (1985). The dysarthrias: Description, diagnosis and treatment. In D. F. Johns (Ed.), *Clinical Management of Neurogenic Communicative Disorders.* Boston: Little, Brown.

Rosenbek, J. C. (1985). Treating apraxia of speech. In D. F. Johns (Ed.), *Clinical Management of Neurogenic Communicative Disorders.* Boston: Little, Brown.

Rosenbek, J., McNeil, M., & Aronson, A. (1984). *Apraxia of Speech: Physiology, Acoustics, Linguistics, Management.* San Diego, CA: College-Hill Press.

Rosenbek, J., Collins, M., & Wertz, R. (1976). Intersystemic reorganization in the treatment of apraxia of speech. In R. H. Brookshire (Ed.), *Clinical Asphasiology: Conference Proceedings.* MN: BRK Publishers.

Rosenbek, J., Lemme, M., Ahern, K., Harris, E., & Wertz, R. (1973). A treatment for apraxia of speech in adults. *Journal of Speech and Hearing Disorders, 38,* 462–472.

Shane, H., & Darley, F. (1978). The effect of auditory rhythmic stimulation on articulator accuracy in apraxia of speech. *Cortex, 14,* 444–450.

Tonkovich, J., & Marquardt, T. (1977). The effects of stress and melodic intonation on apraxia of speech. In R. H. Brookshire (Ed.), *Clinical Aphasiology: Conference Proceedings.* MN: BRK Publishers.

Wertz, R., Lapoint, L., & Rosenbek, J. (1984). *Apraxia of speech: The disorder and its treatment.* New York: Grune & Stratton.

Yorkston, K., & Beukelman, D. (1982). *Assessments of intelligibility of dysarthric speech.* Tigard, OR: CC Publications.

Chapter 7

Treatment of the Prosody Subsystem

Speech signals contain more than just lexical, syntactic, semantic, and articulatory messages. In the full spectrum of spoken language, pragmatic or sociolinguistic and emotional or affective information, ordinarily conveyed by suprasegmental features and prosodic modulations, also contribute to the complexity of these signals. Sometimes used synonymously, the terms "suprasegmental" and "prosody" will be defined here with distinctions relative to their overall vocal effects. Variations in pitch, loudness, silence, and segment duration fall under the suprasegmental umbrella. The coloring, melody, and cadence of speech, better described as rhythm, stress, and intonation patterns, characterize the general features of prosody, which result from interactions of the suprasegmentals. For ease of discussion, only the term "prosody" will be used in this chapter, but it shall represent all the aforementioned speech features. When a speaker normally varies or modulates prosody, the intention may be to impart a certain affective tone to the message. Whereas minor modulations may impart subtle emotional signals, strong prosodic variations may convey more meaningful or purposeful information. Said one way, the words "don't stop" mean to proceed. Emphasized differently, they mean to halt. A sentence may be spoken as a statement or a question, depending on the prosodic features employed. The intonation selected, for example, may engender a calm, receptive response or a defensive, recalcitrant one. As these essential factors suggest, normal speech is constantly subject to and modified by prosodic modulations.

Virtually all patients with motor speech difficulties exhibit prosodic insufficiency to some degree. Germane to these individuals are two of the three primary classes of disturbed prosody: Dysprosody and aprosody. The former implies distortion of any one or more of the general features of prosody, which may at times cause speech to sound abnormally burdened by a thick foreign accent. The term "ataxic prosody" has been applied to this disorder. Aprosody, on the other hand, is a condition marked by a complete absence of prosodic features in spoken language. In the real clinical world, patients rarely emerge with unequivocal and

TABLE 7–1. Capsule Summary of Prosodic Disturbances Commonly Exhibited by Patients with Motor Speech Disorders*

Disorder	Slow Rate	Fast Rate	Variable Rate	Short Rushes	Prolonged Sounds	Prolonged Intervals	Prolonged Pauses	Abnormal Stress	Excess and Equal Stress	Excess Loudness	Reduced Loudness Variation	Pitch Outbursts	Reduced Pitch Variation	Flattened Affect
Flaccid dysarthria	X										X†	X†	X†	
Spastic dysarthria	X										X	X	X	
Hyperkinetic dysarthria			X			X	X			X	X		X	
Hypokinetic dysarthria		X	X	X			X				X		X	X
Ataxic dysarthria	X				X	X	X		X	X		X		
Apraxia of speech	X				X	X	X	X			X	X‡	X‡	

*Note that absence of "X" marks in a column indicates that the abnormal feature in question is *not* typically observed in patients with the disorder shown in the corresponding row.
†With involvement of the Xth cranial nerve.
‡With a phonation subsystem component.
Note: With mixed dysarthria, examine for the features of the components.

total prosodic disability. Rather, most patients present with what may best be diagnosed as dysprosody, which usually contributes significantly to speech unintelligibility.

Focal as well as diffuse lesions of the right cerebral hemisphere, including areas of all lobes, have been implicated in the etiology of dysprosody. It should be noted here, however, that localizing the cause of dysprosody to lesions of the right cerebral hemisphere alone has been challenged by neurolinguists who have demonstrated similar kinds of deficits in patients with left hemisphere disturbances. Notwithstanding such debate, the right hemisphere is generally considered the dominant one in modulating affective language and behavior. Table 7–1 provides a summary of the most commonly occurring prosodic difficulties in patients with motor speech disorders. The exercises in this chapter are based largely on these types of disturbances.

Although speech clinicians now readily acknowledge the important relationship between effective speaking and command of the prosody subsystem, still little diagnostic time may be devoted to the evaluation of prosodic disturbances, and even less may be spent in their remediation. The primary purpose of this chapter is to introduce exercises that may be employed to improve the most commonly observed characteristics of dysprosody in patients with different types of motor speech disorders.

WHEN TO BEGIN THERAPY

As discussed earlier in the text, treatment of prosodic insufficiencies is generally prescribed last in relationship to other speech subsystem disturbances and their management. Delaying such treatment is recommended because gains made during any necessary respiration, resonation, phonation, and articulation exercises usually provide a physiologic backdrop that not only facilitates but also hastens prosody subsystem improvements. On occasion, however, when the motor speech disorder is mild in degree, simultaneous treatment of the articulation and prosody subsystems may prove effective and efficient. Prior to and periodically throughout these exercises, it is wise to render perceptual ratings of prosody and contextual speech abilities on the Speech Characteristics Chart (see Figure 2–2). Such measures are best obtained during conversational speech and contrived oral reading tasks if possible (e.g., paragraphs from a familiar book, *Grandfather Passage* and *Rainbow Passage*). Make certain that all baseline entries on this chart receive the correct activity symbols (BP for prosody and BC for connected discourse) in the appropriate cells of the data column. For tracking the effects of specific subsystem treatments on overall prosody and contextual speech characteristics, the data logged on the chart are tagged in the cell below with the activity symbols P and C, respectively. Let's now proceed with specific treatment recommendations segregated by (isolated) prosodic feature disturbances.

TREATMENT MATERIALS

Assemble the following materials in order to carry out all the exercises recommended in this chapter:

1. See-Scape Device* (see Chapter 3 references and Figure 3–4),
2. Portable tape recorder with V-U meter or sound level meter, which can be purchased for less than $40 at most local stereo-electronic stores,
3. Metronome,
4. Drinking straws,
5. Stopwatch or wristwatch with second hand,
6. Speech Characteristics Chart (Figure 2–2),
7. Prosody Subsystem Behavioral Treatment Chart (Figure 7–1).

Treatment of Pitch Alteration Abnormalities

Patients with apraxia of speech generally do not suffer from vocal pitch disturbances, and even those with a phonation component experience only occasional pitch outbursts. Many dysarthric patients, however, exhibit problems with pitch control, as shown in Table 7–1. Reduced pitch variation (so-called "monopitch") and inappropriate, intermittent pitch outbursts or changes are perhaps the most commonly observed abnormalities for which the exercises below are especially designed. Note that these exercises are not intended as primary treatment for pitch difficulties that may result from laryngeal edema or paralysis. Rather, the approaches below are indicated for patients who exhibit problems with pitch fluctuation and stability as they pertain to general discourse and message intent. It is important to remember that the fundamental frequency of the voice normally varies considerably among individuals relative to age and sex. Even within presumably homogeneously clustered groups of individuals, wide variations occur in this voice parameter. Any manipulations of pitch use should take these facts into consideration so that the objectives of treatment are within the pitch boundaries appropriate to the patient from neurologic, anatomical, age, and sex points of view collectively. As a final note, some clinicians are not favorably disposed to treatment of pitch dyscontrol in dysarthric patients because improvements in this feature of prosody may not enhance speech intelligibility. This clinician, on the other hand, has found that such treatment can and often does contribute to improved speech intelligibility, which after all is a primary goal of speech rehabilitation.

Pitch Control Exercise No. 1

Step 1. To establish baseline pitch discrimination and listening skills, instruct the patient that the task here is twofold: (1) to identify whether pairs of vowels briefly sung by the clinician are the same pitch or different; and (2) if they

---

*Pro-Ed, 8700 Shoal Creek Blvd, Austin, TX 78758.

PROSODY SUBSYSTEM BEHAVIORAL TREATMENT CHART

Patient's name:

Birthdate: Sex:

Speech diagnosis:

Medical diagnosis:

Clinician:

Facility:

Address:

ACTIVITY KEY

Feature:	MEASUREMENT UNIT
1. Pitch (P)	% correct or
	7-point interval scale
	(1 = normal;
	7 = most deviant)
2. Loudness (L)	% correct or
	7-point interval scale
3. Rate (R)	% correct, WPM %, or
	7-point interval scale

Feature:	MEASUREMENT UNIT
4. Basic stress (S)	% correct or
	7-point interval scale
5. Contrastive stress (C)	% correct

Baseline (pre-treatment): B + activity symbol

Comments:

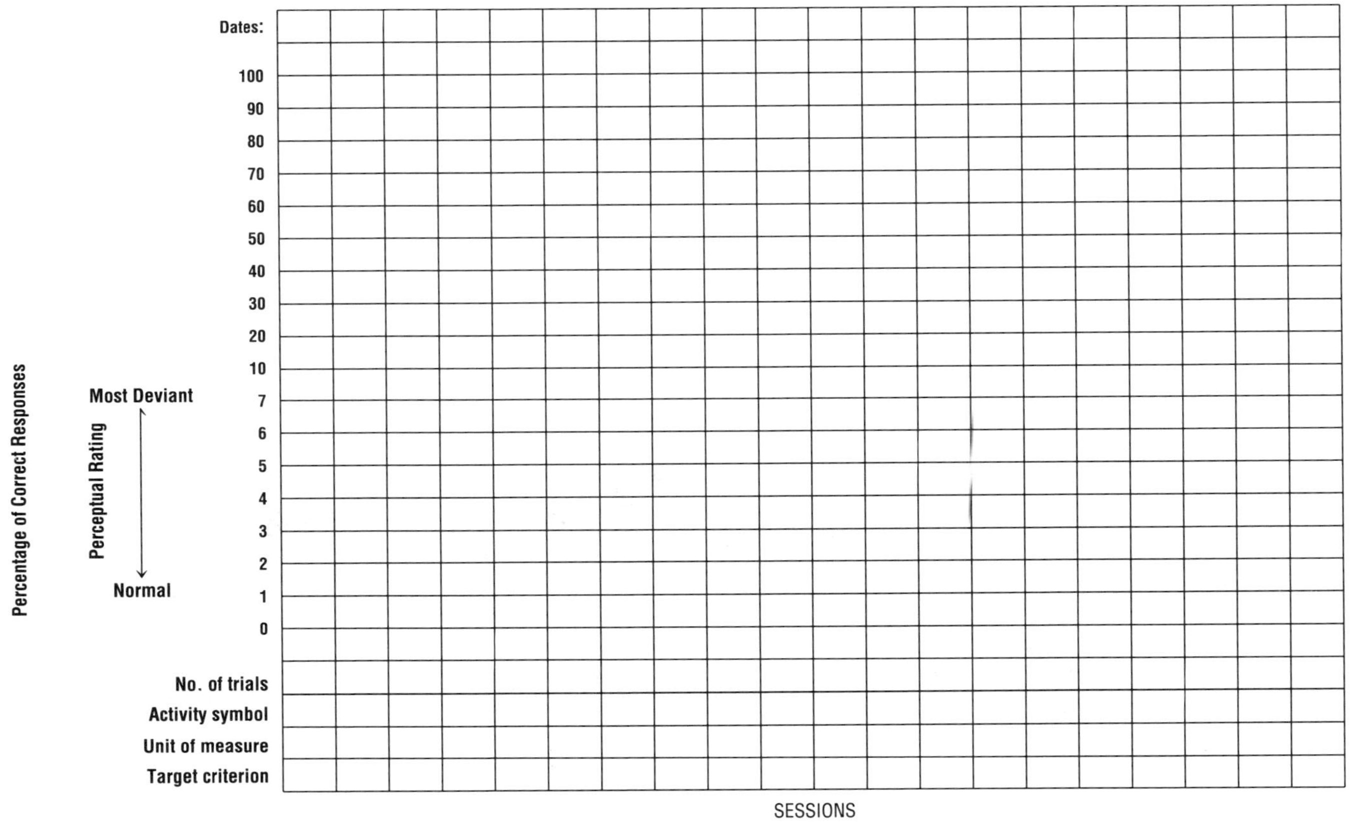

Figure 7–1. Prosody subsystem behavioral treatment chart to be used to log all data collected for the ultimate purpose of measuring treatment effects.

are different and perceived as such, the one that is *higher* pitched must be accurately identified. Before collecting data, allow the patient a practice run by singing a pair of vowels that are grossly different with respect to pitch. Discuss the patient's responses to these stimuli. Provide another example in which the vowel pair are of the same pitch, and discuss the answer again. When it is clear that the patient at least understands the task, commence with the baseline data collection process.

Step 2. Begin with the vowels /a/ and /u/. Sing the /a/ for roughly 3 seconds at a relatively low pitch, followed by the /u/ for the same amount of time at an obviously higher pitch. Solicit the required answers from the patient and record on a notepad whether the responses were *correct* or *incorrect*. The patient, for example, may correctly identify the two sounds as different but fail to specify accurately the one that is higher pitched. The scores would then be 1 correct and 1 incorrect. Repeat this procedure 10 times but select different vowel pairs, periodically and creatively varying the pitch distinctions across the trials to make the tasks perceptually challenging.

Step 3. Tally the total number of correct scores and calculate the percentage score. Enter this baseline result on the Prosody Subsystem Behavioral Treatment Chart (Figure 7–1), making certain to list the number of trials (10) and activity symbol (BP_1) in the respective cells corresponding to the data column. If this score is equal to or less than 75 percent, proceed with Step 4; otherwise advance to the next exercise.

Step 4. Continue with the same basic procedure as in Step 2 above, varying the vowel pairs and the pitch levels used from trial to trial. Be sure periodically to produce pairs that are the same so that the patient is charged with making fine as well as gross pitch discriminations. After each set of 10 trials, tally the total number of correct scores from the notepad, calculate the percentage, and enter this result on the treatment chart accordingly. The activity symbol used to represent these data is "P_1."

Step 5. Continue with this procedure until the patient achieves a mean percentage correct score at least 75 percent improved over baseline or 100 percent correct, whichever is less, over 10 consecutive trials. Calculate the target criterion and enter the value in the respective cell at the bottom of the column on the chart. As in previous subsystem exercises, discontinuation is recommended if after 30 consecutive trials there is no discernible trend of improvement to warrant continuation. Advance to the next exercise as indicated.

Pitch Control Exercise No. 2

Step 1. To establish baseline pitch modulation ability, engage the patient in conversation and tape record the speech sample, which should last at least 5 minutes. If the patient can read aloud a passage from a book or one of the popular standard texts (*Grandfather Passage, Rainbow Passage,* or *Arthur the Rat,* for example), tape record this reading as well, with instructions beforehand that he or she speak most naturally and comfortably relative to pitch, loudness, and phrasing patterns. As a third baseline measure, tape record the patient singing up and down the scale, starting at whatever pitch he or she may choose. Repeat each of these three procedures three times, randomizing the order of their presentation. Review these tapes and on the prosody subsystem behavioral treatment chart record the mean perceptual rating (1 to 7) for each of these three measures, making certain that the correct symbol (BP_{2a}, BP_{2b}, or BP_{2c}, respectively) is used when tagging each baseline entry in the corresponding activity cell. Note that a score of "7" on the chart signifies a marked degree of pitch disturbance, whereas a score of "2" represents very mild difficulty with pitch control. It is important to describe in the comments section of the chart the pitch abnormality characteristics presented by the patient for whom the ratings are rendered. These baseline performances can also serve as data for the aforementioned Speech Characteristics Chart ratings of overall prosody and contextual speech abilities. If the patient scores "3" or worse on two or more of these three baseline measures, proceed with Step 2; otherwise advance to the next exercise.

Step 2. Demonstrate for the patient two vowels sung at grossly different pitch levels. The first can be at the lowest possible pitch accompanied by a low-positioned hand gesture, and the second at the highest within the chest register accompanied by the hand held high above the head to illustrate symbolically the gross difference between these two sounds. Repeat this procedure a few times. Coupled with the preceding exercise, these pitch distinctions should by now be perceptually apparent to the patient; if they are not, the prognosis for pitch control improvement is poor. Ask the patient to try to perform the same task, striving for a low-pitched sound at first, followed by a much higher-pitched one. Encourage use of the corresponding hand gestures during the performance. Score the effort, using the dichotomous *correct/incorrect* scale. A correct score is awarded if the two sounds produced are perceptually at least three whole notes apart in fundamental frequency. Continue with the task until the patient achieves this target criterion on 10 consecutive trials.

Step 3. At the completion of each set of 10 trials, tally the percentage of correct responses from the notepad and enter this result on the treatment chart, making certain to list the date of the session, number of trials (10), and activity symbol (P_2) in the respective cells corresponding to the column in which these data are recorded. Advance as usual and indicated. *Note:* Altering pitch can sometimes adversely affect vocal quality. Be mindful of this possibility and weigh and balance the benefit of pitch practice if it appears to be at the expense of other vocal parameters.

Pitch Control Exercise No. 3

Step 1. Follow the exact same baseline method as in the preceding exercise, and advance to Step 2 if so indicated; otherwise proceed to the next exercise. Note that the activity symbols "BP_{3a}, BP_{3b}, and BP_{3c}" are used to tag these baseline data on the treatment chart.

Step 2. This is the same basic exercise as Exercise no. 2 above, except that here the first vowel is sung at the highest and the second one at the lowest pitch levels possible. Follow the same demonstration, rating, scoring, charting, and advancement criteria used in the preceding exercise. Note that the activity symbol "P_3" is used to identify these treatment data on the chart.

Pitch Control Exercise No. 4

Step 1. To establish baseline pitch range ability, once again have the patient sing up and down a scale in whole notes. This time rate the effort using the dichotomous *correct/incorrect* scale. If at least four of the eight required whole notes are perceptually different from each other, and higher than the lowest note on the "up" side and lower than the highest note on the "down" side of the scale, the performance is rated *correct*. Allow the patient a total of five trials and enter on the Prosody Subsystem Treatment Chart the baseline percentage of correct scores, listing accordingly the date, number of trials, and activity symbol (BP_4) in the corresponding cells of the data column. If this result is equal to or less than 80 percent, proceed to Step 2; otherwise advance as usual to the next exercise.

Step 2. Starting with the lowest musical note possible, sing slowly up the scale in eight whole notes using the vowel /a/ to enable the patient to discriminate the same task ahead. As these notes are sung, use stairstep manual gestures to symbolize the upward pitch progression. Once at the top of the scale, reverse the procedure and sing down in whole notes, this time using the manual gestures to show symbolically the stepwise pitch decline. Ask the patient to try to sing up the scale as demonstrated. Tape recordings can be very helpful for biofeedback and review. Patients who are capable should accompany the pitch changes with corresponding manual gestures as defined above. After each trial, rate the performance using the same scoring procedure described in Step 1.

Step 3. Continue with this method until the patient demonstrates either 75 percent improvement over baseline or a score of 100 percent correct, whichever is less, over 10 consecutive trials. Calculate this target criterion and enter the value in the corresponding cell at the bottom of the data column. After each set of 10 trials, tally from the notepad the percentage correct score and enter the result on the treatment chart in the usual way. Be certain to tag these data with the activity symbol "P_4" in the appropriate cell below the data entry. Advance as usual and as indicated.

Pitch Control Exercise No. 5

Step 1. To establish a baseline, have the patient read aloud one of the passages previously used in testing. Rate the overall performance relative to the pitch modulation characteristics exhibited, using a percentile scoring method. A rating of 100 percent indicates use of exceptional and effective pitch flexibility throughout the passage. Scores that fall below this mark should symbolize respectively poorer pitch modulation control and usage during the oral readings. Allow the patient three different trials, preferably on different passages, and record the mean percentage rating on the Prosody Subsystem Treatment Chart. The activity symbol BP_5 should be listed in the corresponding cell below this entry. Proceed with the next step if this score is equal to or less than 75 percent; otherwise advance to the following exercise.

Step 2. Reproduce on a legal size sheet of paper, in triple space form, one of the reading passages used for baseline testing. Earmark all words in each sentence that naturally, according to the intended message, should be spoken at noticeably different pitch levels, whether higher or lower, than neighboring words. These markings can take the form of up-going or down-going arrows placed above or below encircled target words, as in the following:

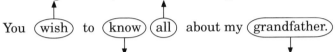

Other creative ways of signaling to the patient when to shift the pitch effectively can be explored, such as color coding target words and writing the target word(s) on the line above if it is to be spoken at a higher pitch, or on the line below if a lower pitch is desired. Demonstrate oral reading of the passage, and briefly discuss the performance along the way, perhaps after each sentence is recited.

Step 3. Request that the patient try the passage next. Each sentence should be judged and discussed independently immediately after it is read aloud. If adequate pitch variability is demonstrated, the sentence is rated *correct*. Failures to modulate pitch accurately according to all the targeted segments of the sentence generate an *incorrect* rating. At the completion of the entire passage, tally the total percentage of sentences produced that were rated correct.

Step 4. Repeat this procedure with the same passage and with other ones until the patient achieves a score that is either 75 percent improved over baseline or 100 percent correct, whichever is less, over 10 consecutive passage recitations. Calculate this target criterion and enter the value in the corresponding cell at the bottom of the data column. After each set of 10 readings, calculate from the notepad the mean percentage correct score and enter the result on the y-axis grid of the treatment chart, making certain to list the appropriate activity symbol (P_5) in the cell at the bottom of the data column. Advance to the next subsection when so indicated.

Pitch Control Exercise No. 6

Note. Practicing pitch modulating control during connected discourse should be introduced next, but need not be rigidly described here. Use of the tape recorder for biofeedback is always helpful.

Treatment of Loudness Control Abnormalities

Normal vocal loudness is influenced by four primary aerodynamic-myoelastic variables: (1) subglottal pressure, (2) glottal resistance, (3) glottal airflow rate, and (4) amplitude of abduction and force of adduction of the vocal folds. As a general rule, increases in these variables transfer proportionally and directly to gains in loudness; decreases induce the opposite effect. Contributing largely to the regulation of these changes are the respiration and phonation subsystems. As such, disturbances of one or both of these subsystems usually cause loudness dyscontrol, a condition that is not unique to one population, as can be seen in Table 7–1. If previously administered treatments of these causally related subsystems have resulted in notable gains, the prognosis for teaching improved loudness control via more direct exercises significantly brightens. Failures at these earlier levels, however, tend to dampen the prospects for improvements at this point in the treatment program. Brief reviews and explanations of the interrelationship between the respiration and phonation subsystems should be offered at the outset so that the patient comprehends the linkage required for success here. Our overall goals are to increase vocal loudness potential, improve loudness variations, and reduce abnormal loudness outbursts.

Loudness Control Exercise No. 1

Step 1. To establish baseline vocal loudness discrimination and listening skills, inform the patient that the task here is twofold: (1) to identify whether pairs of vowels briefly spoken (by the clinician) are of the same loudness or different; and (2) if they are different and perceived as such, the one that is louder must be correctly identified. Note that this exercise is very similar to Pitch Control Exercise no. 1, except that here loudness not pitch distinctions are targeted. For the purpose of practice and discussion, present a pair of vowels to the patient that are grossly different in loudness, and request him or her to respond to them with respect to the above-mentioned task. Discuss the answers and then provide another vowel pair, but this time they should be equally loud. Review the patient's answer again. Once the patient appears to understand the task, start with the baseline data collection process.

Step 2. Follow the same baseline procedural, scoring, rating, charting, and advancement methods as in Pitch Control Exercise no. 1, but substitute "loudness" for the pitch variation stimuli. When entering these baseline data on the Prosody Subsystem Treatment Chart, be certain that the correct activity symbol (BL_1) is used to tag the entry.

Step 3. Follow the same overall treatment methods as in Pitch Control Exercise no. 1, except that here we vary the "loudness" of the stimuli not the pitch. The activity symbol "L_1" is used to represent these data on the treatment chart. Proceed to the next exercise in accordance with the previously defined criterion for advancement. Note that to reduce vocal abuse, the duration of each utterance should be restricted to less than 5 seconds.

Loudness Control Exercise No. 2

Step 1. To establish baseline vocal loudness characteristics, move the patient through the same set of three tasks used in Pitch Control Exercise no. 2. Here, however, the ratings rendered (1 to 7) should correspond to perceptions of "loudness" not pitch control, and each score should be tagged on the treatment chart with the correct respective activity symbol (BL_{2a}, BL_{2b}, or BL_{2c}). Follow the same basic scoring and advancement criteria, naturally making the necessary adjustments for loudness not pitch abnormality descriptions. Be certain to note in the comments section of the treatment chart the specific types of loudness difficulties that the patient initially exhibits.

Step 2.   Follow the same overall procedural, scoring, rating, charting, and advancement methods as in Pitch Control Exercise no. 2. Note that for loud utterances, accompanying hand gestures should be high in the air, and for soft ones the hand is held appreciably lower. Make certain that these treatment data are tagged with the correct activity symbol (L_2) on the chart.

Loudness Control Exercise No. 3

This is the same basic exercise as the preceding one, except that here the first vowel is uttered at a loud level and the second one is spoken softly. Follow the same scoring, rating, charting, and advancement methods detailed in Exercise no. 2, except that all baseline data are represented by the activity symbols "BL_{3a}, BL_{3b}, and BL_{3c}," and the treatment data by the symbol "L_3." Advance to the next exercise as indicated.

Loudness Control Exercise No. 4

Step 1.   Establish baseline loudness variation ability by requesting the patient to prolong the consonant /m/ for roughly 5 seconds at a very soft loudness level. Be sure that the patient *does not* use whispered phonation to accomplish this task. On a notepad, rate the performance either *correct* or *incorrect*. A correct score is awarded if vocal quality is not significantly sacrificed, and the loudness level produced perceptually qualifies as very soft and is maintained throughout the trial. Have the patient repeat the task three more times, increasing with each successive trial the degree of loudness generated; i.e., on the second trial the voice should be soft, on the third it should be relatively loud, and on the last attempt it should be very loud, but not piercing to the ears. Rate each of these trials individually, adjusting the criteria accordingly. Repeat all four levels again to give the patient a second chance to demonstrate baseline skills. At the completion of all trials, calculate from the notepad scores the percentage of correct responses and enter this result on the prosody subsystem behavioral treatment chart in a separate column. Be sure to tag these baseline data with the correct activity symbol (BL_4). If this score is equal to or less than 75 percent, proceed with the next step; otherwise move on to the next exercise.

Step 2.   Use the See-Scape apparatus described previously and a tape recorder with a loudness indicator or a sound level meter. Using a marking pen, draw a line about one-fourth of the way down from the top of the See-Scape tube. Cut a drinking straw into four pieces of differing lengths: 1½, 1, ¾, and ½ inches. Remove the cap of the tube, drop the ½ inch piece of straw on top of the float, and then replace the cap. Position or tape the plastic nasal olive in either nostril, provided each one permits free and unobstructed nasal airflow, and request the patient to prolong the consonant /m/, noting that the float moves in response to the aerodynamic properties of this production, including the level of vocal loudness used. Generally, the speed and degree of float activity are proportional to the loudness level. Instruct the patient to generate loudness sufficient to raise the straw to the line drawn on the tube and maintain it at that level for 5 seconds. Place the V-U meter near the See-Scape apparatus so that the patient can simultaneously glance at the weighted float and indicator for loudness biofeedback. If the production is too loud, the straw will fix at the top of the tube, requiring that the volume be reduced to lower the float into the target area. If the voice is too soft, the straw will not rise high enough, necessitating an increase in loudness to raise the float effectively. Allow the patient to practice for about 1 minute before data collection. When ready the patient is instructed to demonstrate the 5-second task as defined and practiced.

Step 3. On a notepad, rate the effort *correct* if it meets the following criteria: (1) vocal quality is not significantly sacrificed to achieve the target loudness level; (2) the straw remains in the zone of the line drawn or above it, but not in contact with the cap of the tube, for a full 5 seconds; and (3) any deviation of the straw, either too high or low, can only occur once and must be corrected within 2 seconds to the target zone of the tube; otherwise the trial is rated *incorrect*. Repeat the task until the patient achieves a score either 75 percent improved over baseline or 100 percent correct, whichever is less, over 10 consecutive trials. Calculate and enter this target criterion in the corresponding cell at the bottom of the chart. After each set of 10 trials, calculate from the notepad the mean percentage correct score and enter the result in a separate column on the y-axis grid of the treatment chart, using appropriately the activity symbol "L_4" in the cell below to represent these data. Advance when indicated.

Loudness Control Exercise Nos. 5 to 7

These three are identical in methodology to the preceding exercise, except that for Exercise no. 5 the ¾ inch piece of straw is used, for Exercise no. 6 the 1 inch piece, and for Exercise no. 7 the 1½ inch straw. The larger the straw, the more intense the voice must be to achieve criteria. It is advisable periodically to clean the interior of the tube owing to the tendency toward moisture accumulation, which can retard float dynamics and contaminate the data collection process; threading a facial tissue through the tube usually suffices. Make certain that for these three exercises the baseline activity symbols "BL_5, BL_6, and BL_7," respectively, are used, and the treatment data are correspondingly tagged with the symbols "L_5, L_6, and L_7" on the treatment chart.

Loudness Control Exercise No. 8

Step 1. To establish baseline loudness modulating ability, engage the patient in conversation and have him or her describe in detail an action photograph or picture. Using the 7-point interval scale as before, rate specifically the overall flexibility in loudness control exhibited collectively during these tasks. A perceptual rating of "7" may signify either marked reduction in loudness variation (monoloud) or extreme swings in loudness (excess). Less severe disturbances are commensurately rated anywhere along the continuum from "6 to 2." A "1" rating is used when loudness modulations are perceived to be within normal limits. Enter this baseline impression in a separate column on the Prosody Subsystem Treatment Chart, making certain that the activity symbol "BL_8" is used to tag the data. If the patient scores "3" or worse on this measure, proceed with Step 2; otherwise move on to the next exercise.

Step 2. Use the tape recorder with the V U meter and demonstrate once again that the indicator light or needle moves in degree from left to right commensurate with the level of vocal loudness. Vowels, continuant voiced consonants, words, and short sentences may all serve effectively as speech stimuli during this task. Be sure to alter loudness enough for visual biofeedback at many different indicator levels. Deliberately glide in and out of zones on the meter to illustrate both visually and auditorily the effects of loudness modulation during isolated utterances as well as connected discourse.

Step 3. Have prepared on individual index cards the speech stimuli to be used in the exercise. Naturally, try to choose words and sentences that are as meaningful as possible and within the patient's speech repertoire. Shuffle this deck of stimulus cards and present one for practice. Request the patient to produce the sound, word, or sentence with varying degrees of loudness control as demonstrated earlier and measured by the responsive movements of the V-U meter indicator. Allow the patient 1 full minute to practice such variations before the stimulus card is withdrawn. On a notepad, rate the performance relative to the proficiency of loudness modulation demonstrated, using the 7-point scale again as the yardstick of measurement. Present another stimulus card and repeat this procedure until ten 1-minute trials have been permitted.

Step 4. Calculate the mean perceptual rating and enter this result on the treatment chart, making certain to list the appropriate date of data collection, number of trials (10), and activity symbol (L_8) in the corresponding cells of the data column. Continue until the patient achieves a mean perceptual rating at least "3" scale values better than the baseline level or "1," if the baseline score was 3 or 4, over 10 consecutive trials. Calculate and enter this target criterion on the treatment chart, as usual. Remember, as with all other exercises, this one should be discontinued if after 30 consecutive trials there is no discernible improvement trend. Advance to the next exercise as indicated. Note that the loudness modulations generated should not necessarily be prompted or regulated. It is often better to allow the patient to experiment with various levels that feel comfortable rather than to be drilled at predetermined levels.

Loudness Control Exercise No. 9

Step 1. To establish baseline loudness control during connected discourse, engage the patient in conversation about a topic of interest, or if necessary use an action photograph or picture to elicit spontaneous speech. On a notepad, keep track of the time the patient spends using a perceptually soft voice. At the end of 10 minutes of interaction, tally this figure in percentage terms and deduct the score from 100 percent. Enter this baseline value on the treatment chart, using the symbol "BL_9" to represent these data. If this result is equal to or less than 75 percent, proceed with the next step; otherwise move on to the next exercise subsection.

Step 2. Use the tape recorder again and arbitrarily mark off three zones on the V-U meter that are within the loudness range capabilities of the patient. Ideally, the entire range of the meter will be mapped in thirds. From left to right, the first third is the soft voice zone, the second the normally loud voice zone, and the last the loudest voice zone. Engage the patient in discussion again, instructing him or her that the indicator must remain beyond the first zone for at least 75 percent of the time spent talking. Demonstrate that in natural discourse using a conversational loudness level, the indicator generally weaves between the second and third zones for most of the time, slipping down into the soft voice zone at the ends of some statements and when vocal decrescendos have a dramatic communicative effect. As the patient speaks, record as unobtrusively as possible the segments of time during which he or she slips into soft voice. Continue with this interaction, discussing the indicator movements that occur in concert with the loudness levels used to converse with one another.

Step 3. At the completion of 10 minutes of conversation, calculate the percentage of time in which the patient failed to achieve the aforementioned loudness criterion. Subtract this score from 100 percent and enter the result on the treatment chart, making certain to record the correct activity symbol (L_9) in the corresponding cell at the bottom of the data column. Continue with this same method until the patient achieves a score either 75 percent improved over baseline or 100 percent without error, whichever is less, over 10 consecutive minutes of connected discourse. Calculate and enter this target criterion in the corresponding cell at the bottom of the data column. Advance as indicated.

Note. Notwithstanding the likelihood of improvement with these loudness control exercises, especially in patients who have responded favorably to earlier respiration, resonation, phonation, and/or articulation subsystem treatments, some patients may not make significant gains here. In Chapter 5, Case no. 2 illustrates the (potential) usefulness of artificial amplification in a patient who was unable to generate sufficient vocal loudness. Loudness augmentation can be implemented with various other devices to help those who simply do not or cannot benefit from the loudness control behavioral exercises outlined in this subsection.

Treatment of Speaking Rate Disturbances

The rate at which one routinely speaks may influence not only articulatory precision during the production of individual words, but also the overall intelligibility of sentences. Most normal adults speak at an average rate of 150 to 200 words per minute: Somewhere between three and five syllables per second. Oral reading rate tends to be slightly slower. Children use somewhat slower speaking and reading rates. From a phonetic standpoint, the rate of speech is largely dependent on the duration of speech segments or sounds, the number of pauses, and the amount of time spent pausing or in silence. Abnormalities in (1) duration, such as prolonged or shortened sound production; (2) pause time, such as prolonged or shortened intersyllabic or interword intervals; or both may cause the rate to be too slow, too rapid, or inappropriately variable. Table 7–1 shows that difficulty with speaking rate control is a universal problem in patients with motor speech disorders. Incompetence of the articulation subsystem is considered most culpable for these prosodic disturbances, although breakdown of the respiratory, resonatory, and phonatory subsystems may contribute as well. Even if only minimal gains were realized in speech breathing, oral/nasal resonance balance, voice motor control, and/or articulatory proficiency with formal treatment, the bases should provide a springboard for prosodic intervention. When therapy for rate control is indicated, a brief review of the interrelationships between the functions of those subsystems and speaking rate is suggested before initiating treatment. The objectives of these prosodic treatments are (1) to increase rate if the slowness exhibited (a) significantly disturbs speech intelligibility, (b) significantly burdens the listener, and/or (c) can be modified without adversely affecting intelligibility; (2) to decrease the rate if the quickness exhibited (a) significantly disturbs speech intelligibility, (b) does not afford the listener sufficient assimilation time, and/or (c) can be modified without adversely affecting intelligibility; and (3) to train modulation control so that the rate can be effectively and purposefully increased and decreased at the patient's discretion, provided that such stimulation does not adversely affect intelligibility.

Rate Control Exercise No. 1

Step 1. To establish baseline rate discrimination and listening skills, inform the patient that the task here is twofold: (1) to identify whether pairs of sentences read aloud are exactly the same or different with respect to overall rate of presentation; and (2) if they are indeed different and perceived as such, to identify correctly the one that is faster. For practice purposes, read aloud two different sentences, each containing the same number of words (at least 10), which are grossly different in rate. Have the patient differentiate this pair accordingly. Discuss the answers and present another pair of sentences for practice, but this time make the distinctions in rate more subtle, yet obvious. Run through the answers again and then proceed with baseline data collection once it is clear that the patient comprehends the task at hand.

Step 2. Have prepared several different sentences on index cards, each one at least 10 words in length. Randomly assign a fast, slow, or variable speed to each sentence at which it will be recited for discrimination purposes. Shuffle the deck of cards and read aloud the first pair according to their assigned rates. Solicit from the patient the answers to the aforementioned tasks. If the rates are indeed different, the patient ideally will answer that they are not the same and next identify correctly the one that is faster. If the rates of presentation are the same, only one answer is required. All *correct* and *incorrect* responses are rated as such. Repeat this procedure 10 times, selecting for each trial a different pair of sentences from the deck. Tally the total number of correct responses and calculate the percentage score. Enter this baseline result on the Prosody Subsystem Behavioral Treatment Chart, making certain to list the appropriate date, number of trials (10), and activity symbol (BR_1) in the respective cells of the data column. If this score is equal to or less than 75 percent proceed with Step 3; otherwise advance to the next exercise.

Step 3. Continue with the same basic method as in the preceding step. Periodically discuss the patient's correct as well as incorrect responses. Use a notepad to track these scores, and after each set of 10 trials tally and calculate the correct percentage. Enter this result on the treatment chart accordingly. These treatment data are represented by the activity symbol "R_1." Proceed in this way until the patient achieves a mean percentage correct score at least 75 percent improved over baseline or 100 percent correct, whichever is less, over 10 consecutive trials. To identify easily whether or not the patient has achieved this goal, calculate and enter the target criterion in the corresponding cell at the bottom of the treatment chart. Invoke the regular discontinuation rule if necessary. Advance to the next exercise as indicated.

Rate Control Exercise No. 2

Step 1. To establish baseline speaking and oral reading rates, engage the patient in conversation and have him or her read a familiar passage. Tape record these samples. Repeat these tasks with another conversation and reading passage. Replay the tape and count the number of words spoken during each condition (extemporaneous and oral reading) and log the total number of seconds that elapsed while the patient actually spoke in each sample. Average the number of words spoken and seconds that elapsed during each condition. To compute the mean words per minute (WPM), multiply the average number of words for the condition by 60 and divide this figure by the average number of seconds that elapsed during the measures. Thus, if the patient uttered a total of 350 words over the two extemporaneous speaking measures, and the total speaking time was 140 seconds, the mean number of words and seconds equals 175 and 70, respectively: 60 times 175 equals 10,500, which divided by 70 yields a mean WPM score of 150. Perform similar computations for the oral reading data.

Step 2. These scores next need to be converted into percentiles so that the results can be transferred to the grid of the treatment chart. The following arbitrary conversions are recommended: (1) 150 plus WPM equal *100 percent*, (2) 135–149 WPM equal *90 percent*, (3) 120–134 WPM equal *80 percent*, (4) 105–119 WPM equal *70 percent*, (5) 90–104 WPM equal *60 percent*, (6) 75–89 WPM equal *50 percent*, (7) 60–74 WPM equal *40 percent*, (8) 45–59 WPM equal *30 percent*, (9) 30–44 WPM equal *20 percent*, (10) 15–29 WPM equal *10 percent*, and (11) less than 15 WPM equal *0 percent*. These figures assume an average distribution of single, bi-, tri-, and multisyllable words that are spoken with articulatory intelligibility. Whereas unintelligible segments are not computed in the WPM scores, imprecise but fully comprehensible words or sentences are counted. Enter the speaking and reading rate scores separately on the treatment chart, using the activity symbols "BR_{2a} and BR_{2b}," respectively, to tag these data.

Step 3. As a final baseline measure, use the 7-point interval scale to score the rate variability characteristics demonstrated during these samples. That is, if the patient was prone to frequent and marked variations in speed or an unusually flat rate profile throughout the sample, a score of "7" might be applied. Less frequent and milder rate fluctuations or flatness may warrant a score of "2 or 3" on the scale. A score of "1" would symbolize a normal amount of perceived variability. Enter this perceptual rating on the treatment chart in a separate column, making certain to use the activity symbol "BR_{2c}" to tag these data at the bottom of the column.

Step 4. If the patient scores less than 70 percent on either or both of these measures as a result of perceived "slowness," treatments aimed at *increasing* the rate are initially indicated. As such, advance to the steps below in this exercise and continue with Exercise nos. 3 to 6. If the patient scores less than 70 percent as a result of perceived "fastness," which reduced the WPM score because of incomprehensible segments, treatments aimed at *decreasing* the rate to improve speech intelligibility are initially indicated. Thus, skip this exercise and Exercise nos. 3-6 and advance directly to Exercise nos. 7 to 11. Rapid rate may not necessarily result in a reduced WPM score, but the fast pace may be quite taxing to the listener because it is perceptually difficult to follow. Thus, even if the patient does not score less than 70 percent but is judged to need rate reduction therapy to smooth out the prosodic envelope, advancement to Exercise nos. 7 to 11 is still indicated. If the primary rate control problem is neither slowness nor fastness alone, but "excess or reduced variability," as determined by a perceptual rating of "3" or worse, treatments aimed at improving rate modulation are initially indicated. For such a patient, proceed from here directly to Exercise no. 12. If these baseline results do not lend support to the need for rate control therapy at all, move on to the Intonation treatment subsection.

Step 5. To *Increase the Rate of Speech,* begin by explaining to the patient the potential perceptual and sociolinguistic hazards of speaking too slowly. Review the audiotapes made and discuss the overall objective of this exercise, which is to stimulate the fastest rate possible without adversely affecting articulatory proficiency or the listener's ability to assimilate the message. At the outset it is important to discuss the fact that a slower than so-called "normal" rate of speech is usually the therapeutic target for most patients. Before getting started here, it should be understood that aspiring to normally fast rates of control may result in frustration and failure. Be ready to tape record all performances for periodic review and biofeedback.

Step 6. Use the metronome and set it at 150 beats per minute (bpm). Demonstrate recitation of the alphabet, one letter per beat, without time out until the end. Explain that the task here is to stay on beat, as demonstrated, articulating each letter as precisely as possible. Each production will be graded individually as either *correct* or *incorrect*. If the letter is produced on the beat and inherent (baseline) articulatory precision is not discernibly worsened, a correct rating is rendered. Set the metronome in motion and allow the patient to begin at his or her own discretion. Once started, however, the entire alphabet must be performed before a break is permitted; aborting the task prematurely generates incorrect ratings equal to the number of beats that occur without corresponding letter productions. At the completion of the trial, a maximum correct score of 26 (100 percent), or some combination of correct/incorrect scores that equal 26, is possible. Tally either the correct or incorrect productions, whichever is less burdensome, as the patient performs the task. After the trial, calculate the percentage of correct productions and discuss the effort, its characteristics, and the score rendered. Review the audiotape for demonstrative purposes, if desirable. Repeat this procedure until the patient achieves a mean correct percentage of 80 or better over 10 consecutive trials.

Step 7.   At the completion of each set of 10 trials, calculate the mean percentage correct score from the notepad and enter this result on the grid of the Prosody Subsystem Treatment Chart, making certain to list the date, number of trials (10), and activity symbol (R_2) in the corresponding cells of the data column. Invoke the usual discontinuation rule if necessary. Advance to the next exercise in sequence, also designed to stimulate an increase in speaking rate, when indicated. *Note:* If the patient masters this task, experimentation with faster rates may prove worthwhile before advancing to the next exercise. Conversely, failure at this rate demands attempts at a slower speed before abandoning the exercise as useless.

Rate Control Exercise No. 3

Step 1.   Follow the exact same baseline method detailed in the preceding exercise. These data, however, are tagged with the activity symbols "BR_{3a}, BR_{3b}, and BR_{3c}," respectively, on the treatment chart. Advance to the steps below if an increase in rate is still indicated; otherwise proceed to Exercise no. 12, which is designed to train rate modulation control.

Step 2.   Follow the exact same rate increase treatment procedures detailed in Steps 5 to 7 of the preceding exercise, except that for this exercise we have the patient count from 1 to 10, not recite the alphabet, to the beat of the metronome. Note that the speed of the metronome is set at 150 bpm for this task as well. Demonstrate the task by counting from 1 to 10 two times in a row without stopping, allowing only one number per beat. Grade each number individually as either *correct* or *incorrect*. If the number is produced according to and in proper timing with the beat, and inherent (baseline) articulatory precision is not discernibly worsened, a correct rating is rendered.

Step 3.   On a notepad, keep track of the correct or incorrect scores as the patient counts to 10, two times in a row, to the beat of the metronome. Remember that at the completion of the trial a maximum correct score of 20 (100 percent), or some combination of correct/incorrect scores that total to 20, is possible. Follow the same review, scoring, charting, and advancement methods discussed in the preceding exercise, making certain to use the activity symbol "R_3" to represent the data collected and entered on the treatment chart.

Rate Control Exercise No. 4

Step 1.   Again, employ the baseline methods discussed in Exercise no. 2. Tag these data, however, with the activity symbols "BR_{4a}, BR_{4b}, and BR_{4c}," respectively, on the treatment chart. Advance to the steps below if the need to increase rate is still indicated; otherwise proceed to Exercise no. 12, designed to stimulate improvements in rate modulation control.

Step 2.   To further stimulate an *Increase in Speaking Rate,* have prepared individually on index cards well-rehearsed sentences, phrases and passages, that are familiar to the patient. Unique sayings, memorized scripts and songs, the Pledge of Allegiance, the Lord's Prayer, and so forth are excellent material for this exercise. Shuffle the cards, be ready to tape record the performances, and use the metronome again; set it at 150 bpm and select at random one of the index cards for demonstration purposes. Recite the passage to the beat, one syllable per beat continuously until completion. Note that the performance will lack intonation contour and sound automated or artificial. Instruct the patient that this result is a natural consequence of the task, as rate improvement is the main objective here. Also assure the patient that periodic skips of the beat for breathing purposes will not be penalized, so long as these do not disrupt fluidity by occurring too frequently. Lengthy passages, those that may require more than 1 minute to recite, can be broken into desirable segments, perhaps 45 seconds each, separated by brief rest periods. Explain to the patient that the task is to produce one syllable, *not one word,* per beat. That multisyllable words require as many beats to complete their productions must be demonstrated to ensure comprehension of the full task. Discuss the grading system. Each word is to be rated individually as either *correct* or *incorrect*. If the entire word is produced according to and in proper timing with the required number of beats and if inherent (baseline) articulatory precision is not discernibly worsened, a correct rating is rendered.

Step 3.   Set the metronome in motion as usual, and instruct the patient to begin at his or her discretion. Once started, however, the task continues until completion of the passage or the designated rest period. Throughout the performance, tally either the correct or incorrect productions, whichever seems least difficult to track. After the entire performance, calculate the percentage of correctly produced words in the passage. Discuss this result and the characteristics of the trial. Review the tape recording if deemed helpful. Repeat this procedure, randomly alternating the index card in use, until the patient achieves a mean correct percentage of 80 or better over 10 consecutive trials (target criterion).

Step 4.   At the completion of each set of 10 trials, tally and calculate the mean percentage correct score and enter this result on the treatment chart grid, listing accordingly the date, number of trials (10), and activity symbol (R_4) in the corresponding cells of the data column. As usual, advance when indicated to the next exercise in sequence, also designed to stimulate an increase in speaking rate. *Note:* As with the previous rate control exercises, if the patient masters this task, experimentation with faster rates may prove worthwhile before advancing to the next exercise.

Rate Control Exercise No. 5

Step 1. Once again, follow the baseline procedures of Exercise no. 2, except that these results are tagged with the activity symbols "BR_{5a}, BR_{5b}, and BR_{5c}," respectively. Advance to the steps below if the need to increase rate is still indicated; otherwise proceed to Exercise no. 12 for rate modulation stimulation.

Step 2. To stimulate further an *Increased Rate of Speech,* have prepared on index cards many sentences of varying lengths, one sentence per card. Try to design these sentences so that each one is composed of a mixture of mono-, bi-, tri-, and multisyllable words. Whenever possible, construct sentences that may be meaningful to the patient and that contain words within his or her phonetic-linguistic repertoire. In addition, have available standard passages such as *My Grandfather, The Rainbow Passage,* or *Arthur The Rat* for use during this exercise. Familiar reading passages are acceptable as well. Randomly select one of these sentences for demonstration purposes. Read it aloud at a rate perceptually comparable with the one practiced last in the preceding exercise. Discuss the speed of word production and point out that maintaining articulatory proficiency is an important requirement of the performance. For comparative reasons, now repeat the same stimulus at a noticeably slower rate of speech, and review the distinctions between this performance and the previously faster one. Explain the following grading policy for this exercise. Each performance will be tape recorded and timed so that the average number of WPM can ultimately be calculated. Only those words that are comprehensible will be considered in this average; thus, articulatory proficiency, as noted above, is vital to the total score. Imprecision is not penalized provided that the word is intelligible. Have available a stopwatch or wristwatch with a second hand to time each performance.

Step 3. Present the patient with a stimulus card and request that the sentence or passage be read aloud at the same basic rate (or faster, if manageable) as just demonstrated. As soon as the patient begins, start the stopwatch. The clock stops upon completion of the last word. On a notepad, record the number of intelligible words produced. Multiply this number by 60, and divide the result by the number of seconds that elapsed to read the entire sentence aloud. This figure is the "word per minute" equivalent. Use the conversion table in Exercise no. 2, Step 2 to determine the percentile score for the performance. Review the tape recording and score with the patient. Discuss any necessary ways to modify the next trial. Repeat this procedure, periodically switching the stimulus item, until the patient achieves a mean percentile score at least 75 percent improved over the oral reading baseline or 100 percent (150+ WPM), whichever is less, over 10 consecutive trials. Calculate and enter this target criterion in the corresponding cell of the treatment chart.

Step 4. At the completion of each set of 10 trials, tally and calculate the mean WPM percentile from the notepad scores and enter this result on the treatment chart grid, making certain to tag these data with the activity symbol "R_5" in the corresponding cell at the bottom of the column. Advance to the next exercise when this criterion is met, or after invocation of the usual discontinuation rule.

Rate Control Exercise No. 6

Step 1. To establish, once again, baseline conversational speaking rate, follow the method outlined in Exercise no. 2 for the connected discourse measure only. Tag this baseline result with the activity symbol "BR_6" on the treatment chart, and proceed with the step below if required; otherwise move on to the rate modulation (Exercise no. 12) regimen.

Step 2. To stimulate an *Increased Rate of Speech* during connected discourse, engage the patient in conversation about topics of interest. Remind him or her of the importance of maintaining any previous gains made in rate of speech; it must be appreciated that carry-over to extemporaneous use has been the ultimate treatment goal. To track and score the patient, tape record all segments of conversation. The WPM grading criteria adopted in the preceding exercises is used here also. After a 3- to 5-minute sample has been recorded, replay the tape and review the rate characteristics of the performance with the patient. During this analysis, use the notepad to score all correctly produced words. At the end of the sample, compute the WPM score in the usual way. Convert this result into a percentile score using the aforementioned table in Exercise No. 2.

Step 3. Continue with this same basic procedure through a variety of conversational samples until the patient achieves a mean percentile score that is at least 75 percent improved over baseline or 100 percent (150+ WPM), whichever is less, over 10 consecutive minutes of conversation. As usual, list the target criterion on the chart as a handy reference. At the completion of each set of 10 minutes, tally and calculate the WPM percentile from the notepad score sheet and enter the result on the treatment chart grid. Make certain that these data are tagged with the correct date, number of trials (10 minutes), and activity symbol "R_6" in the corresponding cells of the column. Advance to the rate modulation (Exercise no. 12) regimen upon achievement of this criterion, or if the discontinuation rule was invoked here owing to poor treatment effects.

Rate Control Exercise No. 7

Step 1. The baseline data collected in Exercise no. 2 are used to direct this exercise. Use the symbols "BR_{7a}, BR_{7b}, and BR_{7c}" respectively, to tag these data on the treatment chart.

Step 2. To *Decrease the Rate of Speech* begin by explaining to the patient the overall negative articulation and listener perception effects of speaking too rapidly. Review the audiotape baseline samples and discuss the characteristic rate difficulties exhibited by the patient. Describe the objective of this exercise, which is to stimulate a slower rate of speech so as to facilitate (1) articulatory proficiency and (2) decoding of the message by listeners. It is important at the outset of this exercise regimen to explain that most patients benefit when they slow the rate of their speech, because slowing down affords coordinate speech subsystem activities. Mention that in fact slowing the speaking rate will likely increase, not decrease, the average number of *intelligible* words per minute. The key here is the term "intelligible." Speaking rapidly is almost always excessive and unnecessary, especially if the speed burdens the listener and interferes with articulatory precision. The patient must also be taught that this regimen does not aim for a so-called "normal" rate of speech. Rather, the target rate will be somewhat slower than normal. Assure the patient that such overcompensation has proved through experience to be a necessity for most patients whose speech motor difficulties are attributable, at least in part, to rapid-fire rate. Be ready to tape record all performances for periodic review and biofeedback.

Step 3. Use the metronome and set it at 100 bpm. Follow the exact same procedures detailed in Steps 6 and 7 of Exercise no. 2; however, use the activity symbol "R_7" to tag these data on the Prosody Subsystem Treatment Chart. Experimentation with faster rates may be attempted upon successful achievement at this speed, but with caution in that for many patients, faster rates may induce intelligibility breakdown. Advance to the next exercise in sequence when so indicated.

Rate Control Exercise No. 8

This exercise to *Decrease the Rate of Speech* is identical to Exercise no. 3, except that here the metronome is set at 100 bpm and the activity symbols "BR_{8a}, BR_{8b}, BR_{8c}" and "R_8" are used to represent these baseline and treatment data, respectively, on the treatment chart.

Rate Control Exercise No. 9

This exercise to *Decrease the Rate of Speech* is identical to Exercise no. 4, except that here the metronome is set at 100 bpm and the activity symbols "BR_{9a}, BR_{9b}, BR_{9c}" and "R_9" are used to represent these baseline and treatment data, respectively.

Rate Control Exercise No. 10

Step 1. Repeat the baseline method detailed in Exercise no. 2. In addition, using the 7-point interval scale, render a perceptual rating of the degree of rapid speaking rate present during these baseline measures. A score of "7" is symbolic of rapid, nonproficient speech that almost always negatively influences intelligibility. A score of "4" is given for moderately rapid speech that impairs the overall speech proficiency profile. A score of "1" represents perceived normal rate. Proceed with the next step if the percentile score is less than "70," as described in Step 4 of Exercise no. 2, or the perceptual rating is equal to or worse than "3"; otherwise advance to Exercise no. 12 for rate modulation training. Note that the activity symbols "BR_{10a}, BR_{10b}, BR_{10c}, and BR_{10d}," respectively, are used to tag these baseline data on the treatment chart.

Step 2. To *Decrease the Rate of Speech,* prepare the sentence and reading passage material described in Step 2 of Exercise no. 5. Strategically underline some of the words in each sentence and passage assembled. In addition, place slash (//) marks in key locations within each sentence and passage. The underlined words are to be read (even) more slowly than the neighboring words, and where a slash appears the patient must noticeably pause in silence before reading aloud the next word. For example, "My grandfather. You wish to know // all about *my* grandfather. Well, // he is nearly 93 years old, yet // he still thinks as swiftly as // ever . . ." Select one of the sentences for demonstration purposes and read it aloud at a rate perceptually comparable to the one practiced in the last exercise, making certain to increase the duration of both the words underlined and the pauses highlighted by slash marks. Discuss the reading and then repeat the task at a deliberately fast rate, with disregard for the marked segments for comparative review. Explain that for grading purposes each performance will be tape recorded and timed, so that ultimately the average number of WPM can be calculated. It should be made clear to the patient that only words produced intelligibly will be computed in this average, so that attention is focused during practice not only on rate but on overall proficiency.

Step 3. Present the patient with a stimulus card and request that the sentence or passage be read aloud slowly with special adherence to the underlined words and slash marks, as discussed and demonstrated. As soon as the patient begins, start the stopwatch. The clock stops upon completion of the last word. Replay the tape recording for review of the performance with the patient. On a notepad, record the number of intelligible words produced and multiply this amount by 60. Divide the result by the number of seconds that elapsed for the entire reading to derive the WPM equivalent. Use the conversions in Exercise no. 2, Step 2, to determine the percentile score for this performance. Review the score with the patient and discuss the nuances of the performances relative to rate control, speech precision, and overall communication impact. Repeat the procedure, periodically varying the stimulus item, until the patient achieves (1) a mean percentile score at least 75 percent improved over the oral reading baseline level or 80 percent (120 to 134 WPM), whichever is less, over 10 consecutive trials; and/or (2) a mean perceptual rating at least "3" scale values better than the baseline score or "1," if the baseline score was 3 or 4, over the same 10 consecutive trials.

Step 4. At the completion of each set of 10 trials, tally and calculate the mean WPM percentile score from the notepad recordings and enter this result on the treatment chart grid, making certain to tag this entry with the activity symbol "R_{10a}" in the corresponding cell at the bottom of the column. Also, enter the mean perceptual rating on the grid in a separate column, tagging these data with the activity symbol "R_{10b}." Advance to the next exercise when the criteria are met here, or if the discontinuation rule was employed.

Note. Before abandoning this exercise as useless for the patient struggling to adjust speaking rate, take a blank index card and make a slot (1½ by ½ inches) in the center. Use this window to reveal one or two words at a time in a sentence stimulus and try the oral reading task again, moving the card slowly across the sentence as each word is spoken. Slow tapping of a finger or the foot in unison with the words slowly spoken may also prove helpful. Some clinicians find use of a pegboard, pacing board or finger pacing device, similarly useful in decreasing (or for that matter increasing or varying) the rate of speech. For one patient with severe mixed hypokinetic-ataxic dysarthria with co-occurring rapid speaking rate, secondary to a closed head injury, we used small strips of Velcro material to create a pacing device. One strip was wrapped around the patient's index finger and the other around the opposing thumb. When brought into contact with one another by a light pinching force, these rings stick together. The fingers separate the rings with a noticeable drag, owing to the resistance of the Velcro material. The patient practiced the exercise stimuli, pacing his utterances with separation of the Velcro rings. Speaking rate was decreased, although there was no apparent rhythm or pattern to the technique. It seemed that intermittent rather than continuous Velcro separation was all that the patient needed to stimulate rate control. He wore the rings all day long, using them as needed during conversational speaking situations.

Rate Control Exercise No. 11

Step 1. Employ the exact same baseline methods as those used in the preceding exercise. Use the symbols "BR_{11a}, BR_{11b}, BR_{11c}, and BR_{11d}" to tag these data on the treatment chart.

Step 2. Follow the same basic treatment method detailed in Exercise No. 6, except that here stimulation of a *Decreased Rate of Speech* during connected discourse is emphasized, and the criteria for improvement are different. For this exercise, adopt the methods for advancement employed in Steps 3 and 4 of the preceding exercise. All data collected here receive the activity symbol "R_{11a}" (percentile scores) or "R_{11b}" (perceptual ratings). Advance to the rate modulation exercise regimen next in sequence.

Rate Control Exercise No. 12

Step 1. For patients who enter this exercise directly from Exercise no. 2, the baseline data just collected in that exercise serve to direct these events. Patients who have arrived here from either the preceding rate increase (Exercise nos. 2 to 6) or decrease (Exercise nos. 7 to 11) regimen require baseline testing of rate modulation or variability control to determine the need for intervention.

Collect these data by engaging the patient in conversation about topics of interest and having him or her read aloud various sentences, short stories, and familiar passages. Using the 7-point interval scale, render a composite perceptual rating of such control. As specified earlier in Exercise no. 2, a score of "7" might be
offered if the patient exhibits wide, frequent, and injudicious swings in the speaking rate used throughout these samples. Similarly, a markedly flat rate profile,
wherein no signs of variability are displayed, would also warrant a rating of "7."
On the other hand, a less conspicuous moderate rate deficit or flatness is scored a
"4." When a "1" rating is awarded, this score symbolizes a perceived degree of
normal rate variability. If the patient receives a score equal to or worse than "3"
on this scale, advance to the next step. Enter this result on the Prosody Subsystem Treatment Chart in a separate column, making certain to list the activity
symbol "BR_{12}" in the corresponding cell at the bottom of the data column. Proceed directly to the Intonation subsection if rate modulation therapy is not indicated.

    Step 2. To stimulate *Rate Modulation Control,* assemble reading materials
familiar and of interest to the patient such as short stories, quotations, special
passages from the Bible, and so forth. On a copy that can be marked strategically, lace these material stimuli with the symbols ⊢⊣ , ⊢——⊣ , or ⊢————⊣ ,
which require that the words following the symbol be read quickly, at normal
speed, or slowly, respectively. For example, ⊢————⊣ My grandfather. ⊢⊣ You
wish to know ⊢——⊣ all about my grandfather. ⊢⊣ Well, he is nearly ⊢——⊣ 93
years old, yet he still thinks ⊢——⊣ as quickly as ever. He dresses himself
⊢————⊣ in an old black frock coat, ⊢⊣ usually several buttons missing. ⊢——⊣ A
long beard clings to his chin, ⊢⊣ giving those who observe him ⊢————⊣ a pronounced feeling ⊢⊣ of utmost respect . . . and so on. Demonstrate the passage
and discuss the rate variability used. Have ready a tape recorder for biofeedback
of the patient's performances.

    Step 3. Present the patient with a prepared stimulus passage and request
that he or she read it aloud following the speed limit signs accordingly. Replay
the tape recording and analyze the performance with the patient. Perceptually
rate the effort according to the following criteria: (1) a score of "1" is earned if the
patient moves efficiently and accurately from one prompt to the next throughout
the entire trial, demonstrating "normal" rate variability control; (2) a score of "7"
is levied if the patient miserably and consistently fails to exhibit smooth and accurate transitions from prompt to prompt, rendering the effort devoid of rate
modulation control; and (3) scores of "2 to 6" are given in recognition of different
levels of rate variability dyscontrol, with "2," "4," and "6," respectively, representative of mild, moderate, and severe difficulties making the requisite speed shifts.
Repeat this procedure, periodically varying the stimulus, until the patient
achieves a mean perceptual rating at least "3" scale values better than the baseline score or "1" if the baseline score was 3 or 4, over 10 consecutive trials. Calculate and enter this target criterion in the respective cell at the base of the
treatment chart.

    Step 4. At the completion of each set of 10 trials, calculate the mean rating and record this result on the treatment chart, using the activity symbol "R_{12}" to represent these data. Move on to the next exercise in the sequence.

Rate Control Exercise No. 13

Step 1. To establish baseline rate modulation control during connected discourse engage the patient in conversation and render a perceptual rating of such ability. Follow the rating criteria established in Step 1 of the preceding exercise. If the patient earns a score of "3" or worse, advance to the next step; otherwise proceed directly to the Intonation treatment subsection. Remember, these baseline data are tagged with the symbol "BR_{13}" on the treatment chart.

Step 2. Use the tape player to record conversational samples. Remind the patient of the primary objective here, which is to learn to transfer rate modulation control to extemporaneous speaking situations. Discuss the importance of periodically varying the rate of speech. Using examples, differentiate flat, excessive, and normal amounts of rate variability during connected discourse. Have the patient attempt to mimic these differences, and tape record the trials for review. After each set of 10 minutes of conversation, discussion, and tape review, render a perceptual rating of the patient's rate-modulating ability and enter this score on the treatment chart, listing as always the date, number of trials (10 minutes), and activity symbol (R_{13}) in the corresponding cells of the data column.

Step 3. Continue with this method until the patient achieves a perceptual rating that is at least "3" scale values better than the baseline score or "1" if the baseline score was 3 or 4, over 20 consecutive minutes. Advance to the next exercise, designed to improve intonation, when this criterion is met or when the discontinuation rule is invoked owing to poor treatment effects.

Treatment of Intonation Disturbances

Intonation refers to the rise and fall and variability in the pitch of the voice, frequently as they are associated with stress. Intonation patterns in the English language use three different pitch levels; low, modal, and high, as adjuncts of stress and to indicate the purpose or meaning of a message. For example, to emphasize a specific word in a phrase or sentence we generally use higher pitch and increased loudness and duration. To convey a question we usually raise the pitch at the end of a sentence, except when the sentence begins with an interrogative (wh) word, in which case we most often drop the pitch at the end of the question. If, however, such a sentence ends with a rising pitch, it calls for repetition or confirmation of an answer already provided. To make a statement requires that we lower pitch at the end of a sentence to signal finality.

Many patients use inappropriate pitch levels at phrase endings, which tend to obscure the true meaning of the information trying to be conveyed. Patients whose pitch variations are minimal because of narrow range (monopitch) frequently come across (affectively) as unemotional, dull, and detached. Because of the strong interrelationship between intonation, pitch control, and loudness, improvement of impaired intonation is often proportionally contingent on the outcome of the pitch and loudness exercises stressed previously. It is important to note that patients who make minimal gains in these earlier treatments generally fail to succeed with the intonation exercises described below. The objectives of these plans include the use of pitch changes effectively to impart emphasis and convey accurate attitudes, feelings, and intentions. These objectives are also incorporated into the Stress Control treatment subsection presented later.

Intonation Contour Activity No. 1

To practice *statements,* prepare numerous declarative sentences, some simple and some complex, on index cards. Use the numerals 1, 2, and 3 in the margin to the left of the sentence to govern low, modal, and high pitch use, respectively, when reading the sentence aloud. Remind the patient that the most emphasized or operative word is spoken at the highest pitch level, and the last word ends on a low note in a declarative sentence. Failure to adopt these intonation patterns may not only confuse the listener as to the meaning of the sentence, but also limit his or her ability to shift focus to upcoming information. The following sentences are examples of this type of practice material:

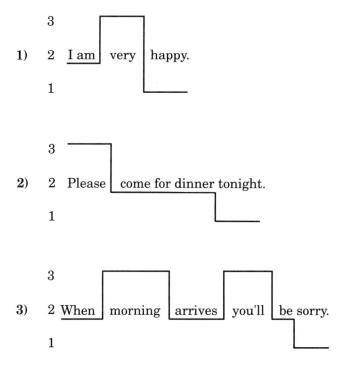

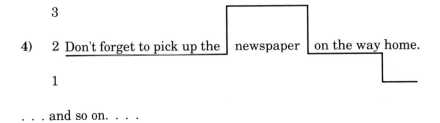

4)   2 <u>Don't forget to pick up the</u> | newspaper | <u>on the way home.</u>

. . . and so on. . . .

Using a tape recorder for biofeedback and altering emphasized words to illustrate how varying intonation patterns may induce slight as well as dramatic influences on sentence meaning may prove useful.

Intonation Contour Activity No. 2

To practice *questions,* prepare sentences in much the same way as recommended above. Remind the patient that a sentence can usually be converted into a question by raising the pitch on the last word or syllable spoken. Sometimes it is necessary to glide from high (3) to even higher (3+) pitch at the end of a sentence that calls for an answer. Patients who struggle with this requirement are often frustrated when listeners fail to respond to their questions.

The following sentences are examples of this type of practice material:

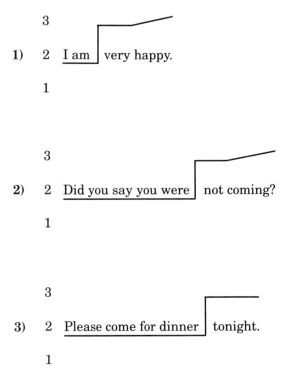

1)   2 <u>I am</u> | very happy.

2)   2 <u>Did you say you were</u> | not coming?

3)   2 <u>Please come for dinner</u> | tonight.

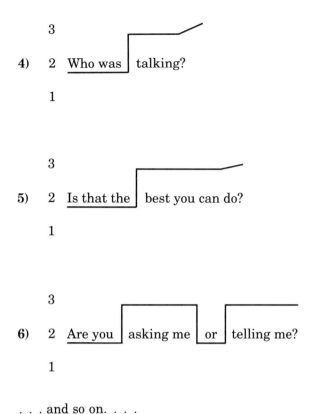

4)   2   Who was | talking?

5)   2   Is that the | best you can do?

6)   2   Are you | asking me | or | telling me?

. . . and so on. . . .

Experimentation with various alternative contours at the ends of these sentences should highlight the importance of the inflections practiced.

Intonation Contour Activity No. 3

To practice *questions* that cannot be answered with yes/no replies but instead require information, prepare additional sentences on index cards. Instruct the patient that for these types of sentences, usually beginning with interrogative (wh) words, the most emphasized words are pronounced at high pitch levels followed by a drop to low pitch at the close. Negative practice can be very effective here, as incorrect pitch use may induce unusual, unexpected deviations from the intended question. A tape recorder is useful for biofeedback and review.

The following sentences are examples of this type of practice material:

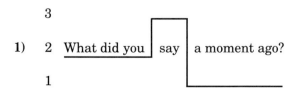

1)   2   What did you | say | a moment ago?

2)

   3

2 <u>What</u> | time | is it?

   1

3)

   3

2 <u>When will you be</u> | coming | home?

   1

4)

   3

2 <u>Why are you</u> | go | ing?

   1

5)

   3

2 <u>Whose</u> | turn is it | to buy dinner?

   1

6)

   3

2 <u>Where do you</u> live?

   1

7)

   3

2 How | come you | always | arrive late?

   1

Intonation Contour Activity No. 4

Sometimes sentences led by interrogative words can be spoken in such a way as to call not for an informative answer, but rather for repetition or confirmation of one already offered. For example, said this way,

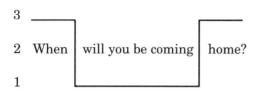

the speaker conveys surprise in response to arrival news from a roommate who was thought to be due home *after* the holiday weekend. Here the rising pitch at the beginning and end of the sentence accomplishes the objective of discovery. Practice variations of this theme with the patient. Include permutations that convert interrogative sentences into rhetorical ones by strategic use of pitch inflections. Meaning to induce his or her own answer, a speaker might query,

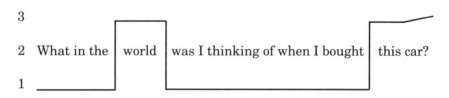

Intonation Contour Activity No. 5

To practice intonation control in *phrases,* long sentences, familiar paragraphs, and passages can be prepared as practice material. To divide these stimuli into acceptable phrases, use slash marks. Curved lines, signaling the need for gradual pitch declinations or glides on single syllables, may also be helpful markers.

The following passages are examples of material that may be constructed for this purpose:

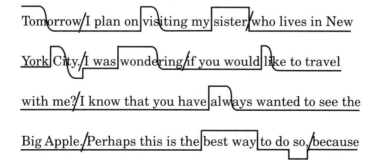

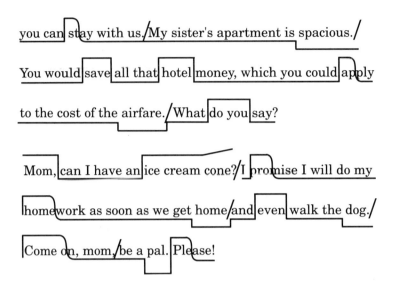

Treatment of Stress Control Disturbances

Syllables, words, and groups of words spoken emphatically, so that they achieve prominence in the message, are considered *stressed*. Normal speakers rarely use stress indiscriminately. Rather, words of the greatest importance to the meaning of the message are emphasized; others remain relatively unstressed, thereby striking a prosodic balance in ongoing speech. Generally, stress is accomplished by increasing the pitch, duration, and loudness of the target. Empirically, adequate pitch control, loudness and duration appear to be indispensable to proper use of stress. In virtually all speaking situations, stress may be placed on more than one target within a sentence or phrase, although one target (of greatest importance) receives the heaviest amount of stress.

Stress patterns differ from one language to the next. Variations in pitch, loudness, and duration in one language that represent standard, logical and emotional usage, with which native speakers identify may be unrecognizable patterns if translated without modification into another language; e.g. Scandinavian in English. As a rule, if the type and degree of stress that a speaker uses evoke negative listener reaction, obfuscate or even change the meaning of the message, or both, stress control intervention is indicated. In Table 7–1 we see, among the abnormal speech features exhibited by ataxic and apractic patients, difficulty with stress control. It should be understood, however, that other types of patients, most notably those with pitch, loudness, and rate dyscontrol features, frequently exhibit associated stress abnormalities as well. Because of the natural prosodic interrelationship between stress use and pitch, loudness, and rate of speech, treatment for *stress* dyscontrol is best delayed until this point in the sequence of prosody subsystem exercises. Of course, all earlier therapy provided, including measures to improve functions of the other speech subsystems, should influence the outcome of the exercises below. Poor results during prerequisite treatment generally cast a shadow on the prognosis for improvement with stress therapy.

Patients who have shown gains in therapy with related subsystem disturbances generally respond favorably to this phase of intervention. The program below is designed to improve stress control in isolated words, sentences, and phrases. In these exercises different symbols are used to designate heavy stress (/), light stress (/), pausing (//), and articulation time (:). The program also introduces the method popularly called *contrastive stress drill.*

Basic Stress Control Exercise No. 1

Step 1. To establish baseline stress control skills, engage the patient in conversation for at least 5 minutes and award a perceptual rating, using the 7-point interval scale relative to the accuracy of the stress patterns exhibited. A score of "7" represents the most deviant degree from normal; a "4" moderate impairment, and a "1" rating denotes normal stress control. Enter this rating in a separate column on the Prosody Subsystem Treatment Chart, making certain to list the date, number of trials (5 minutes), and activity symbol (BS_{1a}) in the corresponding cells of the data column.

Step 2. In addition, prepare on index cards at least 30 common phrases and general sentences (like those below) to be used to measure baseline stress. *Note: Do not* include the diacritical stress symbols on the cards presented to the patient for measures of *baseline* oral reading: (1) Brush // your // teeth; (2) Come in; (3) Turn on // the light; (4) Shut // your // mouth; (5) Get lost; (6) Close // the // door; (7) Take // a // walk; (8) Bread and butter; (9) I have invited // Mary and John // to join us for dinner // this evening; . . . and so on. Keep in mind that slight variations from these recommended stress patterns are permissible provided that the basic meanings are preserved. If the entire sentence is read aloud without error, it is rated *correct;* otherwise an *incorrect* rating is rendered. Enter the mean correct percentage of all baseline trials on the grid of the Prosody Subsytem Treatment Chart, using the symbol "BS_{1b}" to represent these data. If the patient scores less than 75 percent here and/or receives a perceptual rating equal to or worse than "3" on the preceding baseline measure, proceed with treatment in Step 3; otherwise advance to the next exercise.

Step 3. Have ready for use several two-, three-, and four-word phrases that are within the scope of the patient's interests and language skills, no more than three examples per index card, all of which shall include the proper primary and secondary stress marker symbols. Shuffle the deck of cards prepared and draw one for demonstration purposes. If, for example, the phrase "salt and pepper" is drawn, read it aloud for the patient, using the appropriate stress patterns. Then, deliberately produce the phrase with inappropriate stress, such as "salt and pepper" or salt and pepper." Discuss these distinctions and provide another example, such as "don't // stop," which calls for the cessation of an activity. Explain and discuss this production. Now present the same phrase using a different twist of stress, such as "don't stop," which conveys the desire for continuation. Discuss these contrary results and the obvious communicative effects of stress variation, whether intended or not. Provide a sufficient number of examples to ensure the patient's comprehension of the task as well as perceptions of the error patterns.

Step 4.   Be prepared to tape record all patient performances for review and biofeedback. Present a card to the patient that contains three different phrases and request that he or she read one aloud with special adherence to the stress markers. After the reading, discuss the performance and any errors exhibited. Review the tape recording for additional feedback. If stress pattern errors were identified, have the patient repeat the phrase, trying this time to improve on the preceding effort. Discuss the second attempt, permit one more trial if further improvement is necessary, and then shift to another phrase whether or not the third reading was without error. Grade each attempt individually on a notepad as either *correct* or *incorrect,* as defined in Step 2 above. Continue with this procedure until the patient achieves a mean percentage of correct responses at least 75 percent improved over the baseline (BS_{1b}) score or 100 percent correct, whichever is less, over 10 consecutive trials using different phrases. Calculate and list the target criterion in the corresponding cell at the bottom of the treatment chart.

Step 5.   At the completion of each set of 10 trials, calculate the mean percentage of correct responses and enter the result on the grid of the treatment chart in the usual way. Be sure to use the correct activity symbol (S_1) to tag this data column. Advance to the next exercise when the target criterion is met, or as usual if the patient fails to demonstrate an observable trend of improvement after 30 consecutive trials.

Basic Stress Control Exercise No. 2

Step 1.   Employ the exact same baseline methodology used in the preceding exercise. Advance as indicated, noting use of the symbols "BS_{2a} and BS_{2b}" for these data on the treatment chart.

Step 2.   Have ready for use several general sentences of varying lengths, no more than two examples per index card, all of which contain primary and secondary stress markers as well as pause symbols to which the patient will be expected to adhere. Select a sentence for demonstration purposes. If, for example, the sentence, "I plan to order a pizza // not Chinese food // for dinner tonight" is selected, read it aloud and abide by the markers without deviation. Then, deliberately use inappropriate and even bizarre stress patterns when repeating the same sentence for illustrative negative practice. An unconventional reading may sound like this: "I // plan to order // a pizza not // Chinese food for // dinner tonight." Discuss these differences and provide other examples to ensure that the patient understands the task and correct/incorrect distinctions before proceeding with the next step.

Step 3.   Be prepared to tape record the patient's performance. Present a card to the patient containing a stimulus sentence, and request that it be read aloud with careful attention to the stress markers. Follow the exact same procedures as in Steps 4 and 5 of the preceding exercise, making certain that all these data entries on the treatment chart are tagged with the appropriate activity symbol (S_2). Advance to the next exercise as indicated by the treatment results.

Basic Stress Control Exercise No. 3

Step 1. Once again, follow the exact same baseline procedure as in Exercise no. 1, except that here the activity symbols "BS_{3a} and BS_{3b}" are used to represent these data. Advance as indicated by these results.

Step 2. Here we use sentences that teach the patient to embellish the meaning of the message by adding words and stress cues while maintaining the core idea. Moreover, speakers carry out this sort of modification routinely as they converse with one another. Prepare sentences similar to the following, which can be expanded for such practice:

1. Bob wants to improve // his control.
2. My patient Bob // wants to improve // his stress control.
3. My patient Bob // is depending upon me // to improve his stress control.

Demonstrate these sentences for the patient, making certain that the stress markers get their full attention for illustrative purposes. Discuss the transition from one to the next sentence. Then, deliberately alter the sentences with inappropriate stress patterns and review the effects with the patient. Provide other examples before initiating the next step.

Step 3. Be prepared to tape record the patient's efforts. Present an index card containing a string of related sentences with their stress markers and request the patient to read them aloud, focusing on their differences. Each sentence is to be treated individually in the grading policy. Follow the scoring, charting, and advancement methods advocated in Exercise no. 1, Steps 4 and 5, except that here all data entries on the treatment chart are tagged with the activity symbol "S_3."

Basic Stress Control Exercise No. 4

Step 1. Reestablish the patient's baseline stress control status during connected discourse by engaging him or her in conversation. Use the 7-point interval scale, as described in Step 1 of Exercise no. 1, to render a perceptual rating, and enter this result on the treatment chart in the usual way. The activity symbol "BS_4" should be used to tag this finding. Proceed with the next step if this rating is equal to or worse than "3"; otherwise move on to the contrastive stress drills.

Step 2. Tape record the session. Explain that the purpose here is to help transfer any gains made in the preceding Basic Stress Control Exercises to conversational speech. Discuss the value and importance of this shift, and review the principles of the first three stress exercises. Throughout the discussion, deliberately include abnormal stress patterns, informing the patient in advance to be on the lookout for and to tag these segments when they occur. Be certain to provide sufficient samples for identification. Proceed with Step 3 when the patient shows the ability to detect at least 80 percent of the errors over 10 consecutive minutes of conversation. Review the tape recording for feedback and discussion along the way.

Step 3. Request the patient to describe a favorite hobby or activity, concentrating on use of proper stress patterns. Add as a requirement that erroneous stress be placed periodically on segments as negative practice and for discussion. Identify all abnormal stress markers and discuss whether or not they were intended. Repeat these segments until the correct patterns are understood and demonstrated by the patient. Continue with this technique, playing back the audiotape at key times for feedback, until the patient achieves a perceptual rating that is at least "3" scale values better than the baseline score or "1," if the baseline score was 3 or 4, over a period of 20 consecutive minutes of extemporaneous speech. After each 10-minute sample, enter the rating on the treatment chart in the usual way, making certain to tag these data with the activity symbol S_5. Discontinue this activity when this criterion is met or if no observable trend of (additional) improvement occurs after 30 consecutive minutes to justify continuation. In either case, move on to the supplemental activities below before proceeding with the Contrastive Stress Drills. It is helpful to list the calculated target criterion in the respective cell of the treatment chart.

Supplemental Basic Stress Activities

Patients may enjoy practicing the following pairs of sentences, which train vocal expressiveness and ways to alter meaning through creative manipulation of stress and pauses:

1a. Rover, I told you // not to poop on the carpet.
1b. Ro:ver, // I told you: // no:t to poop // on the // carpet. //

2a. Mr. Smith, // your payment is now six weeks past due. // You have 48 hours to make // good on this debt, or we // will turn the account over // to collections.
2b. Mr. Smith, // your payment // is now six weeks past due. // You have // 48 hours to make good on this debt, // or // we will turn the account over to collections. //

3a. He's a // nice man.
3b. He's a n//ice man.

4a. Although an accomplished magician she enjoys doing tricks on street corners to earn a living.
4b. Although an accomplished magician // she enjoys doing tricks on street corners // to earn a living.

5a. She was the stableman's daughter, and all the horsemen knew her.
5b. She was the stableman's daughter, // and all the horse//men knew her.

6a. A man eating shark.
6b. A man // eating shark.

Tape record and review these efforts. Think of other examples, practice them, and then advance to the next section.

Contrastive Stress Drill

Note. Contrastive stress exercises are structured according to a question and answer paradigm as the patient is permitted to speak at a rate with which he or she feels most comfortable. The task requires the patient to place the heaviest amount of stress on the component of the phrase or sentence that signifies the new or most important information requested. Systematically the segment to be stressed is varied on the basis of the clinician-patient interchange and basic discourse rules. To initiate the exercise, the first production usually assumes a neutral, declarative intonation pattern, with all words equally stressed. The entire interactive sequence for a given phrase or sentence constitutes a single trial, after which a *correct* or *incorrect* score is awarded based on the complete performance, not isolated segments. The trial is rated correct if at least 80 percent of the interchange is characterized by adequate and proper use of stress on the target segment(s). The stimuli chosen for this exercise should conform in complexity to the language and overall speech motor control abilities of the patient. The following is an example of how this exercise works:

    Clinician: "The box contained three sweaters." (Read as a statement.)
    Clinician to Patient: "Can you repeat what I just said?"
    Patient Target: "The box contained three sweaters." (Also read as a statement.)
    Clinician: "The box contained three háts?"
    Patient Target: "No: The box contained three swéaters."
    Clinician: "The box contained fóur sweaters."
    Patient Target: "No: The box contained thrée sweaters."
    Clinician: "Did you say, the box contained fóur háts?"
    Patient Target: "No: The box contained thrée swéaters."
    Clinician: "Three háts?"
    Patient Target: "Three swéaters."
    Clinician: "Fóur sweaters?"
    Patient Target: "Thrée sweaters."
    Clinician: "Was it the dráwer that contained three sweaters?"
    Patient Target: "No: The bóx contained three sweaters."

Step 1. To establish baseline, prepare on index cards several different sentences of varying length and complexity within the linguistic-speech motor repertoire of the patient. Without detailed instructions to the patient, read aloud one of the sentences using a declarative tone. Then, initiate an interchange like the example below to measure the stress-contrasting skills of the patient:

    Clinician: "Mary likes Pete."
    Clinician: "Can you repeat what I just said?"
    Patient Target: "Mary likes Pete."
    Clinician: "Did you say, Mary likes Bíll?"

Patient Target: "No: Mary (or she) likes Péte."
Clinician: "Oh, she likes Sám?"
Patient Target: "No: She likes Péte."
Clinician: "Jóe?"
Patient Target: "No: Péte."
Clinician: "Whó likes Pete?"
Patient Target: "Máry."
Clinician: "She hátes Pete."
Patient Target: "No: She líkes Pete."
Clinician: "Whó likes Pete?"
Patient Target: "Máry."

This entire sequence of stress contrasts constitutes a single trial. Rate on a notepad the patient's responses using the *correct* or *incorrect* scoring method. Repeat this procedure with the different stimuli until at least 10 different exchanges are accomplished. Tally the mean percentage of correct responses and enter this result on the grid of the Prosody Subsystem Treatment Chart, making certain to list the appropriate date, number of trials (?), and activity symbol (BC_1) in the respective cells of the data column. Proceed with this exercise if these baseline data are less than 80 percent correct; otherwise the patient has completed the prosody subsystem treatment hierarchy. Here are other sentences or phrases that may be considered for use as baseline material:

1. Apple pie and coffee.
2. Ham and eggs.
3. Suit and tie.
4. Walk the dog.
5. The boy kicked the ball.
6. Let's go to the movie.
7. The shopping mall was very crowded.
8. Driving quickly is always dangerous.
9. Pet the puppy.
10. Little girls like to play with dolls.
11. Politicians kiss babies.
12. Money makes the world go around.
13. Two plus two are four.
14. Bob went to the pet store to buy a parakeet for his mother.
15. Sue won't be coming to dinner.

Step 2. Prepare many sentences and phrases like those above, and have a tape recorder handy to tape all interchanges for review and discussion. Remember to construct these stimuli in accordance with the patient's overall interests and ability levels. Throughout the trials, track the patient's correct/incorrect patterns as inconspicuously as possible on a notepad. At the completion of a trial discuss the performance, both the correct and incorrect productions, and replay the audiotape for biofeedback and further discussion. Calculate the percentage of correct responses for the trial, and review the score with the patient. Repeat this

TABLE 7–2. Capsule Summary of Prosodic Subsystem Treatment Hierarchy*

Feature Dyscontrol	1	2	3	4	5	6	7	8	9
1. Pitch	Discrimination and listening training	Low vs. high vocalizations with vowel pairs	High vs. low vocalizations with vowel pairs	Singing the scale	Variations during oral reading	Practice pitch control in conversation			
2. Loudness	Discrimination and listening training	Soft vs. loud vocalizations with vowel pairs	Loud vs. soft vocalizations with vowel pairs	/m/ prolongations with See-Scape Device and ½ inch straw anchor	Ditto with ¾ inch anchor	Ditto with 1 inch anchor	Ditto with 1 inch anchor	Ditto with 1½ inch anchor	Variations during sounds, words, and sentences with V-U meter
3. Rate:									
a. Too slow	Discrimination and listening training	Recitation of alphabet to 150 bpm of metronome	Counting 1-10 repeatedly to 150 bpm of metronome	Familiar phrases, sentences, and passages recited to 150 bpm of metronome	Unfamiliar phrases, sentences, and passages without metronome	Practice increased rate in conversation			
b. Too fast	Ditto	Ditto at 100 bpm of metronome	Ditto at 100 bpm of metronome	Ditto at 100 bpm of metronome	Ditto, supplemented by pause and duration markers	Practice decreased rate in conversation			
c. Too much/little variability	Familiar reading material with different speed limit symbols	Practice rate modulation in conversation							
4. Intonation	Practice statements with pitch markers	Practice simple questions with pitch markers	Practice complex questions with pitch markers	Practice questions calling for repetition with pitch markers	Practice phrases with pitch markers				
5. Stress	Practice phrases with stress and pause markers	Practice general sentences with primary and secondary stress and pause markers	Practice sentence embellishment with same markers	Practice stress control in conversation	Supplements for vocal expressiveness and meaning alterations	Contrastive stress drills			

*The program begins with an exercise designed to facilitate pitch discrimination and ends with contrastive stress drills.

For 9: Practice in conversation with V-U meter

procedure until the patient achieves a mean percentage of correct responses that is at least a 75 percent improvement over the baseline score or 100 percent correct, whichever is less, over 10 consecutive trials using different stimuli sentences and phrases. As usual, calculate and enter this target criterion on the treatment chart.

Step 3. After each set of 10 trials, calculate the mean percentage of correct responses and enter this result on the grid of the treatment chart, making certain to list the appropriate activity symbol (C_1). Remember that the discontinuation rule is invoked if after 30 consecutive trials the patient fails to demonstrate any observable trend of improvement to justify further practice of the exercise. In either case, upon termination of this regimen the patient has completed the prosody subsystem treatment program.

Note. Some patients, particularly those with apraxia of speech for whom this regimen may prove beneficial, may find it helpful to synchronize finger- or foot-tapping or other pacing activities with the responses. Forceful taps may be simultaneously coupled with productions of those words targeted for emphatic stress. Ultimately, however, such facilitating techniques should be faded as the patient improves stress control.

Table 7–2 provides a capsule summary of the prosody subsystem treatment hierarchy. The suggested readings are relevant to prosodic abnormalities and their treatment.

SUGGESTED READINGS

Barnes, G. J. (1983). Suprasegmental and prosodic considerations in motor speech disorders. In W. R. Berry (Ed.), *Clinical dysarthria*. San Diego, CA: College-Hill Press.

Caligiuri, M., & Murry, T. (1983). The use of visual feedback to enhance prosodic control in dysarthria. In W. R. Berry (Ed.), *Clinical dysarthria*. San Diego, CA: College-Hill Press.

Crystal, D. (1969). *Prosodic systems and intonation in English*. London: Cambridge University Press.

Fairbanks, G. (1960). *Voice and articulation drill book*. New York: Harper & Row.

Fisher, H. B. (1975). *Improving voice and articulation*. Boston: Houghton Mifflin.

Gorelick, P., & Ross, E. (1987). The aprosodias: Further functional-anatomical evidence for the organisation of affective language in the right hemisphere. *Journal of Neurology, Neurosurgery, and Psychiatry, 50,* 553–60.

Haynes, S. (1985). Developmental apraxia of speech: symptoms and treatment. In D. F. Johns (Ed.), *Clinical management of neurogenic communicative disorders*. Boston: Little, Brown.

Kent, R., & Rosenbek, J. (1982). Prosodic disturbances in neurologic lesion. *Brain and Language, 15,* 259–291.

Kent, R., & Rosenbek, J. (1983). Acoustic patterns of apraxia of speech. *Journal of Speech and Hearing Research, 26,* 231–249.

Lehiste, I. (1970). *Suprasegmentals.* Cambridge, MA: M.I.T. Press.

Luria, A. R. (1970). *Traumatic aphasia: Its syndromes, psychology, and treatment.* The Hague: Mouton.

Minifie, F. D. (1973). Speech acoustics. In F. Minifie, T. Hixon, and F. Williams (Eds.), *Normal aspects of speech, hearing and language.* Englewood Cliffs, NJ: Prentice-Hall.

Murry, T. (1983). Treatment of ataxic dysarthria. In W. H. Perkins (Ed.), *Current therapy of communication disorders: Dysarthria and apraxia.* New York: Thieme-Stratton.

Rosenbek, J. C. (1985). Treating apraxia of speech. In D. F. Johns (Ed.), *Clinical management of neurogenic communicative disorders.* Boston: Little, Brown.

Rosenbek, J., & LaPonte, L. (1985). The dysarthrias: Description, diagnosis, and treatment. In D. F. Johns (Ed.), *Clinical management of neurogenic communicative disorders.* Boston: Little, Brown.

Ross, E. D. (1981). Functional-anatomic organization of the affective components of language in the right hemisphere. *Archives of Neurology, 38,* 561–569.

Ross, E., & Mesulam, M. (1979). Dominant language functions of the right hemisphere? Prosody and emotional gesturing. *Archives of Neurology, 36,* 144–148.

Ryalls, J. (1988). What constitutes a primary disturbance of speech prosody? A reply to Shapiro and Danly. *Brain and Language, 29,* 183–187.

Weintraub, S., Mesulam, M., & Kramer, L. (1981). Disturbances in prosody: A right-hemisphere contribution to language. *Archives of Neurology, 38,* 742–744.

Wilson, D. K. (1979). *Voice problems of children.* Baltimore: Williams & Wilkins.

Yorkston, K., & Beukelman, D. (1981). Ataxic dysarthria: Treatment sequences based on intelligibility and prosodic considerations. *Journal of Speech and Hearing Disorders, 46,* 398–404.

Index

t indicates table

Boredom, 36, 69, 74
Botulinum A toxin injection, 141
Brain damage, 4, 5
Breathing
    connected speech, 72–77
    exercises for, 50–54
    manipulation of mechanism of, 47
    patterns of, 59
    relaxation and, 50, 51
Breathing rates, slow speech, 63, 64
Broca's area, 4, 5
Bromocriptine (Parlodel), 142
Bulbar palsy, 6, 85

C

Carbidopa (Sinemet), 142
Cards, cue, 243
Case(s); *see* Illustrative case(s)
Cerebral hemorrhages, 2
Cerebral infarction, 2
Cerebral ischemia, 2
Cerebral thromboses, 2
Cerebrovascular accidents, 2
Characteristic differences between patients,
    187–191
Chart(s)
    metronomic mobility treatment, 224
    for motor speech planning treatment, 269
    for phonetic subsystem, 146, 158, 159
    for prosody subsystem, 307
    for resonation subsystem, 105
    for respiration subsystem, 44, 47, 78–80
    speech characteristic, 27–29, 90–92
    strengthening, 210
    tone improvement, 196
Charting of progress, 23
Chlorpromazine (Thorazine), 142
Clinical steps prior to treatment, 15–20
Clinician, 17
Clonazepam (Klonopin), 142
Clostridium botulinum, 141
Cogwheel rigidity, 194
Connected speech, exercises for, 120, 121
Connected speech breathing, 72–77
Consonant(s), 251–262
Consonant-vowel (CV) syllable, 71
Consultation with attending physician, 147
Contextual speech exercise, 156, 157, 167
Contrastive stress drill, 339–342
Cranial nerves, 204
Criteria
    for advancement and discontinuation of
        treatment, 24–27
    less strict experimentation with, 110
Criterion, target, 25–27
Crossbar for tongue, lip, and jaw strengthening,
    206–208
Cue cards, 243
CV; *see* Consonant-vowel
CV syllable combination exercises, 271–273
CV syllable sequence exercises, 270, 271
Cyst, 3

D

Dabul's Apraxia Battery for Adults, 263
Damage to frontal lobe of brain, 4, 5
Degenerative diseases, 3
Demyelinating diseases, 3
Dentures, poor fitting, 211
Design
    therapy intervention, 19
    treatment, types of, 20
Device, pacing, 326
Diagnosis, differential, 15
Diazepam (Valium), 142
Differences between patients, 187–191
Differential diagnosis, 15
Diphthongs, 251
Discontinuation of treatment, criteria for, 24–27
Disorder(s)
    idiopathic, 3
    metabolic, 2, 3
    motor speech, 37
    neurologic voice, 136–185
    speech, etiologic agents of, 1–3
    treatment based on severity and type of, 33, 34
Disturbances
    intonation, 328–334
    of speaking rate, 316–328
    stress control, 334–342
Drill, contrastive stress, 339–342
Drooling, 131
Dworkin-Culatta Oral Mechanism Examination,
    263
Dysarthria, 5–13, 27; *see also* Ataxic dysarthria;
    Flaccid dysarthria; Hyperkinetic dysarthria;
    Hypokinetic dysarthria; Mixed dysarthria;
    Spastic dysarthria
    articulation subsystem and, 188–190
    connected speech breathing exercises and, 73
    selection and sequence of treatment for, 27–32
Dysarthric patients
    goal of therapy with, 30
    hierarchy of subsystem treatments for, 31, 32
    neuromuscular impairments and, 16
    respiration subsystem disturbances in, 43t
    treatments, objectives, and methods for, 76t
Dysdiadochokinesia, 9
Dyskinesia
    tardive, 3
    pharmaceutical intervention and, 142, 143
Dysmetria, 9
Dysphonia, 147
    ataxic, exercises for, 176–181
    hyperkinetic, 181, 182
Dyspraxia, 1; *see also* Apraxia; Apraxia of speech
Dysprosody, 303–305
Dysrhythmia, 9
Dystonia, 13
    pharmaceutical intervention and, 142, 143

E

Edentulous patients, 211
Encephalitis, 2
Ethopropazine (Parsidol), 143